CALLING THE SHOTS

Calling the Shots

Why Parents Reject Vaccines

Jennifer A. Reich

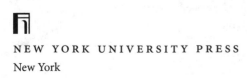

NEW YORK UNIVERSITY PRESS

New York

NEW YORK UNIVERSITY PRESS
New York
www.nyupress.org

© 2016 by New York University
All rights reserved

ISBN: 978-1-4798-1279-0

For Library of Congress Cataloging-in-Publication data, please contact the Library of Congress.

New York University Press books are printed on acid-free paper, and their binding materials are chosen for strength and durability. We strive to use environmentally responsible suppliers and materials to the greatest extent possible in publishing our books.

Manufactured in the United States of America

10 9 8 7 6 5 4 3 2 1

Also available as an ebook

For Jonas, Lilia, and Harrison
And Dave. Always.

CONTENTS

ACKNOWLEDGMENTS

Spending the better part of a decade engaged on one research project generates a sizable number of debts. I am lucky to have a community of friends and colleagues who have generously provided feedback on many drafts of this book at various stages. Daniela Kraiem, Jennifer Lois, Jonathan Wynn, Laura Carpenter, Joanna Kempner, Rene Almeling, and Andrew London each provided detailed comments on the manuscript alongside years of friendship. Anna Kirkland, Sara Shostak, Kristin Barker, and Meika Loe offered useful suggestions throughout. As this book was taking shape, Anna Muraco, Claire Decoteau, Carole Joffe, Forrest Stuart, Tracy Weitz, Amy Wilkins, Wendy Simonds, Joya Misra, Linda Blum, Chris Bobel, Orit Avishai, John Dale, Paula Fomby, Betsy Lucal, Jessica Fields, Shari Dworkin, Judy Reaven, Lori Helmstetter, Vikki Katz, Kevin Roy, Annette Lareau, Miranda Waggoner, and the amazing women of the National Advocates for Pregnant Women, including Jeanne Flavin, Lynn Paltrow, and Farah Diaz-Tello, helped me think through the questions presented and opportunities for nuance. Neighbors and friends too numerous to name have talked with me about this research, shared their ideas, and provided much-needed encouragement; I hope they know who they are and how grateful I am. Being a part of the HPV workgroup that created *Three Shots at Prevention* and working closely with Steve Epstein, Julie Livingston, Keith Wailoo, and Laura Mamo helped me immensely to develop this work. This book is better for the conversations I had with students, faculty, staff, and alumni at the University of Denver, the University of Colorado, and the other institutions that invited me to discuss this research. Melissa Pace and Traci Jones have cheered me on throughout.

This project has traveled with me across three institutions. It began at the University of California, San Francisco, where I received encouragement from Dan Dohan and Claire Brindis. All my colleagues at the University of Denver, and especially Nancy Reichman, Hava Gordon,

Lisa Pasko, Jennifer Karas, Lisa Martinez, Pete Adler, Seth Masket, Lisa Conant, and Randall Kuhn, helped me to develop this project in countless ways. At the University of Colorado Denver, I have received support from all of my colleagues and am particularly grateful to Keith Guzik, Stacey Bosick, Terri Cooney, and Anne Libby. Emily Williams and Tracy Kohm have helped to disseminate my research. The residents at Children's Hospital Oakland (class of 2000–2003) and hospitalists at Children's Hospital Colorado, and especially Dan Hyman, tolerated my questions and shared their experiences and passion with me, which was a huge help. Ellen Rodgers, Becca Bolden, and Tom Albert helped with transcription. The DU Faculty Research Fund and PROF Award program funded portions of this research.

Ilene Kalish has been a stalwart supporter of this project for as long as I have been working on it and has been an exceptional editor. She saw the potential early and has provided equal measures of feedback and encouragement. Thanks to her, Caelyn Cobb, and the staff at New York University Press for everything they have done to make this book better.

My family has offered me insight into the meanings of disease, risk, care, and responsibility in countless ways. Stephanie Reich and Seth Brindis have served as both cheerleaders and clipping service. John Reich, Nancy Gottlieb, Mark Christman, Jo Scudamore, Alisa Scudamore, and Vicki Reich have provided encouragement, discussion, and dispatches on vaccine politics from around the world. Doug Scudamore, whose miraculous transplant gave us all an extra fifteen years together but left him immune-compromised, reminds me always of fragile meanings of health and our shared responsibility for each other. Grandmothers Gladys Scudamore, who was born during the flu pandemic of 1918; Isabella Terrill, who overcame polio as a child but lived with permanent disability; and Violet Reich, who survived the Holocaust and a revolution, but lost so many and so much, each inspire me to think harder, feel more deeply, and remember what's at stake in these discussions.

Dave Scudamore has endured almost two decades of living with my research, which expands into most aspects of our life. I suspect that this study was harder on him than any of my others have been. I hope he knows how much I appreciate his patience—with my travel, tales of anti-vaccine activism, and endless medical questions—and faith in me. My children, who have grown up under the shadow of this book, have taught me more than anyone. Jonas was born as I began data collection, so I was choosing vaccines for him at the same time I was listening to why others rejected them. This book followed Lilia and Harrison from preschool to middle school and high school, respectively, and brought us all new questions about the meanings of health, risk, and community along the way. From allowing me insight into the experience of being a parent making healthcare decisions to dialoguing with me about their own ideas and experiences, they have generously offered their wisdom, humor, insight, and willingness to live with my laptop perpetually on the kitchen table.

Last, but not least, I am most thankful to the parents, physicians, attorneys, researchers, and policy makers—those in this book and others who shared with me their ideas and experiences more informally—for trusting me with their perspectives. Although there is, at times, great distance between their views, I know they all share a desire to see children thrive. I hope they believe that their trust in me was well-placed and that we can find ways forward to creating a just world for everyone's children.

Introduction

Minutes before the phone rang that Sunday evening, Tim was feeling good. His three-year-old daughter, Maggie, who had been diagnosed with leukemia months before, had survived multiple rounds of chemotherapy, lumbar punctures, and surgery to implant her port to make the next two years of treatment easier. Treatment had not been easy, with six hospital admissions, weeks in a local children's hospital, missed holidays, and the pain of the treatment itself. Now she had a three-week break from treatment to stay home with her parents and ten-month-old brother.[1] Tim was excited about what he called the "vacation from chemotherapy." But then the phone rang.

A few days before, Maggie had been at a local hospital with her mother and brother for a lab test. Another patient at the hospital had been infected with measles, and unknowingly exposed those around her to the disease. The patient, a woman in her forties, had been infected by a stranger during a winter trip to Disneyland. As we now know, that outbreak infected about 150 people from twenty states and the District of Columbia, as well as travelers from Mexico and Canada (who subsequently infected more than 150 others in their home countries[2]). Although Maggie had been vaccinated before her cancer diagnosis, her immune system was indisputably compromised; she was also most vulnerable to serious complication. Her baby brother was simply too young to be immunized. The next two weeks would be a process of watching, waiting, and avoiding contact with others—not the "vacation" they had hoped for.

Tim and his wife, Anna, were panicked. "My biggest fear is that I'll lose my child, or that she'll become deaf," Anna explained at the time. "My family has been through enough with cancer. I don't want her to go through anything else."[3] Focusing her frustration on the large number of unvaccinated people implicated in the Disneyland outbreak,[4] Anna imagined for a moment what she would say if she were facing a parent who opted not to vaccinate her children and increased risk to kids like Maggie:

"Your children don't live in a little bubble. They live in a big bubble and my children live inside that big bubble with your children. If you don't want to vaccinate your children, fine, but don't take them to Disneyland."[5]

Tim, a pediatrician, went further. Rather than imagining what he would tell a parent who rejects vaccines, he penned an open letter, "To the Parent of the Unvaccinated Child Who Exposed My Family to Measles," in which he expressed his frustration that both of his children were exposed to a disease that had been deemed eradicated from the United States in 2000. Written initially for the blog he keeps about his daughter's care, it was passed along to others by a nurse and subsequently reprinted multiple times, shared more than 1.3 million times on social media, and widely read.[6] Some even felt compelled to reply.

Megan was one. A self-described naturopath, writer, stay-at-home mom, and cofounder and president of a nonprofit organization that focuses "on orphan care and poverty alleviation in Africa," Megan says she has "developed the habit of researching everything from the toothpaste we use to the toilet paper we wipe our butts with." Her blog describes how her information gathering "prompted us to throw out our microwave, ditch the gluten, sugar, milk, pork, and genetically modified foods, burn our medicine cabinet, wear our kids, breastfeed our babies, recycle our trash, up the probiotics, unschool our kids, and rip up the CDC's vaccination schedule."[7]

Speaking directly to Tim, but citing "the creators of the hysteria" and "measles propaganda," Megan described the reasons for her frustration with Tim: "That you do not respect my choices, that you think my unvaccinated child is the only one who threatens yours, and that you would insinuate that my child should be sacrificed on the altar for your child." Calling vaccines artificial immunity that has upset the natural order of disease and naturally occurring immunity, Megan reiterated that she has the right to decide what is best for her children and what risks she and other parents might choose to take:

> When we take our child to a place like Disneyland, or any other public place for that matter (including a hospital), we assume the risk that we might come into contact with a sick person, someone who hasn't washed their hands, a kid who has picked their nose, or rides that have not been properly sanitized between each use.

Megan replied directly to Anna and Tim's insistence that as members of a community, children live in the same large bubbles, retorting, "It is not fair to require that my child get vaccinated for the benefit of yours or to force my child to live in a bubble so that yours doesn't have to."[8]

Other parents shared her view, some more vocally than others. Jack, a cardiologist and father of two unvaccinated children, was among the loudest. Addressing Tim and Anna, he insisted, "It's not my responsibility to inject my child with chemicals in order for [a child like Maggie] to be supposedly healthy. . . . I'm not going to sacrifice the well-being of my child. My child is pure." Jack too challenged claims that vaccines promote health, arguing instead that disease is good for people: "We should be getting measles, mumps, rubella, chickenpox, these are the rights of our children to get it. . . . We do not need to inject chemicals into ourselves and into our children in order to boost our immune system."[9] Also responding specifically to the notion of shared responsibility and individual parental rights, Jack made clear that he is comfortable in his commitment to rejecting vaccines, even if his child were to infect another child who became gravely ill. "It's an unfortunate thing that people die, but people die. I'm not going to put my child at risk to save another child."[10]

The measles outbreak at Disneyland in December 2014 and the subsequent online feuds about the vulnerability of one child and the rights of parents of other children reflect many of the existing tensions about vaccines. As Megan's and Jack's responses illustrate, parents who reject vaccines distrust claims of safety and necessity, believe that disease is natural in a way vaccines are not, and identify their primary role of parents as superseding obligations to others. They also make clear that they are experts on their own children—able to assess and manage risk—and thus uniquely qualified to decide what their children need.

For the past decade, I have followed vaccine refusal from the perspectives of those who distrust vaccines and the corporations that make them, as well as the health providers and policy makers who see them as essential to ensuring community health. In an effort to tell the story of vaccines and explore the tensions between these views, I sought out a variety of key perspectives. I started with parents, and was careful to include those who opted out of vaccines completely and others who consented to select vaccines on a schedule of their own choosing. Children whose parents challenge vaccine recommendations are most likely to be white, have a college-educated mother, and a family income over $75,000. For the most part, this is what the parents in this study look like too. Only about 15 percent of parents in this study are fathers, since children's healthcare decisions are overwhelmingly maternal terrain. (I detail the sample in appendix A.)

I then broadened my view by conducting in-depth interviews with pediatricians to learn how they address parents' questions about vaccines and strategize vaccinations in their own practices. Physicians serve as intermediaries between expert knowledge and individual experience, and are present at critical moments in families' lives.[11] Since many parents referenced their trust in complementary health providers, I sought out those perspectives as well, interviewing chiropractors, naturopathic doctors, and other lay healers, most of whom disapprove of vaccines.

To understand vaccine risk and liability, I interviewed attorneys who work in the federal Vaccine Injury Compensation Program (VICP), a relatively unknown branch of the federal claims court that is tasked with compensating any person who is adversely affected by a vaccine. Paid for with a tax on every vaccine in the country, this court system—with only eight special masters and fewer than a hundred attorneys—was designed to be nonadversarial and able to compensate individuals quickly to ensure faith in public health. The perspectives of those who develop vaccines, set federal guidelines, work in county health departments, and research vaccine policy are also important, and I interviewed many of those who have positioned themselves as leaders on this topic, writing books on alternative vaccine schedules or in support of federally established ones, or who advocate for or against vaccine mandates.

To add complexity to this discussion, I observed meetings of organizations opposed to vaccine mandates, pediatric lectures for doctors by doctors about vaccines, community events for parents about vaccines, meetings of the Institute of Medicine about vaccine safety, and conference calls of federal vaccine advisory boards. I also analyzed hundreds of e-mails, newsletters, and blogs from different stakeholders, including parents.

Disagreements about vaccines raise larger questions. To what degree are we obligated to protect the most vulnerable members of our communities? Where are the limitations of our individual liberty? What defines good parenting? What counts as expertise? What do we owe others? These questions do not reside on the political left or right. They surround us always, but largely remain unheard. The parents I studied question, modify, or outright reject vaccines because they see them as unnatural, as tainted by the profit motives of big pharma, as inadequately tested and regulated, or as unnecessary for illness prevention. These parents engage in what we might call *individualist parenting*, expending immense time and energy strategizing how to keep their children healthy while often ignoring the larger, harder-to-solve questions around them. They tend to focus on the subjects of their own expertise: their own children. In the 1970s, when most of these parents were children, schools required vaccination against seven vaccine-preventable illnesses. By 2014, evidence of vaccination against thirteen vaccine-preventable illnesses became required for kindergarten attendance, with more recommended in adolescence. As the number of recommended vaccines has increased, resulting in more boosters and as many as two dozen shots by age two,[12] even parents who don't reject vaccines altogether have started to question their safety and necessity and seek modifications of the schedule.

I am a mother of three children with much in common with the parents who participated in this study. Although we have made different decisions about vaccinating our children, the same questions surround us—at children's birthday parties, in long-term care facilities visiting relatives, in hospitals, on international flights, on college campuses that require immunization for incoming freshmen, and in the homes of people in our communities. These questions feel pressing as I think of the newborn babies in my family, my father-in-law, who was immune-compromised after a transplant, or my friends infected with HIV.

Most people engaged in this debate believe passionately in the correctness of their positions for or against vaccines, and believe the other side to be woefully misinformed, and possibly even dangerous to their children and families. In this book I aim to fill the middle ground between them by providing a better understanding of how different people approach vaccines and make sense of the meanings of risk, benefit, and obligation in the context of vaccines—something that carries both individual and collective consequences. This does not mean that I equally support all positions and interpretations. Rather, I believe that if we can trace the points of disconnect between these positions, we can improve our thinking about vaccine choice, and ultimately public health.

The Triumph of Modern Medicine

Immunizations against childhood illnesses are touted as one of the greatest achievements of modern medicine and are credited with drastically reducing, or virtually eliminating, incidences of polio, diphtheria, measles, mumps, rubella, haemophilus influenzae type b (Hib), tetanus, whooping cough (or pertussis), and more recently varicella (chickenpox) and rotavirus in the United States. Vaccines improve life expectancy and lower healthcare costs.[13] About 90 percent of children in the United States receive most of what federal advisory groups define as the key childhood immunizations, even if they do not receive all.[14] This high rate owes its success to compulsory immunization laws, passed in all fifty states, which require children to provide evidence of immunization before enrolling in schools or childcare settings.[15] These laws have been around in their current form since the 1960s, with every state having one by 1981.

As mentioned, the number of vaccines that are required for school attendance has increased significantly between the 1970s, when there were seven, and 2014, when there were about sixteen spanning into adolescence. These can result in as many as twenty-four to twenty-six shots by the time a child is two years of age. A child can potentially receive up to six shots during one doctor visit, although there is no set upper limit (and some vaccines may be combined into fewer injections).[16] Despite the virtual elimination of many infectious diseases in the last two decades, vaccines have become controversial. Celebrities opposing vaccines have continued to posit a link between vaccines and autism, and outbreaks of measles, which had been eradicated from the United States in 2000, are seen with increased frequency. Although relatively few parents reject vaccines, 25 percent of parents in one nationally representative survey shared the view that children's immune systems could become weakened by too many immunizations.[17] Even more parents report concern about the pain of injections.[18] Vaccine choices also reflect parents' relative levels of trust in biomedicine and practitioners, parents' perceptions of necessity, and fear of unknown long-term side effects, with which children who did not consent to the vaccine would have to live.[19] The parents I interviewed and observed for this book who choose to reject medical advice on vaccines also communicate more widely held anxieties about vaccine safety. Often, they express disbelief in the claims that a high proportion of a community needs to get vaccines to protect its members. They insist that children's bodies should be treated as unique rather than uniform. They also express distrust in the commercial production of vaccines and the regulatory agencies that oversee them.

This last point is not a small issue. Vaccines are currently manufactured by for-profit pharmaceutical companies. Five transnational companies (GlaxoSmithKline, Sanofi Pasteur, Merck, Pfizer, and Novartis) manufacture most of the world's vaccines, with fewer than ten companies manufacturing any. This is a significantly reduced number from four decades ago, when there were at least seven times as many companies working to develop, produce, and distribute vaccines.[20] These companies are not public health agencies and are driven by profits. Recently, we have seen vaccine shortages due to contamination in manufacturing, miscalculations in production and equipment replacement, and dysfunction in systems of payment and distribution.[21]

Outside the vaccine context, there are many examples of malfeasance or neglectful practices by pharmaceutical companies. We can see these issues in the recent example of Vioxx, a widely used drug Merck manufactured to treat arthritis or chronic pain that was withdrawn from the market in 2004 because of increased risk of heart attack and stroke in users; in problems with the blood thinner Heparin, which was contaminated during manufacture in China, killed eighty-one people in the United States, affecting hundreds more worldwide; in multimillion-dollar settlements; or in recalls because of contamination or production incompetence in products ranging from lifesaving medications to Children's Tylenol.[22] Pharmaceutical companies engage in other questionable practices, including repackaging and repurposing medications to avoid the expiration of profitable patents that would allow more affordable generics to be produced or applying for expedited FDA approval with limited data or follow-up.[23] The current vaccine arrangement, in which states mandate the consumption of a for-profit health product, stokes parental skepticism. So while this book focuses most heavily on those who reject medical advice about vaccines, it also examines anxieties about health, risk, and medical care that are more widely shared. Although some may dismiss these parental fears about vaccines as simply people who just don't understand how vaccines work, it behooves us to take their concerns seriously. As this book will show, when parents opt out of vaccines for their children, we are all affected. Our public health is at stake.

Vaccines as Public Health

Vaccines are a cornerstone of U.S. public health policy, which aims to protect the health and well-being of an entire population. For example, public health campaigns include efforts to ensure safe drinking water, inspect food, or monitor air quality, all of which would be difficult for an individual to accomplish alone on his or her own behalf. Public health campaigns also require individuals to give up some personal liberty or freedom to protect the well-being of the population. Sometimes public health campaigns limit individual preferences for the good of the individual or to save costs to those in the community. For example, the state can compel me to pay taxes to fund fire departments because, even though individuals might protect their homes or businesses with smoke detectors and fire extinguishers, they remain vulnerable if a neighbor's house burns quickly and spills over to their own property. Because nineteenth-century fire brigades were once private entities that would refuse to put out uninsured properties (a practice that led to uncontrollable fires), U.S. cities began to fund civic fire departments.

In some ways, public health law can be similarly justified, as it constantly aims to balance the distributive effects of a rule to improve the lives of members of a community against the cost to their individual freedoms. This can even take the form of compromising individual bodily integrity or privacy, as seen, for example, in legal requirements for directly observed therapy for tuberculosis; court orders to take anti-psychotic drugs; legal mandates to report sexually transmitted infections; or state power to quarantine individuals who might present infection risks.[24] These interventions benefit individuals, just as vaccines provide benefit to the child who receives them. Federal estimates are that vaccines prevent about 1.4 million hospitalizations and 56,300 deaths for each birth cohort that receives them.[25] This clearly shows individual benefits from vaccination, alongside public health costs that would be shared collectively. Yet the state's response to individuals who do not want to partake in lifesaving interventions is complicated; it requires finding a balance between preventing widespread infection that would detrimentally affect others and compelling an individual to consume a pharmaceutical product he or she may not want.

Understanding public health requires a keen understanding of the points where individuals have compatible or conflicting interests and needs. One such point is "herd immunity" against infectious disease. When a person receives a vaccination, she has a far greater chance of being protected from that illness—receiving individual benefit—but also helps to protect others in the community who are vulnerable to infection. Some vaccines benefit only the individual, like that for tetanus, which is a disease that is not contagious but results from exposure to a toxin in the environment that causes neurological damage and death and is difficult to treat. However, the majority of required vaccines do not just protect the child who receives inoculation, but also prevents exposure of life-threatening illnesses in the disabled, the aged, the immune-compromised, the infants too young to be vaccinated, and the pregnant women whose fetuses could be devastated by these illnesses, as well as those few individuals who did not gain immunity from a vaccine they received.[26]

If a community-level immunity rate, known as herd immunity, of approximately 85–95 percent (depending on the disease) is maintained, virtually all members of the community are protected from infection. It is impossible to create immunity in 100 percent of a population. With herd immunity, diseases are blocked from reaching those who would be at risk by those who are vaccinated. As an example, if Child A has measles and Child C is unvaccinated, Child B is a fully vaccinated intermediary who protects Child C from infection. This is even more effective when a high percentage of the population are fully vaccinated, creating more Bs to protect the occasional C. Public health mandates to require vaccination for school attendance—where children are in dense quarters and likely to share risks of exposure to disease—aim to increase the numbers of vaccinated children who can protect that vulnerable Child C and buffer the risk of infection from the infected Child A. Herd immunity can absorb only a small portion of the population failing to vaccinate. Therefore, the philosophy of herd immunity holds that the only exemptions should be for those who cannot safely receive vaccines because of a medical condition or because they are too young, or those for whom vaccines do not work. Essentially, those who can be vaccinated and generate immunity will help to protect the most vulnerable in their community. Parents who reject vaccines for their children benefit from herd immunity, but refuse to contribute to it, making them free-riders to other children's immunity.

Estimated Herd Immunity Thresholds for Vaccine-Preventable Diseases

Disease	Transmission mode	R0[a]	Herd immunity threshold[b]
Diphtheria	Saliva	6–7	85%
Measles	Airborne	12–18	83—94%
Mumps	Airborne droplet	4–7	75—86%
Pertussis	Airborne droplet	12–17	92—94%
Polio	Fecal-oral route	5–7	80—86%
Rubella	Airborne droplet	5–7	80—85%
Smallpox	Social contact	6–7	83—85%

Source: CDC, "History and Epidemiology of Global Smallpox Eradication," CDC.gov, 2003, http://www.bt.cdc.gov/agent/smallpox/training/overview/pdf/eradicationhistory.pdf.
[a]Number of new infections per infected person (known as R0).
[b]Percentage of population to be vaccinated to achieve community immunity.

Public Health in the Age of "Have-It-Your-Way" Medicine

Vaccines are intended as a uniform healthcare intervention—provided at about the same age in similar doses to all children. A federal advisory group of experts recommends a schedule of when vaccines are to be administered, which is usually accepted by professional medical organizations like the American Academy of Pediatrics, and enforced through state laws. The federal Advisory Committee on Immunization Practices (ACIP) comprises experts in vaccinology, immunology, pediatrics, internal medicine, nursing, family medicine, virology, public health, infectious diseases, and preventive medicine, and a consumer representative who provides perspectives on the social and community aspects of vaccination; the committee examines all research on vaccine safety and efficacy when making the schedule.[27]

The creation of an expert-informed schedule that states and professional organizations adopt makes state vaccine schedules safe and effective, and distribution relatively inexpensive and efficient. Yet the parents with whom I spoke instead see this schedule as impersonal and imprecise, providing a "one-size-fits-all" vaccine routine that may not be appropriate for their children. Even among parents who support vaccination, more than 20 percent do not agree that following the recommended vaccine schedules is the safest course for their children.[28] In short, there is limited faith in the official schedule.

We live in an age of personalization. A fast-food restaurant's catch-phrase promising that you can "have it your way" is emblematic of this. We see heightened efforts to personalize medical care to meet the needs and desires of the individual. This might include new methods of identifying individual risk of developing certain diseases, to genetically testing embryos before implantation for particular characteristics, or calculating risk of future health challenges. Although companies are beginning to offer racial and biological analyses of individual genetic material, and pharmaceutical companies promise to create personalized medicine that could eventually match drugs to individual personal genetic profiles, these innovations have yet to hold major practical uses or even hit the market.[29] Still, their development has contributed to a vocabulary of individualized medicine that shapes expectations of care and supports understandings of our bodies as unique.

From this understanding, health itself comes to be defined by personal choices and behaviors, often through consumption and risk management.[30] We understand that we must actively manage our lives, work hard, behave morally, and avoid calculable risk through informed decision making.[31] The individual in a "regime of self" is expected to actively shape her or his life through active health choices, with socially defined good choices becoming the cultural norm against which an individual's morality might be evaluated.[32] (The condemnation of smokers or overweight people illustrates this as well.) From this springs the ideology of individualist parenting.

A commitment to individualist parenting contributes to heightened demands for personalized attention from institutions, including schools, tutoring centers, volunteer organizations, therapeutic courts, and, for our purposes, healthcare systems and providers. There are a great many reasons that enhanced abilities to focus on individual learning styles and needs, health risks, or skills are beneficial and hold the promise of assisting individuals in reaching their full potential. Although individualized care does not necessarily yield better health outcomes, it may create a more positive experience of healthcare.[33] When it comes to vaccines, parents face both a social understanding that responsible parents vaccinate their children and an expectation that good parents advocate for their children and their individual needs. As they perceive their child's needs and bodies as unique, the parents I spoke with and observed view the state's efforts to compel vaccine use for the good of the community as unacceptable. Instead, they insist that as parents they have the right to make individual choices for their children.

Rhetoric of individual preference proliferates in these parents' efforts to define themselves as good parents who want what is best for their children. This insistence on individualism directly contradicts the goals of public health, which expects parents to absorb a measure of risk to their own children in order to protect others in the communities in which they live or travel. Yet, as others have observed, parents often insist that they "should be 'empowered' to pursue their own self-interest as a condition of their rights (and obligations) as consumers of public resources," which places their desires for their own children ahead of others.[34] Ultimately, I will argue in this book that the emergence of an ideology of individualist parenting, which prioritizes individual choice for one's own children over community obligation, ignores how some families with fewer resources have fewer options, but face increased risk of illness.

The Limits of Parents' Rights

Parental concern for vaccine safety is not new. In fact, the power of the state to compel vaccines comes from a 1905 U.S. Supreme Court decision in which a father did not want to vaccinate his child against smallpox. When the father was fined for failing to participate in the mandatory vaccine program, he refused to pay the fine and appealed his case. In the decision of *Jacobson v. Massachusetts*, the Court ruled against the father and clarified that the state is entitled to use police powers to protect public health. Highlighting the duty to protect community health, the decision states, "It was the duty of the constituted authorities primarily to keep in view the welfare, comfort and safety of the many, and not permit the interests of the many to be subordinated to the wishes or convenience of the few." In doing so, the state's power to require individuals' participation in public health campaigns, even when they disagree, was set. (The *Jacobson* decision was notably also used to justify involuntary sterilization in 1927, further defining and refining state powers to act on the bodies of its citizens.[35])

Despite the articulation of the state's right to compel participation in vaccines and other health programs, the United States maintains a strong ideological commitment to parental authority and individual autonomy. Every state has a mechanism that allows parents to opt out of required vaccinations. All states allow exemptions for medical reasons, almost always as verified by a medical provider. All states except West Virginia, Mississippi, and, as of 2016, California allow parents to exercise an exemption for religious beliefs, defined relatively broadly in most states, and not subject to verification. About eighteen states also allow exemptions based on philosophical, personal, or conscientiously held beliefs.[36] Exercising exemptions vary in process and requirement; some states require parents who claim philosophical or personally held beliefs against vaccines to apply those beliefs to all vaccines. Other states do not view as contradictory parents' claims that they object to only certain vaccines, allowing parents to pick and choose which vaccines they want for their children. Some states require more cumbersome documentation for exemptions, including signatures from two parents, notarization, or extensive explanation, or countersignature from a medical provider, while other states simply require a signature on a form. Colorado, where I conducted my interviews with parents and providers, is a state that allows exemptions for medical, religious, or personal beliefs and requires little documentation. Colorado has among the highest rate of personal belief exemptions.[37] This state is an ideal place to examine the multifaceted meanings of vaccine uptake and refusal among parents as they craft their own solutions with less legal regulation, but nonetheless communicate the same anxieties expressed by parents around the country, whose choices may be more constrained.

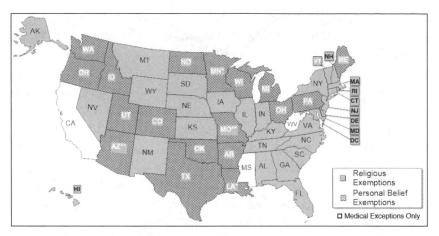

States with personal belief exemptions, religious exemptions, or medical exemptions. Reproduced from National Conference of State Legislatures, http://www.ncsl.org/research/health/school-immunization-exemption-state-laws.aspx.

The Uneven Landscape of Parental Choice

Public health scholars divide children who have not received all vaccines required for school attendance (but who do not have a medical reason to avoid vaccines) into two groups. On one side, there are the children who are undervaccinated because they lack consistent access to medical care. These children are more likely to be children of color, have a younger mother who is unmarried and does not have a college degree, and live in a household near the poverty line. Children on the other side—those who are unvaccinated because of parental choice—look significantly different. They are more likely to be white, have a mother who is married and college-educated, and to live in a household with an income over $75,000; they also tend to be geographically clustered.[38] What this means is that the choice to opt out of vaccines is almost exclusively made by families with the most resources and represents a fairly privileged parenting practice. These differences reflect broader schisms in how families with different resources have access to choices.

The "choices" families make exist within a public policy context that structures requirements. For example, school attendance is legally required but can be avoided through adherence to paperwork and certification; complementary health providers or birth attendants are outside

mainstream healthcare, often accessible only to those with private resources; work policies may inhibit or facilitate breastfeeding. Childhood
vaccinations are legally required for school attendance, but parents can
avoid these by filing forms for exemptions. Each of these regulations or
requirements is enacted for the good of the entire community, but also
allows alternatives so individuals with resources can exercise choice. As
the sociologist David Cheal suggests, "Family members define their proj-
ects with reference to personal desires, rather than public goals, and they
are free to implement them to the limits of their resources."[39] Clearly,
not all families are equally able to assert their preferences. Illustrating
this, Colorado, which has among the most liberal legal frameworks for
opting out of vaccines, until recently punished welfare recipients whose
children were not fully vaccinated.[40] As families exercise their choice to
opt out of vaccines, signing a form that entitles their unvaccinated child
to attend school, they do so as educated parents with privilege—and
without fear of public sanctions. In so doing, they also insist that they
are the experts on their children and uniquely qualified to decide what
they need.

Claiming Parental Expertise

The relationship between medical experts and parents has a long and
contentious history. Early twentieth-century physician-authored texts
highlighted mothers' ignorance about caring for children and the need
for parent education. Doctors dispensing scientific and medical advice to
women developed a practice of "scientific motherhood," which "refined
and redefined what it means to be a good mother, a proper mother."[41]
Throughout the twentieth century, women differentially embraced,
challenged, or ignored the tenets of scientific motherhood, reflecting
differences in class, ethnicity, family immigration history, experience,
education, and region.[42] By the mid-twentieth century, mothers had
become savvy consumers of professional advice, and professionals needing patients, from Dr. Spock on baby care to Dr. Dick-Read on natural
childbirth, began including mothers' own insights and experiences
in their "expert" advice. The medical historian Rima Apple suggests
that this communicated approval of women's views on childrearing
and birthing, which reinforced women's confidence as mothers and

empowered them to question medical authority.[43] These transformations happened as an emerging women's rights movement grew, yielding the women's health movement. That movement further challenged the role of the expert as it provided support for natural childbirth, facilitated the Boston Women's Health Book Collective's publication of *Our Bodies, Ourselves*, and saw the formation of La Leche League to provide feminist support for breastfeeding. These cultural forces repositioned expertise as residing within the individual, and women began to see expert advice as mere suggestions to incorporate into their own mothering practice. The market of parent-driven advice books exploded just as patients newly insisted on being able to shop for medical providers. This then forced physicians, particularly in obstetrics and pediatrics, to innovate in their practices in order to compete for paying patients.

Experts often encourage parents to become independent and self-efficacious, even to use online sources of information to become educated on an issue. In some realms, they design programs specifically to empower low-income or vulnerable groups to participate fully and advocate for themselves and their children.[44] In education and health-care specifically, efforts to "empower parents" to manage their children's asthma, diabetes, medications, learning disabilities, or education are ubiquitous. Most assume that empowering parents will lead them to choose for their children what experts believe is correct and will improve outcomes. However, much research on empowered parents, including studies of charter schools, school choice, or chronic disease management, show that the most privileged parents remain the most empowered to advocate for their own children, often furthering inequality. Parents with resources are most able to demand services, more likely to view providers as contributing advice rather than dictating behaviors, and less likely to be reported to state agencies like child protective services. They also receive more respect from providers as potential partners in their children's care.

In arenas as diverse as medicine, mental health, law, education, business, and food, self-help or do-it-yourself movements encourage individuals to reject expert advice or follow it selectively.[45] Avoiding experts and their institutions is possible in many of these realms. Vaccines, however, require a gatekeeper to administer them, forcing structured interactions between parents who reject expert advice and the professionals who control access to medical technologies that parents at times may want or need.

Vaccines are not the only medical issue where patients demand individualistic treatment. The emphasis on individual choice reflects much of the rhetoric of U.S. women's health movements, including calls for greater challenges to mainstream medical advice.[46] Campaigns for abortion access in the United States, a procedure that also requires access to services though medical gatekeepers, claim, "My body, my choice." The historian Rickie Solinger suggests that in the context of abortion, the vocabulary of choice is too often reduced to images of "women shoppers selecting among options in the marketplace" without concern for the larger power relations at stake.[47] This form of "choice feminism" lays the backdrop for women's individual choices for their children's healthcare. Freedom from compulsion (in this case from vaccine requirements) rather than access to resources to create widespread access to care becomes the political goal.[48] As individual preference becomes synonymous with freedom, the unequal ability to exercise choice, particularly around state policy, is obscured.

Most parents who oppose vaccines are not part of a political movement. In the United States, a handful of organizations and grassroots groups politically mobilize against vaccine mandates, gain celebrity spokespersons and extensive media coverage, even as no similar movement exists to create equity in access to pediatric care. Those who reject expert advice on vaccines are not necessarily conservative or liberal, with a wide array of political affiliations and views of the state. They are generally well-intentioned parents committed to assessing the individual benefits of vaccines for their individual children and wanting to choose for themselves, without state mandates or expert advice proscribing their freedom of choice. As parents decide what is best for their children, they overlook—or explicitly deny—how their choices can be costly for other people's children.

Individualist Parenting and the Culture of Mother-Blame

Parents generally want their children to succeed, but their ability to facilitate their success is shaped by access to resources. The sociologist Annette Lareau shows how middle-class and affluent families embrace an ideology of "concerted cultivation," where they aim to actively manage their children's lives so they might become successful adults who can outperform others.[49] This takes a variety of forms, from adult-organized play, to management of homework, to advocacy in schools. The overarching goal is to manage children's development so they will be successful and to optimize their personal opportunities. Concerted cultivation is a class-based ideology that inspires cumbersome practices that fall more heavily on mothers than on fathers and differentially transmits advantage to children.

Regarding parents' vaccine choices, children's healthcare is intense and largely, although not exclusively, maternal terrain.[50] In fact, cultural expectations of mothering have become increasingly demanding—of time, energy, and money.[51] While there is evidence that this ideology of intensive mothering has permeated the lives of mothers at all socioeconomic levels, this experience of motherhood is marked most intensely as that of middle- and upper-class mothers, who have the material and cultural resources to invest most heavily in their children's development and most intensely fear their children's downward mobility.[52] Women receive cultural encouragement for this kind of individualist management. In prenatal care, for example, they are directed to develop birth plans because they are told they are entitled to consume information and services.[53] As mothers, they are told it is their obligation to manage risk and pursue success for both themselves and their children. Mothers are responsible for the physical, emotional, and psychological health of their children; healthy children symbolically represent good mothering, just as mother-blame proliferates in the lives of women with sick children.[54] In these ways, the tenets of scientific motherhood are reframed in a market economy, where informed mothers become consumers with a plethora of individual choices awaiting them.

This work of individualist parenting is overwhelming—both time- and resource-intensive. Yet there is also evidence that mothers acquire a sense of accomplishment from their ability to care for their children and take pride in crafting their sense of self as experts. We can see examples of this in research about "natural mothers" who reject consumerism, homeschooling mothers who dictate the pace of their families' lives, or women who breastfeed their children—sometimes for many years—as a commitment to their children's well-being. Each of these practices is more readily available to women with private resources.[55] In the case of vaccines, parents choose to reject vaccines they do not trust in an effort to maximize their children's long-term health. As they do, they claim expertise over their own children and what they see as their unique bodies, even as they refuse to acknowledge how other parents may not be equally able to do so.

Much of the research on parents who refuse vaccines for their children focuses on what parents think, often according to surveys or focus groups. Although I too share an interest in understanding what parents think, I aim throughout the book to put these views in a cultural, historical, and social context. I argue that these views represent broader cultural trends that support a view of medicine as personalized and individualized. These views are rooted in ideas about middle-class and affluent parenting that expect parents to heavily invest in their own children, even at a cost to others. This ideology of individualist parenting is tightly bound to economic and social trends that privatize individuals and their bodies into informed consumers. Parents tout their commitment to informed individual choice as a way of expressing their commitment to their children, which overrides a commitment to community responsibility and social justice.

Overview of the Book

In searching for a full range of perspectives, I aimed to find sites of contested meanings about what vaccines are and whether and how they should be used. What are their symbolic meanings? How do they convey different notions of individual choice and collective responsibility? How do views of vaccines communicate perceptions of family, science, authority, and the state? I also identify the points of disconnect and place these different views in conversation. At times, I bring in the social history of certain diseases to add context to parents' views. My goal is to paint complex pictures of the meanings of disease, risk, fear, and health that are woven through all disagreements about vaccines. As a technology that provides individual benefits and risks, enforced by the state, and administered on young children's bodies, vaccines allow us to explore these complex and contradictory meanings and to examine challenges to expertise, choices of consumption, and the ways these dynamics are structured by privilege. In each chapter, I weave parents' concerns, physicians' experiences, and the meanings of vaccines, with an eye to the role of the state in mediating these meanings and experiences.

First, I provide a broad historical overview of vaccine policy and controversy, including how vaccines were created and came to be legally required for school entry. Because vaccine mandates arose in the 1960s as a way to increase funding and provide access to low-income children, I point to the meanings of community health and access, even as vaccine mandates are no longer perceived this way. I also highlight significant moments when consensus about vaccines as a good and safe technology broke down. Each vaccine's invention has raised different issues about health, risk, necessity, and the relationship between citizens and the state. As such, this chapter provides a chronology of vaccine development so readers can better understand how these unique histories have led us to where we are today.

Beginning in chapter 2, I show how parents define themselves as experts on their own children, best qualified to evaluate vaccine risk and benefit claims. Parents filter information from myriad sources—books, websites, research, peers, providers, or their own intuitions—to weigh claims of risk of disease against the risk of the vaccine itself. They expend energy and resources assessing whether their children are at greater risk for complications from vaccination. Promoting an expectation that all parents should actively challenge medical experts to advocate for their own children, despite the unequal ability to do so, they reject vaccines when they perceive that risk outweighs benefit. Chapter 3 examines how parents define their sense of themselves as experts on their children and then deploy that parental expertise to argue that vaccines are unnatural, creating inferior immunity. Chapter 4 builds on these views and presents parents' perceptions that vaccines represent a voluntary introduction of chemicals into children's bodies. Drawing on the celebrity-led march to "Green Our Vaccines," the controversy over thimerosal, a mercury-based preservative that was until recently used in vaccines, and the now-discredited claims that vaccines can cause autism, I elucidate how some parents see vaccines as toxic and thus harmful.

Unlike other self-directed health movements, vaccines require physicians to serve as gatekeepers—to provide vaccines as well as the documentation needed to access childcare and educational settings. Parents generally believe that medicine as practiced—with busy providers who have limited time with each patient—hinders practitioners' ability to understand each child as unique and prevents them from serving as advocates. Chapter 5 examines how pediatricians view their role as medical experts in their work with parents who claim competing expertise. Chapter 6 looks at parents' resistance to what many call the "one-size-fits-all" schedule of vaccinations and how they rework or reject the timing and dosage of vaccines. Using their own sense of expertise, parents demand slow or alternative vaccine schedules for their children against the illnesses they believe require protection at a time they view them as most relevant. As parents engage these processes, they do so with physicians who are differentially supportive of their claims as experts.

Disease risk intrinsically involves uncertainty. Chapters 7 looks at how parents aim to manage risk through intensive parenting practices that are resource-intensive and both claim and reproduce privilege, which include natural living, breastfeeding, and careful preparation of food. They also manage risk by enacting imagined gated communities from which they can control social exposure to those they believe might carry disease. Through these efforts to manage uncertainty and mitigate risk, I suggest, parents feel compelled to invest significant resources as a way of ensuring their children's safety when they reject vaccines as well as maintaining a sense of control over their children's well-being. In chapter 8, I take a close look at the criticism parents who opt out of vaccines face and how they manage social disapproval. This chapter engages the broader cultural meanings of vaccine refusal, from interactions with doctors whom parents see as disapproving, to possible legal and institutional sanctions, including from healthcare providers, schools, or public health agencies. Examining their perceptions of disapproval allows us to better understand the meanings of autonomy, compliance, and consent in medical encounters and the ways parents' claims of expertise and authority do not always prevail. Finally, I return to the public health goal of herd immunity to demonstrate how parents understand claims of community obligation but do not prioritize it in their decisions, as well as how providers broach the topic with their patients' families. In examining perceptions of state regulation and public health goals alongside parents' desires to assert their own expertise, I show how perceptions of disease and risk reflect structures of race, class, and social distance.

Striking a Balance

Many books exist about vaccines, and there is much public debate about them. Yet each discussion seems to stake out and fortify one particular view. Some provide both historical and contemporary understandings of vaccine controversies. Yet, because they write with such certainty of their positions, they portray the parents who resist vaccines as foolish or ignorant at best, and sometimes even delusional or selfish. Correspondingly, the writings of those who oppose vaccines generally, or policies that mandate vaccines specifically, provide no more nuance and yield little ground to those who have experienced infectious disease firsthand or who have expertise built on the scientific method and decades of systematic research.

I am not neutral on whether vaccines are good or bad. I have opted to follow all mainstream medical recommendations and have fully vaccinated my own children. I do so because I trust that vaccines are mostly safe and I accept that we can each absorb minimal risk to protect those in our community who are most vulnerable. I support policies that encourage efforts to broadly vaccinate the population and protect public health. I also very much like and respect the parents I spoke with who laboriously question vaccines and medical recommendations, and who aim to do the best for their children. I know that these families will not agree with everything I argue in this book, but I hope they feel respected. I also accept that not all stakeholders will agree with my analysis, but I do hope this book can encourage better discussions of public health, community obligation, and individual choice. As we ideally find a place of mutual understanding, and even some common ground, perhaps we can then move together toward policies that support everyone's children, not just our own.

1

The Public History of Vaccines

Most histories of vaccines in the United States begin with the story of smallpox, a disease feared for its gruesome symptoms, high fatality rate, and ability to spread quickly. As the historian James Colgrove describes,

> Its symptoms began with chills, aches, and fever, then progressed ominously to nausea, vomiting, and difficulty breathing. About a week after infection, bright red pustules developed on the victim's face and hands, and then spread to cover the entire body. Eventually the pustules dried and itched intensely, scabbed over, and fell off. About one out of four victims died; those who survived were usually scarred for life and often blinded. Children, who were generally more vulnerable to infectious disease, died from the condition more often than did adults, but it struck young and old alike, and without regard to social class.[1]

To save people from this deadly disease, a procedure called variolation was developed. Variolation is a term that refers to the controlled transfer of active smallpox lesions, taking the scabs or pustules from an infected person and placing them under the skin of an uninfected person with a lancet. This technique had long been practiced in Asia and Africa. Although British travelers reported seeing variolation through the seventeenth century, British doctors were unwilling to adopt it as practice. Credit for its eventual widespread use in England is usually assigned to Lady Mary Wortley Montagu, who in 1718 encountered the practice while traveling through Turkey with her husband, a British ambassador. Having survived the disease but witnessing its ravages, Montagu demanded that her son receive variolation by the embassy surgeon, and later, in 1721, she insisted he demonstrate the technique to the British physicians while variolating her daughter. As word spread, interest grew; experiments on the safety of variolation were performed on six prisoners, and later, on orphans, and those proving successful, the Princess of Wales asked to have her daughters variolated.[2] Owing to new popularity and the tightly organized practice of medicine in Europe, variolation became widespread.

Historical evidence shows that variolation was often accompanied by other now-dubious rituals that health providers encouraged, including fasting, bleeding, purging, and mercury consumption.[3] Variolation was risky and actually could *cause* the highly contagious disease it aimed to prevent, or communicate other infections, including tuberculosis, syphilis, or hepatitis. Two to three percent of people variolated died from complications. Even so, these fatalities were ten times lower than from the dreaded smallpox infection.[4]

Variolation reached the American colonies around 1721. Among its early champions was the Reverend Cotton Mather, who saw a smallpox epidemic erupt in the Boston area after a traveler arrived from the West Indies. Panicked, Mather tried to recruit physicians in the area to begin variolation, but was only able to convince Dr. Zabdiel Boylston to variolate anyone who wanted it. Variolation remained controversial in the colonies and as the disease spread through the largely uninoculated population, Mather and Boylston were viewed with increasing suspicion. In 1721, with smallpox infecting more than half of the twelve thousand residents of Boston, the men fought allegations that they were responsible and used statistics to defend themselves and educate the public: while 14 percent of people naturally contracted the disease, only 2 percent of variolated patients became infected.[5] In the following years, variolation became more popular in Europe, owing in large part to the data Mather published after the Boston smallpox epidemic. Although slow in the colonies, variolation received a boost during the Revolutionary War. After the American troops, stricken with smallpox, were unable to seize Quebec from British troops, who had all been variolated, Commander George Washington, himself a survivor of smallpox, required variolation of American troops.

Edward Jenner, a popular English physician, had heard stories of how Gloustershire's milkmaids were protected from smallpox because of their exposure to cowpox, which although similar to smallpox, was not harmful to humans. He theorized that cowpox could also be transmitted through variolation, but without the risks presented by using actual smallpox matter. In 1796 Jenner found a milkmaid with pox on her arms. Using these lesions, Jenner inoculated an eight-year-old boy.[6] Although he developed fever, loss of appetite, and aching for more than a week, he made a full recovery. Two months later, Jenner inoculated the same boy with fresh smallpox material. The boy did not become ill, suggesting he was protected by the initial variolation. Jenner's efforts to publish the results of this study were unsuccessful, but drawing on the Latin for cow, *vacca*, Jenner coined the term *vaccination* to describe the procedure of variolation with cowpox matter (rather than the more virulent smallpox) and published his theory and single result in a booklet he distributed. Jenner was not able to locate additional volunteers for his study, but other physicians he contacted were willing to try vaccination. They confirmed that cowpox vaccination protected against smallpox with less risk than variolation with smallpox material had presented to the inoculated.

Jenner sent vaccination material to other physicians, who often shared it with colleagues. Finding its way to New England, vaccination became popular, gradually replacing variolation, which became prohibited in 1840.[7] Jenner never sold his discovery, spent his own money to create and distribute stock of vaccination and information, and was known to vaccinate the poor in his town for free. At great personal cost, Jenner gave up his lifestyle as a physician and family man to become "a missionary to vaccination."[8] He was ridiculed and harangued throughout his life, both by colleagues who suggested that his growing fame was undeserved, and by popular critics who feared that his distribution of vaccination might lead to unknown complication, including humans sprouting animal parts, as a popularly reproduced cartoon shows.

Jenner's influence was indisputable on both sides of the Atlantic. Thomas Jefferson wrote to Jenner in 1806, "Medecine [*sic*] has never before produced any single improvement of such utility. . . . You have erased from the calendar of human afflictions one of its greatest. Yours is the comfortable reflection that mankind can never forget that you have lived."[9]

Jenner was not the first to recognize that cowpox prevented smallpox. He was not the first to use variolation from cowpox material, either. Yet Jenner was the first to systematically study the issue and to create widespread change through a public campaign. He helped to provide a framework for understanding how germs caused disease, challeng-

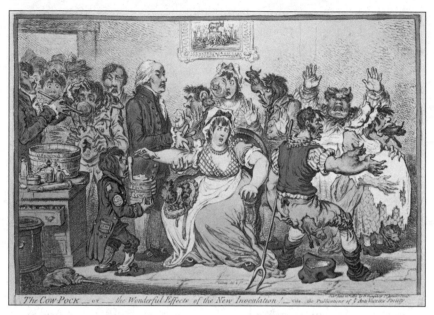

This 1802 cartoon, "The cow-pock—or—the wonderful effects of the new inoculation," by the British satirist James Gillray, expressed anxieties about the risks of vaccination, including that recipients might sprout cow parts. Library of Congress Prints and Photographs Division, reproduction number LC-USZC4–3147, call number PC 1—9924, http://www.loc.gov/pictures/item/94509853.

ing widely held views that illnesses were the result of spirits, miasmas, evil, or even moral failings.[10] As such, the early nineteenth century saw the first compulsory vaccination laws for smallpox, often in response to outbreaks.

In 1813 the U.S. Congress passed and Jefferson's successor President James Madison signed into law "An Act to Encourage Vaccination." This law established the first National Vaccine Agency, even requiring the U.S. Post Office to carry mail weighing up to half an ounce for free if it contained smallpox vaccine material. The goal of the act was to "preserve the genuine vaccine matter, and to furnish the same to any citizen of the United States." Cities or townships also passed their own laws to require vaccines. In so doing, they hoped to protect their neighborhoods or townships from disruptive quarantines and to limit fatalities. Localities expected that individuals would participate out of a sense of public duty, but retained the authority to levy taxes against those who refused.

For example, in 1820 the residents of North Hero, Vermont, voted to institute a tax to pay for the vaccination of all the town's residents after cases of smallpox were diagnosed in the area. Dan Hazen, though present at the town meeting where the tax was approved, did not vote for it and refused to pay it. In response, the town constable seized Hazen's cow and sold it to raise the payment. Hazen sued, leading to a ten-year legal battle that ended when the state's Supreme Court upheld the confiscation. This is one of the first articulations in the United States of the state's power to require vaccines and the willingness of the state to punish those who resist. It was not, however, the last.[11]

Expansion of State Power

Rates of smallpox rose with compulsory school attendance, which brought children into close quarters. In 1823 Boston became the first city to require evidence of vaccination for school attendance, with Massachusetts adopting its own law in 1855. Several other states followed by passing their own laws or developing new public health agencies and infrastructure to combat infectious disease. Thus, by the late 1890s, school attendance and mandatory vaccination laws had become linked. Courts also ruled that school boards, which hold no legislative power, may enact rules for public health, particularly in times of outbreaks, and that state legislatures may also give school boards such powers, providing legal support for these laws.[12]

Enforcement, however, was uneven. Teachers, principals, and school personnel were then, as they are today, largely uninterested in public health enforcement. Public health agents sporadically checked, and often discovered that fewer than half the children in a school might be vaccinated. On such instances, those agents might return and vaccinate all children who lacked a smallpox scar. In New York, for example, in 1894, fifty-six vaccinators from the health department distributed twenty-seven thousand vaccines to schoolchildren. In these ways, the state remained committed to compulsory vaccination and expended resources in support of those goals.[13]

Vaccines effectively limited outbreaks, which, in turn, fed complacency. Many people who had never experienced a smallpox epidemic became reluctant to undergo a procedure they viewed as unpleasant, risky, and of questionable necessity. As the legal scholars James Hodge and Lawrence Gostin suggest, "Since the vaccine has worked, why should individuals continue to be subjected to the harms of vaccination unless there exists an actual threat of disease in the community?" Those "who continued to press for vaccine were characterized as abusive, untrustworthy, and paternalistic." Resisting vaccines, they argue, was equated with fighting government oppression.[14] Suspicious of this new role for the state, organizations opposed to vaccinations grew in the second half of the nineteenth century.

Opponents distributed flyers and pamphlets, lobbied legislatures for the repeal of compulsory vaccination laws, filed lawsuits, and sought to discourage the use of vaccines. Their rhetoric rested on two linked claims: that vaccination was dangerous and unnecessary, and that legal compulsion to vaccinate was a violation of the country's foundational belief in individual liberty. In support of the first claim, they pointed to legal cases for illness or wrongful death caused by vaccines and circulated stories of medical complications. They also alleged that health departments falsified death records to mask vaccines as the cause and refused to share information about the risks. Although they were vehemently opposed to vaccination, their claims were grounded in reason.[15] As those against vaccines weighed the risks of inoculation, they did so in the context of a disease that had become rare by the end of the nineteenth century.[16]

For the second claim—that these laws violated individual liberty—the anti-vaccination groups opposed midnight raids, forced vaccination, and the quarantines that often destroyed the livelihood of owners and workers, sometimes enacted only because of the theoretical risk of infection or refusal to be vaccinated, rather than actual infection. They also argued that the new role of the state violated fundamental American values. Both these claims formed the basis for legal challenges.

Legal Challenges to State Power

Compulsory vaccination laws were, in fact, challenged in many court cases. After years of contradictory decisions from lower courts, the U.S. Supreme Court in 1904 considered whether requirements for vaccination were constitutional. In the landmark case of *Jacobson v.*

Massachusetts (1905), the Supreme Court heard a challenge to the Massachusetts compulsory vaccination law. The state law allowed "the board of health of a city or town, if, in its opinion, it is necessary for the public health or safety," to "require and enforce the vaccination and revaccination of all the inhabitants." The law also specified that anyone "being over twenty-one years of age and not under guardianship [who] refuses or neglects to comply with such requirement shall forfeit $5."[17]

Henning Jacobson, a minister who had emigrated from Sweden when he was thirteen and who lived in Cambridge, Massachusetts, challenged the legal requirement to be vaccinated or revaccinated. Although there was an outbreak at the time, he refused the vaccine for himself and was subsequently fined five dollars (about a hundred dollars today). He insisted that as children, both he and his older son had become ill after being vaccinated and he thus did not want to be revaccinated. He also refused to pay the fine.

Jacobson presented fourteen arguments against vaccination, including the general lack of safety, lack of efficacy, probability of harm, and his own experience of becoming ill after vaccination. More generally, he argued that "a compulsory vaccination law is unreasonable, arbitrary and oppressive, and, therefore, hostile to the inherent right of every freeman to care for his own body and health in such way as to him seems best."[18] Claiming that the laws violated his constitutional liberty interests, which he believed supported the right to bodily integrity, Jacobson insisted that the law was unconstitutional. He also reiterated his commitment to his religion and his objection to the use of cowpox in vaccines, asking, "Can the free citizen of Massachusetts, who is not yet a pagan, nor an idolator, be compelled to undergo this rite and to participate in this new—no, revived—form of worship of the Sacred Cow?"[19]

The lower courts who ruled against him and later the U.S. Supreme Court found his fourteen facts to be immaterial to the legal question at hand. In 1905 the U.S. Supreme Court ruled against Jacobson. In a 7–2 decision, the Court articulated a more narrow view of individual liberty, and clarified the rights of the state to enforce public health. The decision posits,

> The liberty secured by the Constitution of the United States does not import an absolute right in each person to be at all times, and in all

circumstances, wholly freed from restraint, nor is it an element in such liberty that one person, or a minority of persons residing in any community and enjoying the benefits of its local government, should have power to dominate the majority when supported in their action by the authority of the State. It is within the police power of a State to enact a compulsory vaccination law, and it is for the legislature, and not for the courts, to determine in the first instance whether vaccination is or is not the best mode for the prevention of smallpox and the protection of the public health.[20]

The decision did not simply limit individual liberty, but also confirmed a shared community obligation embodied in vaccine requirements. The decision continues,

Society based on the rule that each one is a law unto himself would soon be confronted with disorder and anarchy. Real liberty for all could not exist under the operation of a principle which recognizes the right of each individual person to use his own, whether in respect of his person or his property, regardless of the injury that may be done to others.[21]

This decision makes clear that police powers are not absolute. Public agents must demonstrate public health necessity and not be exercised in "an arbitrary, unreasonable manner" or go "beyond what was reasonably required for the safety of the public." This includes the requirement that there be a reasonable relationship between the intervention and the legitimate public health goal. Additionally, the police powers of the state may not be used in ways that are oppressive, arbitrary, or absurd in consequence, or increase health risks.[22]

Enforcement of vaccines and the expanding role of the state in supporting intervention into private lives cannot be viewed outside the historical context in which states were developing health departments, sanitation boards, and new institutions. This new role of the state as a protector of the public reflected the optimism of the Progressive Era. The ethos that the state can compel individuals toward behaviors they might not otherwise choose for themselves or their children for the good of the community was reaffirmed in other U.S. Supreme Court decisions, including decisions that upheld Congress's right to limit child labor (*Hammer v. Dagenhart*, 1918), states' rights to compel school attendance (*Zucht v. King*, 1922), and even the power of the state to force involuntary sterilization of those deemed unfit to reproduce (*Buck v. Bell*, 1927). The logic also facilitated passage of state laws banning interracial marriage, allowing quarantine, and establishing Prohibition. In short, the Progressive Era was marked by a willingness to limit individual rights and liberties for the perceived health of the community.[23]

This era also saw multiplying numbers of specialists and governmental agencies in healthcare, social work, family life, and education, advising individuals on how to live, eat, parent, and birth.[24] Highlighting the new role of experts who aimed to reform civil society, Colgrove notes, "Expert knowledge formed the basis on which these reformers based their claim to be better qualified than parents to judge the well-being of children."[25]

With police powers and an intense focus on preventing disease, some newly empowered public health entities saw it as their duty to protect public health at all costs. Often relying on coercive methods, state health departments were known to sweep through neighborhoods, looking for incidence of disease and inoculating those in the area. In some areas, the inspectors attempted to forcibly remove children from their homes or vaccinated individuals at gunpoint.[26] In others, they aimed to enact quarantines around the homes of those who were ill. Other cities tried to inspect train stations for boarding passengers who were ill, require vaccination before leaving, or ban public gatherings.[27]

Over time, enforcement of vaccination requirements waned, as did occurrences of smallpox. Simultaneously, anti-vaccination sentiment strengthened. Smallpox was less common, and a milder version of the disease (variola minor) appeared in 1897, which made fear of the vaccine stronger than fear of the disease. The U.S. Public Health Service (a precursor to the Food and Drug Administration) gained powers to inspect vaccine manufacturers, which made vaccines safer but also revealed how microorganisms such as the lethal tetanus bacilli could contaminate them.[28]

There was also broad-based distrust of the state, fueled in part by populist social movements, disapproval of Supreme Court decisions like *Jacobson*, and the Red Scare of 1919, which made communitarian campaigns suspect. The anti-vaccine movement was diverse and in-

cluded homeopathic practitioners and the new specialty of chiroprac-
tic medicine, both of which rejected the necessity of vaccines, as well
as Christian Scientists and anti-vivisectionists, who objected to animal
experimentation. Parents whose children had died or been harmed following vaccination also joined the movement. In the early twentieth
century, states began to repeal mandatory vaccine laws or to pass ballot
initiatives to limit state powers around vaccines.

Diphtheria and the Voluntary Use of Vaccines

The twentieth century brought about a "bacteriological revolution,"
with new understandings of germs, new vaccines, and an evolution in
research.[29] Scientific methods became more rigorous and organized,
in part supported by the newly created departments of health. These
innovations in healthcare, including vaccines, further shaped a popular belief that science could overcome disease. One such disease was
diphtheria, which was the first widely used vaccine for which the state,
lacking mechanisms of enforcement, persuaded parents to use.

Diphtheria, seldom seen today in the United States, is a bacterial infection of the upper respiratory system, spread easily through airborne
droplets. Its bacteria produce a toxin that attacks the body, which commonly causes sore throat, inflammation of the throat and lymph nodes,
and sometimes swelling of the heart, damage to kidneys, and neurological weakness or numbness. Its hallmark feature and what makes it so
dangerous is a thick gray pseudo-membrane that develops in the back
of an infected person's throat, often blocking the airway. The death rate
before treatment was as high as 50 percent, most often in young children
and in adults over forty years old.[30]

The first breakthroughs in treating diphtheria came in the 1890s,
when researchers in Europe found that blood serum from an infected
animal contained antitoxin that could be injected into those afflicted to
help them recover. Researchers soon discovered that mixing antitoxin
with small amounts of the toxin could produce immunity against the
disease for several years. Published in 1913, these results led to the first
vaccine against diphtheria. Along with the subsequent invention of a
skin test to confirm immunity, either from exposure or successful vaccination, these innovations facilitated more reliable research.[31]

World War I delayed vaccine innovation in Europe (where both discoveries were made), and testing fell primarily to two New York researchers, William Park and Abraham Zingher, who began testing the efficacy of the vaccine in ways that illustrate how different research practices were at the time. First, they tested it on children in orphanages, giving them the vaccine and then the Schick skin test, which would show evidence of immunity. With successful results, they took their research to the public schools, where enthusiastic school officials sent letters home asking for parental consent to participate in a larger study.[32] Some also included letters—written in English, Italian, and Yiddish—to reassure parents that unlike smallpox, toxin-antitoxin could not make children sick.[33] With principals' endorsements, about 75 percent of families consented.[34] Schick tests were given to each student; those not immune were immunized. The researchers created a group of ninety thousand inoculated and now immune children, whom they could compare to a group of ninety thousand children whose parents refused participation.[35] The goal of testing the vaccine on children was driven by the reality that children were the ones most vulnerable to the disease and thus, the ones who would most benefit.

Anti-vaccination activists remained distrustful of government-sponsored health programs and highlighted how children were being used as guinea pigs. In 1919 a poorly prepared vial of toxin-antitoxin led to six deaths, and more than fifty people became ill.[36] Other tragedies occurred after toxin-antitoxin had frozen in transit or was contaminated by serum from a sick animal.[37] Yet these complications were rare and largely manageable and correctable. Nonetheless, objections continued, including from those who opposed the use of animals to collect blood serum, and chiropractors who opposed vaccines as polluting children's naturally healthy bodies. In less organized ways, parents felt uneasy about vaccination, were unsure whether diphtheria vaccination was redundant to smallpox vaccination, feared adverse reactions, or believed that good nutrition would protect their children.

Rather than compelling its use, the trend was instead to continue efforts to persuade parents that the vaccine was lifesaving and safe. In collaboration with insurance companies, the New York City Health Department in 1929 created the Diphtheria Prevention Commission, which launched an aggressive marketing campaign to convince parents to get their children vaccinated. Metropolitan Life Insurance Company, for example, working closely with researchers and serving its own financial self-interest, distributed thousands of pamphlets to its policy holders touting the benefits of diphtheria vaccination. Magazines like the *Saturday Evening Post, Ladies' Home Journal,* and *Good Housekeeping* also promoted it.[38] The New York Health Department mailed letters to almost a quarter of a million new mothers urging them to vaccinate their babies against diphtheria. More than three thousand posters were hung in retail stores, movie theaters added trailers to encourage vaccination, and eighty-five thousand leaflets in foreign languages were distributed. The city even hung a two-hundred-foot illuminated sign at Broadway and Twenty-Third Street, among the biggest ever seen in New York. The campaign succeeded; more than 292,000 children received immunization and the city's death rate from diphtheria was cut by almost half.[39] The size and influence of this coordinated effort—between corporations, government, and media—cannot be underestimated.

Between 1900 and 1930, life expectancy increased from forty-seven to sixty years.[40] This rapid change speaks to advances in sanitation, clean water, clean milk supplies, and other public health interventions, but vaccines played a role.[41] The successful diphtheria campaigns transformed American understandings of medicine generally and vaccines specifically. First, the diphtheria vaccine was really the first systematic use of the germ theory and communicated the utility of this new understanding of bacteria. Second, it transformed expectations of how science and medicine should be practiced, thereby adding significant prestige to these fields in new ways.[42] Unsurprisingly, these changes mirrored the transformation of the profession of medicine, from an idiosyncratic system of training to one that was centrally controlled and increasingly composed of elites.[43] By the 1930s, it was clear that toxin-antitoxin provided only temporary coverage and that healthy carriers—that is, people who carry the disease but show no symptoms—could facilitate outbreaks. Researchers developed a new vaccine based on a weakened form of the bacteria, still in use today. In so doing, they created what the sociologist Jacob Heller calls "the vaccine narrative," that is, the public consensus that as preventative care, vaccines represent an unequivocal good.[44]

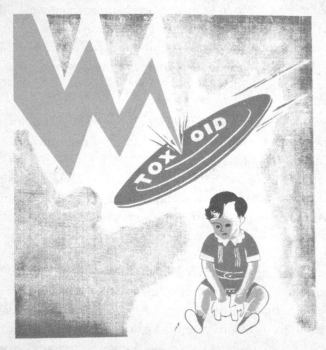

Poster from the Chicago Department of Health on the dangers of diphtheria, c. 1936–1941. Chicago Department of Health, Illinois WPA Art. Library of Congress Prints and Photographs Division, reproduction number LC-USZC2–5171, call number POS—WPA—ILL .01 .D56, no. 1, http://www.loc.gov/pictures/item/98508392.

In addition to building trust in science and medicine, diphtheria shaped the modern understanding of vaccines. Rather than focusing on community obligation, as the smallpox vaccine had, diphtheria was marketed to individuals for individual benefit. As Colgrove explains,

> Instead of protecting the community from imminent peril, citizens were urged to take action in order to move their community toward a state of perfect health. Because toxin-antitoxin was relatively safe and painless, health officials could appeal more directly to individual self-interest, without asking people to subordinate their well-being, or that of their children, to the good of the community.[45]

The success of appealing to individuals generally and mothers specifically, rather than to community responsibility, continues to inform how vaccines are promoted.

Finally, efforts to advertise the diphtheria vaccine, alongside growth in professions committed to child and family health, became part of the new enterprise of health education. Civic groups joined efforts to make health consumption central. As the head of the American Public Health Association explained in 1927, "Health is a saleable commodity. . . . Mere laws to enforce health do not create change."[46] People could be taught to avoid illness, to make better choices to promote their families' health, and to consume products identified (usually by the manufacturer) as health-promoting. Most of this marketing targeted mothers, who were faced with a plethora of expert advice on feeding, childrearing, well-baby care, and consumption of new items like vitamins, toothpaste, and vaccines, as seen in the poster reproduced here.[47] Public health promoters were so convinced of the superiority of their methods that some argued that deaths from diphtheria could be seen as a sign of child neglect. For example, a representative of the American Child Health Association stated in 1926, "The time will come when every case of diphtheria will be an indictment against the intelligence of parents . . . and it will not be many years before every death from diphtheria will be referred to a coroner's jury for investigation for criminal responsibility."[48] Together, the notion that good parents seek out vaccines and trust experts took hold.

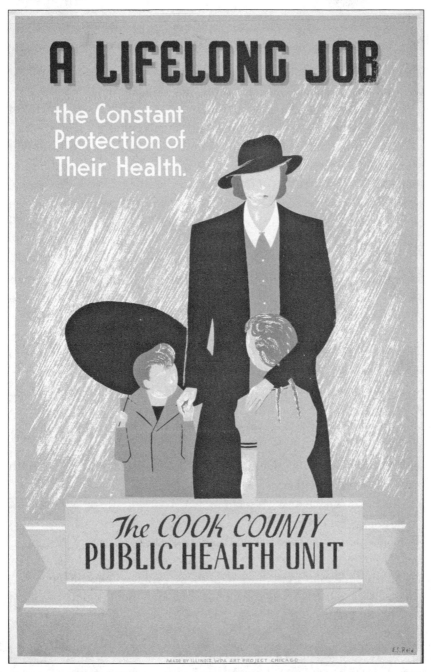

Poster from the Cook County Public Health Unit, c. 1936–1941. Illinois WPA Art Project. Library of Congress Prints and Photographs Division, http://www.loc.gov/pictures/collection/wpapos/item/98513455.

Professional Dominance and the New Public Health

This new ethic of health promotion created new challenges to and for doctors, who saw themselves as the only legitimate practitioners of care. The battle over a particular public health law provides an example of how these issues played out. The goal of the Sheppard-Towner Act of 1921 aimed to reduce maternal and infant mortality. At the time, infant mortality rates were 10–20 percent for the first year of life and higher than 30 percent by the age of five, with poor families disproportionately affected.[49] Death in pregnancy and childbirth, a leading cause of death of women at the time, was also a significant issue. This law aimed to address these issues by allocating $1 million in federal funds annually for five years to support public health programs in states and localities, most particularly in rural and low-income communities where rates were especially high. Specifically, the funding would support health clinics, which would hire doctors and nurses to educate and care for pregnant women and their children, provide funding for visiting nurses who would care for and educate new mothers and pregnant women in their homes, train midwives who would remain in those communities and provide care. It would also provide infrastructure for vaccination. Additionally, funds would be used to produce educational materials on nutrition, hygiene, and parenting. In short, the law and its funding aimed to improve the health of women and children, particularly those with the least access, by deploying the new science of children's health promotion and parent education.

The American Medical Association (AMA) vehemently opposed the bill, arguing that it represented a form of socialism. Despite these objections and the fact that the bill represented the first federal investment in social welfare, it passed easily by a vote of 279 to 39 in the House and by a similarly wide margin in the Senate.[50] The program was implemented, but when the bill was to be reauthorized in 1926, the political tides had changed and the AMA, after strongly lobbying against it, saw its defeat. In doing so, the AMA repositioned medical doctors as the centerpiece of health promotion and care, discredited women providers, who, it argued, were not serious about public health, and significantly limited the role public health nurses, midwives, or community health educators could legitimately play.[51]

The fight over Sheppard-Towner influenced how vaccines would be funded and distributed. Public health practitioners and policy makers saw vaccines as the best way to promote community health. As a result, they aimed to immunize as many people as possible as quickly as possible, which meant providing public vaccine clinics and vaccines for free. These methods undermined the interests of physicians, who aimed to control patient education as a one-on-one experience conducted in their private practice settings and their ability to charge for their services and expertise. Editorials of the era advised government officials to save resources for those who most need them by refusing free services to those most able to pay. By 1930, public health leaders were brokering compacts with physicians. The health departments would not provide free vaccine if doctors provided them at discounted rates, often during special hours when parents could drop in with their children. This arrangement did not lead to higher rates of vaccination, but did generally give physicians ownership of vaccination. The American Academy of Pediatrics, which formed in 1930, began making recommendations about routine childhood vaccinations in 1934, and has largely been responsible for overseeing those recommendations since.

Through the 1930s, medicine alongside scientific research with new, more rigorous methods continued to grow. Perhaps the greatest innovation that led to significant goodwill for medicine was the advent of antibiotics, which made it possible to treat the wounds of soldiers in World War II as well as an array of infectious diseases, including sexually transmitted infections. As the sociologist Paul Starr explains, "the advent of antibiotics and other advances gave physicians increased mastery of disease and confirmed confidence in their judgment and skill."[52] Building on American success over infectious disease, researchers set their sights on other childhood diseases, often with mixed results.

Pertussis and the Changing Expectations of Research

Pertussis, or whooping cough, has always been hard to vaccinate against, but worthy of attention. Known as a killer of babies, pertussis is caused by bacteria that infect the upper respiratory tract. In the first stage of infection, bacteria cause fever, coughing, congestion, and aches. Worsening over ten days, the infected are highly contagious, though antibiotics will help. As infection takes hold, the bacteria release toxins that enter the cells in the tissues and alter cell function, essentially reprograming those cells to reproduce the toxin, which interferes with breathing; the result is a cough with a unique whooping sound. During the second stage of the disease, the bacteria are mostly dead, making antibiotics ineffective. The second phase can last up to ten weeks, and is sometimes known as the hundred-day cough. Pertussis is most dangerous to babies under one year, whose airways are narrow and more easily obstructed; currently in the United States, about half of infected infants will be hospitalized. From 1922 to 1931, about 1.7 million cases of whooping cough were reported in the United States, causing about seventy-three thousand deaths. In the 1940s, pertussis killed about three thousand children a year.[53]

Efforts to create a vaccine against pertussis began in 1906, when German scientists first isolated the bacteria. *Bordetella pertussis* was a difficult organism to grow in a petri dish and did not easily infect mice or other laboratory animals, making testing difficult. By 1931, more than a dozen laboratories had developed versions of vaccines against pertussis, but no scientific consensus existed about which formulation was best or what the appropriate dosing or timing might be.[54] In the United States, two vaccines won the endorsement of the American Academy of Pediatrics. The first was tested on Illinois schoolchildren, but without sound controls in place, which had become the professional standard.[55] The second, developed by Pearl Kendrick and Grace Elderling, used more than four thousand children under the age of five years whose parents had volunteered them during the Great Depression.[56] Using a whole cell that was alive, but weakened, to create an immune response against the dreaded disease, Kendrick worked with another researcher, Margaret Pittman, to improve standardization of the vaccine in manufacturing, including the discovery that thimerosal was the best preservative for the vaccine.[57] Other studies showed that vaccines given in combination created a synergistic effect that improved the immune response of both vaccines. As such, pertussis, packaged with diphtheria and a vaccine against tetanus, became widely available by the early 1950s as the DPT injection.[58] This vaccine was imperfect and, as we will see later in this chapter, its side effects increasingly became a source of concern to parents and providers. Yet it was also successful in preventing pertussis, lessening symptoms in those infected, and creating new expectations for scientific rigor and large-scale testing of new vaccines. These standards set the stage for the race to find a vaccine against polio.

State, Charity, and Corporations: The Race for the Polio Vaccine

Vaccine lore usually identifies the polio vaccine as one of the great successes of science. And yet polio was a disease with relatively low rates of morbidity and mortality, with about 90 percent of those afflicted having few or mild symptoms; it also killed fewer children than measles, diphtheria, or pertussis.[59] Yet polio was feared because in about 1 percent of cases, those infected would become permanently crippled; it also spread easily. Poliomyelitis, known also as the disease of infantile paralysis, showed no preference for race, class, sanitation, or neighborhood. The paralysis of thirty-nine-year-old Franklin Delano Roosevelt, a politician and businessman from a privileged background who would go on to become president, illustrated this and reminded others of the randomness and cruelty of the disease.

During the summer of 1921, while vacationing at his summer home off the coast of Maine, Roosevelt woke with a fever and weakness in his legs. Weeks later he was diagnosed with polio. Roosevelt was reluctant to accept that the diagnosis of paralysis was permanent and sought out different treatments and modalities. He also lived with pain. Accounts detail how Roosevelt imagined that his political career was over but refused to accept the limitations of his disease, using braces, swimming, strengthening his upper body, and adapting modalities to accommodate his disability. He was deeply committed to defeating polio, not just his own, but the disease in general.[60] In 1938 Roosevelt and his former law partner Basil O'Connor founded the National Foundation for Infantile Paralysis (NFIP), which provided care for victims of polio and funded a search for a cure or vaccine. Rather than drawing on family wealth, as most foundations did, the NFIP instituted the March of Dimes, where people all over the country were encouraged to contribute small denominations of money that would collectively fund the national battle against polio. The campaign drew on parental fear, public sympathies, and aggressive marketing through film, radio, and print media, with the face of a president crippled himself by the disease out in front. The

March of Dimes made the search for a polio vaccine a national priority, even as polio did not represent the largest health risk at the time. By 1954, the eight largest health charities raised over $140 million; the NFIP accounted for almost half of those funds.[61] Faith in the nation, which had stood by its people through the Great Depression, and in science, which brought penicillin, was also high. In the postwar years financial investment in biomedical research, newly seen as a valuable national asset, increased quickly in both the public and private sectors.[62] These factors undoubtedly set the stage for the development of the polio vaccine.

The NFIP funded research and brought together top national researchers to share information. One such group determined that there were three types of polio virus, making it clear that a successful vaccine would need to work against all three. The Harvard researcher John Enders, who would later win the Nobel Prize, made a significant breakthrough in 1949 when he cultured the virus and showed that it could grow in non-nerve tissue, which established that the vaccine could work systemically.[63] These discoveries paved the way for the development of two polio vaccines: one developed by Jonas Salk using a killed virus and another using a live but attenuated virus that was weakened by serial passage through cultures until it could no longer cause disease but could still inspire immunity. The latter vaccine was developed in its most successful form by Albert Sabin. It is worth noting that others were developing a similar strategy at the time, including Isabel Morgan, who successfully immunized monkeys with a killed virus vaccine in 1949, and Hilary Koprowski, a pharmaceutical researcher without funding from the NFIP who first successfully tested a live vaccine on institutionalized children.[64] Although children in institutions had been the subject of vaccine research before, in the post-Nuremberg era, Koprowski's research findings, developed outside academe in a commercial lab, enjoyed a chilly reception and his vaccine never became widely distributed.[65] This detail crisply illustrates the power of the NFIP as a national charity to shape science and scientists' careers. With the NFIP's commitment to a killed virus vaccine over a live attenuated one, Salk's vaccine went forward.

Jonas Salk began testing his vaccine first, with parental consent, on institutionalized children who had already had polio to measure antibody response, and then subsequently on institutionalized children who had not had polio, with permission of the state. Although small-scale, with only 161 participants (and ethically questionable by today's understandings of informed consent in research), these initial trials proved successful.[66] With the enthusiastic support of the NFIP and during a widespread outbreak of polio in 1952, Salk laid the groundwork for what would be the largest clinical trial in history.[67]

In 1954 the NFIP began enrolling schoolchildren to test the polio vaccine. Believing so strongly in the vaccine, Salk and O'Connor of the NFIP argued they should not give placebos to children. Salk explained in a letter to O'Connor that he would feel "that every child who is injected with a placebo and becomes paralyzed will do so at my hands."[68] After heated disagreement, the field study went forward with a compromise that only 41 percent of children would receive placebo, but that it would be a double-blind study—where neither researchers nor participants knew whether they were receiving the vaccine or a placebo injection.[69] The rate of polio diagnoses at the time was about 50 per 100,000 per year. As a result, the study would have to be very large to observe effects. Within a year, 1.8 million children had enrolled in this study. With constant news coverage, more than 90 percent of Americans knew about the trials and waited eagerly for results.

In April 1955, the announcement came: the vaccine was 90 percent effective against types 2 and 3 of the polio virus and between 60 and 70 percent effective against the more virulent type 1. The Salk polio vaccine worked. Salk, sharing little credit with colleagues and staff, became a celebrity-scientist who erroneously appeared to work in isolation. Salk was interested in patenting the polio vaccine, but was unable since he had merely synthesized existing scientific methods and had not actually created anything new. Yet his modest public response and insistence that the people owned the vaccine ensured continued public faith. As he told a reporter, "There is no patent. Could you patent the sun?"[70] Within hours of the announcement, six pharmaceutical companies, many that had produced vaccines for the trial, were granted licenses to commercially manufacture the vaccine. This perhaps marks one of the first significant mergers between public research and for-profit pharmaceutical production.[71]

Almost immediately, problems arose. The first major problem was the lack of clarity in how the vaccine would be distributed and who

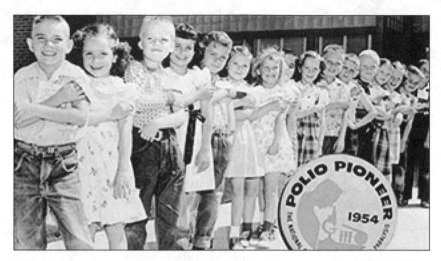

"Polio Pioneers" participating in the field trial. March of Dimes, http://marchofdimes. areavoices.com/files/2012/03/Polio-Photo.jpg.

would decide. Unlike diphtheria, which public health officials worked hard to persuade parents they wanted, the polio vaccine was in high demand. Parents not surprisingly wanted the vaccine for their children, particularly as summer polio season approached. The NFIP had committed funds to all six companies to buy vaccines to distribute to states so they could offer free vaccines to first- and second-grade children, the age group polio most often struck. After companies filled that order, no one was sure how much vaccine would be available or how it should be distributed. Should it be sold to private physicians? Should city and county health agencies be guaranteed a certain portion? The vaccine was most effective when given in a three-shot series. Yet it could be rationed to give out fewer shots to each child to spread it more broadly. It was clear that there would be inadequate stock to satisfy demand, but the next steps were not so clear. Despite the goodwill that led to the creation of the inactivated polio vaccine (IPV), confusion over how the vaccine would be distributed, whether those with political connections or wealth would be given priority, and even who had authority to decide created distrust among consumers.[72]

Parents and local authorities voiced concern about equitable distribution of the vaccine, and some urged the federal government to step in and manage distribution, in part to make sure it remained available to poor urban children. Yet others passionately opposed the government entering the vaccination program. The American Medical Association, which had aggressively campaigned against President Harry Truman's plan to create a national healthcare system, ferociously objected and in 1955 passed a resolution opposing any purchase or distribution of vaccines by the federal government except for those who were too poor to pay for it themselves (and presumably too poor to pay private physicians). Similarly, the American Drug Manufacturers Association lobbied against federal involvement. Drug companies argued that the Salk vaccine belonged to them and insisted that if it were "socialized," they would have no incentive to develop new products, which would be harmful to the country.[73] Although the Canadian government began manufacturing the Salk vaccine, which proved safe and cheap, Americans went a different direction. With a diffuse fear of communism as a backdrop, Congress authorized funds to give to states to buy vaccines, but refused to prescribe methods by which vaccines would be distributed, except to note that it was to go to people under the age of twenty years, pregnant women, and those who could not afford them.[74]

Just over two weeks after the Salk trials had been nationally celebrated, confidence in the vaccine suffered a blow. Reports of paralytic polio in those who had recently received the Salk vaccine emerged. Government investigators traced the outbreak to vaccine produced by Cutter Laboratories, which had not adequately inactivated the vaccine in the manufacturing process. Among the children who received the 120,000 doses from the two defective pools of vaccine, about forty thousand had minor symptoms, including headache, stiff neck, fever, and muscle weakness. Others were more seriously affected: fifty-one were permanently paralyzed and five died. The Cutter vaccine also led to outbreaks of polio: 113 people in the children's families or communities were paralyzed, and five more died. By most accounts, it was one of the worst pharmaceutical disasters in U.S. history.[75]

The Cutter Incident harmed consensus about the vaccine, but it did not destroy it; demand for the vaccine remained high in the first year, with more than five million people receiving it.[76] Unfortunately, supply remained limited, particularly after new safety testing was implemented, and questions of what constituted equitable distribution continued. Doctors believed they should be allowed to buy as much vaccine as needed to meet the demands of paying patients and should not be bound by the age limits set by local officials who continued to prioritize vaccination for those between the ages of five and nine years. Parents, community groups, school officials, and others complained of unfair distribution, and argued that no private physicians should get any vaccine until all children had the opportunity to receive it in school or community settings. These questions remained unresolved and further eroded trust in public vaccine policy.

Supply increased the following year, and questions of distribution disappeared, particularly as demand had flattened. Suddenly, vaccine promoters had to find new ways to communicate the importance of vaccination. Even without age limits and with ample availability, demand did not rise. The NFIP hosted social events like the "Salk Hop" for teens, aggressively publicized the vaccine, and even enlisted celebrity sponsors to promote it. In late 1956, the NFIP commissioned a survey, which showed that demand for the polio vaccine had dropped because there was widespread belief that (1) victory over polio had been achieved as rates of the disease had dropped; (2) adults did not need the vaccine, which protected against a childhood disease (as the name "infantile paralysis" indicated); and (3) it was no longer necessary. This latter perception reflected the reality that the incidence of polio had gone from 38,000 in 1954 to 5,500 in 1957, owing in part to the vaccine itself.[77]

Limits of the Salk Vaccine

The Salk vaccine had limits. Rates of polio in 1958 began rising despite widespread vaccination. However, unlike patterns of disease before the vaccine, which showed no favoritism by neighborhood, income, or race, the resurgence appeared to cluster in poor neighborhoods and mostly among nonwhite residents who lacked access to private physicians and consistent medical care. The Salk vaccine, while safe and effective, also did not provide lifelong immunity, raising questions as to whether a fourth shot should be recommended.

Albert Sabin, a researcher who had developed a polio vaccine made from live but weakened virus, had always been critical of the NFIP's quick embrace of the Salk vaccine. A live vaccine, he argued, worked better and provided long-lasting immunity in a way the inactivated polio vaccine (IPV) could not. Sabin wanted to test his vaccine, which would not be possible in the United States, given the high rates of use of the Salk vaccine. Returning to his country of birth, Sabin provided his oral vaccine—eaten on a sugar cube—to 15 million Russian children to demonstrate that it was safe and effective. Despite the NFIP's opposition, by 1962, the Sabin oral polio vaccine became licensed and ready for manufacture and distribution in the United States.

The oral polio vaccine (OPV) was preferable for several reasons: it could be more easily administered since it did not require hypodermic needles, which made mass vaccination possible; it conferred immunity in days, rather than months, which meant it could be used in response to outbreaks; and since the attenuated virus would pass through the digestive system and be excreted by the child who was vaccinated, others would potentially be exposed and receive some immunity as well, which would potentially support community health. It also did not need the multiple boosters the Salk vaccine required.[78] By the mid-1960s, with the support of several medical organizations, OPV became the preferred polio vaccine in the United States and abroad.

Vaccine Injury and the Duty to Inform

Despite its ease of use, OPV had one serious shortcoming. By the end of 1962, it became clear that in rare cases, the inactivated polio virus could revert to its active form and cause paralysis. Most often in adults and most commonly with the first dose, polio from vaccination happened in about one case per 2.6 million doses (but one per 520,000 first doses).[79] Unlike the Cutter Incident, these cases resulted not from a failure in manufacture of the vaccine, but from the design of the vaccine itself. In two significant legal cases, *Davis v. Wyeth* (1968) and *Reyes v. Wyeth* (1974), courts considered how a vaccine manufacturer might be liable in a case where the vaccine itself—even when perfectly manufactured—carried risks and how those risks should be communicated to consumers. In the first case, a thirty-nine-year-old man attended a mass vaccination clinic, and despite recommendations that adults over thirty should not receive OPV, was given it anyway, without warning of the increased risk his age presented. In the second, an eight-month-old baby was given OPV and developed paralytic polio; her parents had not been advised of the risks the vaccine carried. In these two important cases, courts ruled that the vaccine manufacturer Wyeth Laboratories had a duty to warn consumers of risk. If the manufacturer could not warn the recipient directly of the possibility of an adverse outcome, including paralytic polio, it was to ensure that whoever gave the vaccine did so.[80]

The American Academy of Pediatrics, along with other public health organizations, argued on behalf of Wyeth that it would be impractical to warn every recipient of a vaccine of minuscule risk that might result and would undermine trust in vaccines. Reiterating "the right of the individual to choose and control what risk he will take," including the risk of paralysis, appellate courts rejected these arguments as paternalistic. As the polio vaccine moved forward, there was a choice for consumers to make: the IPV was safe but did not provide long-term protection in all children, and the OPV was very effective, but could in fact cause polio in rare cases.[81] Without a clear role for the state, communicating risk to the public or moving forward with a coherent plan became a challenge.

Social Justice and the Return of Compulsory Vaccine Laws

That changed in 1964. At that time, the CDC formed the Advisory Committee on Immunization Practices (ACIP), which became—and remains—responsible for coordinating recommendations for routine vaccination and advising private physicians.[82] In so doing, the CDC claimed a central role in national vaccination policy. Even with vaccine developments in the 1950s, those who suffered disease tended to be poor and live in communities of color. As such, the federal government needed to find ways to infuse new funds into existing vaccine programs against childhood diseases, funding that supported broader goals of addressing "the trinity of poverty, education, and disease" set out by the Kennedy, and then Johnson, administrations.[83] These new funds would focus on intensive but temporary community immunization programs. The Vaccination Assistance Act, as it moved through Congress in 1962, faced only a few objections. Christian Scientists wanted assurance that vaccines would not become compulsory. CDC officials assured them that the bill did not contain any language about compulsion and that the federal government had no power or authority to require vaccines, since that power resided with states and localities. The American Academy of Pediatrics wanted assurance that this bill would not pull patients away from their private practices into community programs. The bill passed and the CDC began organizing conferences to seek feedback on best vaccine practices and policy.

After polio, vaccine researchers found new ways to conquer old diseases, including a vaccine against measles in 1963, mumps in 1967, and rubella in 1969. These were not the same feared and dreaded diseases of smallpox or polio, even as measles killed more children each year than had polio.[84] They were nearly universally experienced, with about three to four million people infected in the United States each year; of those, between four hundred and five hundred died, forty-eight thousand were hospitalized, and another thousand developed chronic disability. Measles, for most people, is a mild illness. However, children can develop more serious complications like pneumonia, ear infection, diarrhea, deafness, brain swelling, intellectual disability, or, in rare instances (about one in 1,000), death; infection can also cause miscarriage or premature birth.[85] Mumps, once a ubiquitous childhood illness, is also relatively mild, commonly with fever, headache, muscle ache, loss of appetite, and most characteristically, swollen glands under the ears or jaw. Mumps, which lasts seven to ten days, is uncomfortable. Complications are rare but more serious in teens and adults, including testicular or breast swelling, sterility, or more serious secondary infection. German measles (rubella) is also a minor childhood illness, perhaps the most innocuous of them all. It presents with a rash, low fever, and symptoms of a bad cold and lasts a few days. Yet its ramifications in the community are significant. Women exposed to rubella early in pregnancy face high rates of birth defects in their children, including blindness, deafness, heart damage, cataracts, internal organ damage, and intellectual disability. Before vaccination, rubella was the leading cause of congenital deafness in the United States.[86]

A vaccine against rubella addressed two major problems. First, in years of rubella outbreaks, many babies were born with birth defects. Calculating the risk of birth defects from exposure before vaccine is difficult, with estimates ranging from 20 to 50 percent, but the disease clearly caused problems.[87] Second, women in the 1950s would come to hospital review boards to request an abortion because they had been exposed to rubella early in pregnancy. Abortion at the time was often available only for medical necessity, to be determined by a hospital review committee. There was no way to verify rubella exposure, so committee members relied on subjective judgments. The AMA opposed abortion, and many doctors feared that women made false claims of rubella exposure to obtain an abortion.[88] A vaccine held the promise of solving this.

As the rubella vaccine was licensed, questions of how to distribute it emerged. Unlike other vaccines, the goal of the rubella vaccine was to protect fetuses, not children. Targeting only adult women who intended to become pregnant or even teen girls was unlikely to be successful in preventing exposure. Yet the vaccine did little to improve the health of the person receiving it, since the disease's symptoms were so minor to the infected. The question became then whether it was acceptable to introduce risk to the individual receiving the vaccine for the goal of protecting community (and fetal) health. This was a new problem for vaccines, which were almost always marketed as providing benefit to the person inoculated. Even as the rubella vaccine contradicted this logic, Americans in the post-polio era largely trusted vaccines and saw them as lifesaving technologies. Capitalizing on this goodwill, the United States rejected a strategy of targeting the vaccine to those whose fetuses would most benefit, and instead adopted a strategy of universally vaccinating children—some who would eventually become pregnant, others who would encounter pregnant women around them.

Fairness and Access

As new vaccines became available in the 1960s and 1970s, questions of how they should be distributed continued to arise. Vaccines remained more available to high-income children, even as the clear goal was to eliminate childhood illnesses for all children. In part, this was due to the reality that the new measles vaccine, licensed in 1963, was very expensive. The 1962 Vaccination Assistance Act had created a pool of federal funds that states and localities could use to buy and dispense vaccines against polio, diphtheria, pertussis, and tetanus. Although states could use funds for newer, more costly vaccines, doing so would exhaust funds sooner. For example, measles vaccine often cost twice that of all the others combined. The tension between private practice control and public health distribution grew.

In 1964 the ACIP, the new federal advisory body on vaccines, recommended that "immunization should be carried out as indicated by private practitioners and through well-child [clinics] of established public health programs."[89] This commitment to private practice medicine was notable, but ignored the reality that children in low-income neighborhoods without access to regular care received vaccines the least. Since measles was seen as more of a nuisance than a feared disease, that vaccine was a lower priority for public health clinics, which distributed between 50 and 70 percent of childhood vaccines.[90]

Beyond vaccines, healthcare at this time was thriving. In 1965 Congress passed into law Medicaid, which would provide healthcare to low-income individuals, and Medicare, which would provide healthcare to seniors and the disabled. These programs joined a broader War on Poverty, comprising a series of health and welfare programs aiming to help the American poor. This was notably an era of state expansion not seen since the New Deal. As the country prioritized helping the poor, it became clear that poor children were less than half as likely to be vaccinated as wealthier children and three times less likely to see a private physician.[91] Unlike other health inequities, large numbers of unvaccinated children could potentially spread infectious disease, and this created perceptible risks to the broader community. Nearing global eradication of smallpox, public health leaders set their sights on measles and prioritized vaccination as the best tool to battle it. Policy and resources followed.

First, an infusion of resources focused on vaccinating poor children. Head Start, Volunteers in Service to America (VISTA), public health service clinics, neighborhood clinics, and other organizations set out to, among other goals, vaccinate children. By 1967, the federal government had established a reminder system to notify parents of babies that they should seek out vaccines. Sent in both Spanish and English, the notice also asked parents to send a reply card to update agencies on their children's vaccination status.[92]

Second, ongoing questions of how to monitor vaccine uptake continued. During the campaigns to promote the Salk polio vaccine, the National Foundation for Infantile Paralysis argued that vaccines, like charitable giving, should be voluntary.[93] Bills in the early 1960s to require vaccination all failed. Yet, as the federal government newly prioritized immunization, states again considered compulsory vaccination laws. By 1968, half of the states had laws requiring evidence of vaccination for school attendance. There was evidence that these laws worked. In one notable example, a measles outbreak infected children in Texarkana, a city that straddles both Texas and Arkansas. Texas had no vaccine requirements for measles, while Arkansas did. Children in Texas experienced measles at twelve times the rate of neighboring kids in Arkansas.[94]

By 1974, forty states required evidence of vaccination for school attendance. Individuals with vaccine-preventable diseases, according to the historian Elena Conis, were increasingly portrayed in the media as "as a monolithic category whose members were uniformly threatening to the health of American families."[95] By 1981, all states had passed compulsory immunization laws. These laws became the backbone of U.S. vaccine policy. Although it does not match contemporary perceptions, compulsory vaccine laws were in fact created to increase public access to vaccines and were framed under the social programs of the Great Society, as a means of working toward social justice. The relatively rapid passage of these laws was not particularly controversial, underscoring how widely Americans accepted vaccines as a technology of health promotion. Polls from this time period suggest that many Americans—as many as 25 percent—did not know that their state had a compulsory vaccine law; most also expressed that they planned to have their children vaccinated anyway.[96]

Requirements and Exemptions

Unlike laws from the smallpox era, laws in the 1960s and 1970s contained exemptions for children whose parents held religious beliefs opposed to vaccination. These exemptions resulted from the lobbying efforts of Christian Scientists, but were in some places broadly written to be inclusive of other faiths as well. How these exemptions should be interpreted proved complicated. Legal questions through this era revolved around whether parents must belong to an organized religion, whether they could be expected to demonstrate the sincerity of their beliefs, and whether exempting some children created increased risks to others. A series of lawsuits helped carve the multiple meanings of religious exemption, most of which led to liberal interpretations of the laws to allow broad use.[97] Yet the relatively quiet expansion of school attendance laws, which made school personnel the unwilling enforcers of public health law, reflected the general consensus that vaccines were good and enforcement would not be difficult. This consensus would face challenges that would lay the groundwork for today's vaccine controversies.

Swine Flu, Liability, and the Rise of Distrust of Vaccine

Influenza—or flu—is miserable and occasionally life-threatening, even to healthy people. In part, the risk flu presents depends on the strain of flu in circulation. For example, the influenza pandemic of 1918 killed at least 20 million people in one year and lowered the life expectancy for that year by ten years. Unlike other strains, the 1918 strain also killed an unusually high number of young and otherwise healthy people. Other strains are milder, but each flu season brings the fear that this year's strain will be more like the 1918 swine flu strain than other more passive versions.

This was the fear that reigned in 1976 when an army cadet at Fort Dix in New Jersey died suddenly of flu. A culture of that virus revealed that it was a strain closely related to the one that caused pandemic in 1918. Given that soldiers live in close quarters, the risk of that virus moving through the troops was significant. As military, CDC, and New Jersey Health Department workers began examining other soldiers, they found that more than two hundred of them had been infected.[98] The federal government had several choices. Agencies could prioritize vaccinating anyone at high risk for infection, as the Public Health Service was inclined to do. They could focus solely on federal employees, including soldiers; or they could support universal immunization against a possible pandemic. President Gerald Ford assembled leaders in vaccination and infectious disease—including Sabin and Salk—to weigh in on a strategy.

The Advisory Committee on Immunization Practices (ACIP) weighed the evidence and decided on a broad-reaching vaccine program. As one member summarized the consensus, "If we believe in prevention, we have no alternative but to offer and urge the immunization of the population."[99] The government could also have chosen to manufacture flu vaccine and hold it in stockpile. Instead, the ACIP opted to order the vaccine from private pharmaceutical companies and distribute it. President Ford held a press conference, with both Sabin and Salk by his side, and unveiled the National Influenza Immunization Program (NIIP).

The program faced one significant barrier: companies were unwilling or unable to manufacture the vaccine because they could not obtain insurance coverage against possible liability from the vaccine. In response, the U.S. Congress passed legislation authorizing the federal government to assume liability on behalf of the companies.[100]

Before the Fort Dix soldiers were infected, questions of liability were already circulating. Lawsuits from individuals who contracted polio from the Sabin vaccine, and those compensating victims of the Cutter Incident had already raised these questions. As David Sencer, former CDC director, and Donald Millar, director of the NIIP, recall, in January 1976 the CDC supported legislation that would compensate individuals harmed or damaged as a result of immunizations licensed by the federal Food and Drug Administration (FDA) and recommended by the ACIP: "The rationale given was that immunization protects the community as well as the individual (a societal benefit) and that when a person participating in that societal benefit is damaged, society had a responsibility to that person." The surgeon general's office rejected the proposal "with a handwritten note, 'This is not a problem.'"[101] Faced with no way to acquire an adequate supply of vaccines, Congress indemnified the pharmaceutical companies and also required they develop informed consent forms that would warn flu vaccine recipients of potential side effects of the vaccine.[102] Some felt that this form was unnecessarily alarmist, but as a condition of legal protection, it went forward.

The NIIP immunized 45 million people in ten weeks. That fall, three people died of cardiac arrest shortly after vaccination. Although the deaths were ruled coincidental, they did little to engender trust in the program. By December, the CDC had reports that more than fifty people who had been recently vaccinated showed signs of Guillain-Barré syndrome (GBS), a rare neurological disorder, and though often fleeting, can cause paralysis in those affected. Within weeks, with these adverse effects noted and few cases of swine flu actually in circulation, the program halted. By the end of the swine flu program, the federal government saw more than four thousand injury claims totaling $3.5 billion.[103] About two-thirds of these were withdrawn or were unsuccessful, but in the years following the end of the program, the federal government paid out about $20 million in compensation.

The NIIP was expensive. However, the legacy of the failed National Influenza Immunization Program is ongoing. First, the program generated negative publicity for the vaccine and led Americans to distinguish between flu vaccine and other infectious vaccine-preventable diseases. Although most people believed that other illnesses required vaccination, surveys following the swine flu campaign showed that flu vaccines were widely perceived as less safe and less necessary, perceptions that continue today.[104] Second, the NIIP crafted new expectations of informed consent. Following the program, federal agencies continued to carve out policies on informed consent for vaccination. The subcommittees charged with considering the ethics of vaccination found that while informed consent is important, it must necessarily look different for vaccines than for other medical procedures. Since so many people received vaccines, the opportunities for interaction between provider and recipient were more limited. As Colgrove explains, "Because immunization was sponsored by the government on behalf of society, individuals were under special obligations to participate." The risks of vaccines were also seen as lower than in other medical interventions requiring informed consent.[105]

Core questions remained about how individuals should be notified of potential risks and side effects of vaccination. Who should be responsible for notifying recipients and what should be communicated? The outcome was that in 1977 the CDC developed a series of forms that would be included with all vaccines that were administered in public health clinics. These forms would describe the disease, provide estimates of the effectiveness of the vaccine, and list possible side effects and recommendations for those for whom the vaccine was not appropriate. The form would be given to patients or their parents who would be asked to sign it.

The forms were controversial. Public health officials felt that they were unnecessary at best, particularly where vaccines were required, and likely to scare people out of participating in vaccination. Some noted that few people read the form and that it was "a cumbersome time-consuming and useless ritual."[106] Studies of patients were not much more encouraging: many said they did not read the form or did not understand what it said, and few could answer questions about the vaccines or diseases they prevent after reading and signing the form. Although the forms satisfied no one, they nonetheless in 1978 became required for use with all publicly distributed vaccines.

Enforcing Public Health: School Attendance and Vaccine Requirements

Vaccines against childhood illnesses gained a considerable boost in the 1970s, even after the swine flu debacle. In addition to passage of school attendance laws mentioned above, Jimmy Carter's inauguration in 1977 brought with him a national recommitment to childhood immunizations. With an infusion of federal funds and an ambitious goal to vaccinate 90 percent of children, vaccination was again a priority. These goals also called on schools to begin enforcing school attendance laws that were on the books, but seldom used.

Compulsory vaccine laws, to be enforced by school personnel, were easier to craft in law than enforce in practice. First, laws compelled multiple vaccines—about seven in the 1970s—so school staff had a harder task than they had when earlier laws expected them to simply verify a pockmark from a smallpox vaccination. Schools generally lacked additional resources to allocate to the task of verifying medical records. Second, educators were loath to remove children from school, even those whose parents could not locate the requisite paperwork. School personnel, including those with a financial incentive to increase student attendance, were largely reluctant to push kids out. Third, questions emerged as to whether immunization records were part of confidential student records and thus could not be shared with health departments. This concern was eventually addressed by the federal Office of Education, which allowed health departments to review records, but also defined healthcare and education as separate spheres with separate interests.[107]

Legal challenges by parents continued to test the limits of the religious exemption. In general, courts were sympathetic to vaccine requirements, ruling that laws without religious exemptions were constitutional.[108] However, the initial expectation that a parent exercising a religious exemption needed to belong to a recognized church or religion or would need to demonstrate their adherence to a religion that held a position against vaccination faded; Jews, Catholics, and chiropractors successfully challenged their exclusion from religious exemption. Unfortunately, schools often became the respondent in these cases, forced to defend these laws, despite their lack of control over them. In general, vaccine rates remained high anyway, representing people's view of vaccines as lifesaving.

Mandates, Compensation, and the Continuing Challenges of Preventing Pertussis

As mentioned earlier, pertussis is a dangerous disease for infants, is highly contagious, and remains a challenging bacteria to vaccinate against. By the 1950s, the vaccine created by Kendrick and colleagues had become widespread, even as it was flawed. The rigorous testing the researchers had conducted raised the standards for what would count as compelling research and, as mentioned, set the stage for polio research as well as other new vaccines in the following decades, including MMR. But even with this high level of testing, pertussis vaccines had problems.

Almost immediately after development and licensing, reports of rare but serious complications following vaccination arose. In 1933 a Copenhagen study referenced two deaths following vaccination. In 1948 another study reported fifteen admissions over a nine-year period to Boston Children's Hospital for seizure following vaccination with DPT, even as the vaccines were made by different companies. A Swedish study in the 1950s found 36 neurological reactions, including 13 deaths, out of 725,000 children who were vaccinated with DPT. Independent British studies through the 1940s and 1950s found the vaccine to be effective, but did note occurrence of encephalopathy (brain injury) and neurological damage, and thus did not recommend its use in areas with low rates of pertussis.[109] It is worth noting that several studies have since questioned the causal relationship between reported complications and the vaccine.[110] What is most important for our purposes is to understand that perceptions of a relationship between whole-cell pertussis vaccine and disability transformed vaccine politics, policy, and practice in the United States and elsewhere.

By 1975, federal advisory groups noted these complications and called for a reformulation of the vaccine, specifically to develop an acellular vaccine, one that was made from killed bacteria and would likely be safer. These safety concerns led to declining rates of vaccine use in the United Kingdom and Japan, and rising rates of pertussis infection.[111] By 1980, Japanese researchers had developed a new acellular vaccine against pertussis, but their efforts to communicate the process and safety of the new vaccine to U.S. researchers were unsuccessful. In the United States, most manufacturers were not motivated to develop a new vaccine, since the existing whole-cell pertussis vaccine was inexpensive to manufacture, while plans for a new vaccine were vague.

Formal Creation of a Compensation System

The complications from pertussis vaccines led to lawsuits against vaccine manufacturers. Recognizing how risk of liability might affect the vaccine market, the American Academy of Pediatrics issued a policy statement in 1977 explaining that society had an obligation to compensate those few who were injured in the course of complying with state laws on vaccination and should create a compensation program. Lawsuits against vaccine manufacturers continued, and pharmaceutical companies responded in two ways: they drastically hiked the cost of vaccinations or they withdrew from the market completely. For example, the cost of the DPT vaccine rose quickly from $.17 per dose to $11 per dose, while the number of companies that made that vaccine dropped from eight to one.[112] Some of the departure from the vaccine market occurred following litigation from polio injury, not pertussis. Nonetheless, laws to require vaccination for school attendance were pointless if supply remained unreliable and shrinking.

The idea for a compensation program was not entirely new. California had by 1977 created its own state-run compensation system to pay for medical care and rehabilitation services for anyone harmed by a vaccine.[113] The federal indemnification of vaccine manufacturers during the 1976 swine flu program provided another example of how such a program could operate. In 1980, the U.S. House of Representatives asked the Congressional Office of Technology Assessment to examine the possibility of creating a federal compensation system for vaccine-related injury.[114] The report needed to address which vaccines would be covered, what kinds of injuries would be included, and whether there should be a cap on awards. One barrier to calculating the costs and benefits of such a program was the lack of a system for recording the occurrence of adverse reactions. Although the CDC had set up a hotline in 1978, where parents could call and report adverse reactions without medical verification, the reports were vague, incomplete, and of little use to policy makers.[115] In 1981 the AAP further developed its position in support of a compensation program and detailed a plan for what elements such a program should contain. However, President Ronald Reagan and his administration's goal to reduce the role of the federal government in regulatory life served as a significant barrier to developing the system, and the proposal stalled.

Public sentiment was also turning. A 1982 exposé, *Vaccine Roulette*, aired on an NBC-affiliated television station in Washington, D.C., and changed views of vaccine safety in significant ways. This Emmy-winning show presented parents' heartbreaking stories of their children's disability after vaccination with little background or context. By most accounts, this show communicated that vaccines were more dangerous than the diseases they prevent. The program brought attention to vaccine injuries in ways that had not been publicly acknowledged before.

The airing of *Vaccine Roulette* connected parents who had, in isolation, seen their children develop seizures, neurological disorders, or signs of brain injury after vaccination. Parents who watched the show who believed that their children had been injured by the DPT vaccine called the network, which put them in contact with each other, and they began to organize politically.[116] First called Dissatisfied Parents Together (DPT), the group would eventually become the National Vaccine Information Center, now the largest organization in the country committed to eliminating vaccine mandates. This organization, comprising parents who were largely well-educated and middle-class, including a former federal attorney, was well-positioned to demand change.[117]

More generally, distrust of the DPT vaccine increased. Parents had filed two vaccine-related lawsuits in 1978; by 1986, about 250 had been filed.[118] As lawyers began advertising their services to parents who believed that their children had been harmed by vaccines, that number continued to grow, with approximately a hundred new vaccine lawsuits filed each subsequent year, totaling more than $3.5 billion in potential costs and damages.[119] In contrast to these sizable suits, the U.S. vaccine market in 1981 was about a $2 billion industry. Accused of marketing a defective product or failing to warn consumers of the potential risks, companies saw little reason to continue making vaccines. In short, potential liability outweighed potential profits.

In 1983 the AMA convened its own task force and in consultation with pharmaceutical companies, issued guidelines on the components of a national vaccine injury compensation system, including complete protection from liability for manufacturers. Parents vocally opposed liability protection, arguing that without the risk of punitive damages, companies would have no incentive to ensure a safe product. Meanwhile, Reagan continued to oppose any legislation that broadened the role of the government and instead hoped that tort reform would solve this issue.[120]

In 1986 U.S. Representative Henry Waxman, a California Democrat, sponsored legislation that he hoped would provide a compromise. With bipartisan congressional support (and an addition that allowed pharmaceutical companies to export drugs not approved in the United States to other countries where they had been approved, which satisfied manufacturers and Reagan), the National Childhood Vaccine Injury Act of 1986 (NCVIA) passed into law. The centerpiece of the NCVIA was a compensation program to provide monies to those harmed by routinely used vaccines. Funded by a tax on every vaccine in the country, the system provides compensation for lost earnings, costs of care, expenses, pain and suffering, attorneys' fees, and death. Since it was a no-fault system, claims were intended to be processed in a manner that would be "expeditious and fair," with a lower standard for proving causation than would be the norm in a tort claim, making the system more generous to those injured. Those who had been injured before the passage of the NCVIA could apply retroactively. Although the law did not provide total protection from liability, it did require plaintiffs to exhaust the remedies available through the vaccine injury compensation program before filing a liability claim in court.

In addition to crafting the compensation program, the NCVIA also required manufacturers to improve the safety of vaccines and to collect better information about vaccine injury. This latter goal was met by the creation of the Vaccine Adverse Event Reporting System (VAERS), a voluntary, passive reporting system administered by the CDC and the Food and Drug Administration (FDA). The VAERS allows anyone to report an adverse reaction to a vaccine, but does not require anyone to report reactions. To meet the former goal, the Institute of Medicine (IOM), an independent panel of experts empowered by Congress as part of the National Academy of Sciences, reviewed scientific knowledge to identify known possible injuries from vaccines. Injuries from polio, for example, were easier to identify since someone who received the vaccine subsequently developed polio. However, making decisions of causality with more diffuse or wide-ranging symptoms proved more challenging. The IOM did find that although the relationship was somewhat unclear, there was sufficient reason to believe that in rare instances, the whole-cell pertussis vaccine caused adverse reactions. By 1990, about 80 percent of claims made to the compensation system were for the pertussis component in the DPT shot.[121] Within a year, the FDA licensed new acellular vaccines against pertussis, which distributed with tetanus and diphtheria as DTaP, proved to be safer, albeit providing shorter immunity. Claims to the compensation system for pertussis injuries almost immediately declined. The NCVIA attempted to create a compromise between parents who were concerned about vaccine safety and wanted compensation for those injured, the physicians who supported immunization in their practice, and the for-profit corporations who were willing to manufacture the nation's vaccines, so long as they assumed no liability should something go wrong. This law represented this compromise, though there is little evidence it ever satisfied any of these groups.

Persistent Inequality

The disparities policy makers attempted to solve with vaccine mandates persisted. Although by 1990, 90 percent of children received vaccines before entering school, vaccination rates in very young children lagged, with only about one-third of preschoolers receiving all recommended vaccines.[122] Vaccine-preventable diseases returned, and measles surged to the highest levels in more than a decade, particularly in low-income neighborhoods. An increasing number of Americans had no insurance, but even children with private insurance were relying on public clinics, since private insurance companies in the early 1990s often did not cover routine immunization.

President Bill Clinton attempted to make healthcare reform the centerpiece of his administration. One law, which, like the president's healthcare bill, failed, would have provided free vaccines to all children, irrespective of income. Instead, a compromise bill expanded funding for vaccines for Medicaid-eligible children and created a national immunization tracking system. In 1994 Mississippi became the first state to require physicians to participate in vaccine registries; other states soon followed. The failure of universal access but passage of laws to increase monitoring illustrate the political willingness to track vaccine use, but not resolve inequality. None of these laws increased consensus that vaccines were safe or necessary.

Growing Unease and Fears of Autism

Following the new and seemingly safer DTaP vaccine, new vaccines were added to the recommended schedule, including vaccines against haemophilus influenzae type B (Hib) in 1990 and hepatitis B (hep B) in 1991. Hib, a common childhood illness that causes bacterial meningitis, was not particularly controversial. Hepatitis B, which vaccinates against a virus transmitted through bodily fluids often through intravenous drug use or sexual contact, was. Since babies face little risk of hep B infection, parents argued they could not see why infants should absorb the risk of the vaccine to protect against potential adolescent or adult risk behaviors in which they could not imagine their children participating. Public health providers countered that targeting vaccination to at-risk groups is seldom successful and adolescents and young adults do not regularly access care. The growing vaccine schedule, with varied perceptions of necessity, fed a growing sense of distrust.

The historian James Colgrove suggests that the growing unease with vaccines in this era cannot be viewed outside the context in which everything from nuclear power plants to HIV/AIDS demanded individual consideration of risk. Understanding the likelihood, the severity, and what possible benefit justified those risks became an American obsession. Vaccines presented risk, but certain features magnified concern: they primarily affected children, they were manmade and not naturally occurring, and they were forced, owing to school attendance laws.[123] Further, the women's health movement and advocacy in responses to diseases like AIDS created health activists in a way not seen before, where laypeople could successfully challenge scientists, physicians, and public health experts, and even affect the outcome of research.[124] Concerns about vaccine safety increased, but the greatest emerging controversy was around whether vaccines could increase risk for autism, a complex neurobehavioral disorder that impairs social interaction and communication, rising in frequency.

In the United States in the mid-1990s, there was growing concern about environmental sources of toxicity, including lead and mercury. In 1997 Congress passed the Food and Drug Modernization Act, which streamlined approval of new drugs and devices, increased patient access to experimental drugs, and among other things, required the FDA to make public a list of foods and medications that contained mercury (the latter coming from an addition by one legislator concerned about the high levels of mercury in fish).[125] The law, intended to get lifesaving drugs to market faster, increased parental anxieties that vaccines were inadequately vetted and contained potentially toxic levels of mercury.

The FDA asked manufacturers to report what levels of thimerosal, a form of ethyl mercury used as a preservative, vaccines contained. This proved challenging since vaccine administration varied dramatically. The Environmental Protection Agency (EPA) published guidelines for acceptable levels of methylmercury, but the FDA had none for vaccines, which contained ethyl mercury. Although no single vaccine carried enough mercury to be of concern, the cumulative dose from multiple vaccines could potentially exceed the guidelines set forth by the EPA. The FDA convened a panel of leading vaccine researchers to consult on the issue. The details of this process are explored in chapter 4, including the findings of several large studies that found no causal relationship between thimerosal and autism. In 1999, arguing both that thimerosal was not dangerous and that it would be responsible to exercise precaution, the U.S. Public Health Service and the American Academy of Pediatrics issued a joint statement calling for manufacturers to cease the use of thimerosal in childhood vaccinations. Thimerosal was removed from all vaccines, except for flu shots, by 2001.

In the United Kingdom, the vaccine-autism link originated in 1998, when the prestigious British medical journal the *Lancet* published a study written by a group of physicians who treated twelve children for gastrointestinal abnormalities and autism. The article hypothesized that the MMR vaccine caused gastrointestinal illness, which in turn caused autism. Just before the article's publication, the lead author and gastro-enterologist Andrew Wakefield held a press conference to announce the study's findings. New attention in the United States, combined with media coverage of Wakefield's study, and aggressive congressional hearings held by Senator Dan Burton of Indiana, whose grandson was diagnosed with autism, all contributed to parents' concerns. By 2004, most of Wakefield's collaborators had denounced their findings from the *Lancet* article; in 2010 the journal retracted the article. Wakefield's medical license was also revoked in the United Kingdom for misconduct. Wakefield moved to the United States, where he found support for his efforts to connect autism with vaccines. His efforts are also often identified as the leading contributor to the resurgence of measles, which had been eradicated in the United States and the United Kingdom until recently.

Continuing Tensions between Individual Rights and Public Health

The history of vaccine development and policy responses in the United States establishes a few key questions, issues, and tensions that become apparent in the thinking of the parents, providers, researchers, and policy makers in this book. The first point that it is important to make is that vaccines are both a technology for individual benefit and a tool to protect community health. This dual use complicates how we understand informed consent, because something that might be primarily for the community good carries some risk to the individual.

Unlike other medical interventions, infectious disease creates risk for others. Law has not been successful in resolving these tensions, which become magnified when distrust in science and scientific expertise grows.

Second, vaccine uptake is reasonably high when Americans see vaccines as lifesaving and lower when vaccines seem unnecessary. The power of these perceptions becomes most visible with the advent of the flu vaccine, where parents communicate a view of flu vaccines as less necessary than, say, polio vaccines. As additional vaccines become licensed—against chickenpox (varicella), human papilloma virus (HPV), or seasonal influenza—the argument that all vaccines are equally important becomes less convincing.

Third, our vaccine history reveals a core tension between vaccines' significance as a public resource and the reality that it is a product produced by for-profit corporations. During smallpox, we saw an unsuccessful effort to monopolize the Jenner vaccine.[126] More recently, the advent of new very expensive vaccines—including two against HPV—reveals profit motives. Vaccine supply, quality of production, and yield are left to for-profit corporations to determine. Even though most significant vaccine developments have benefitted from public funding, particularly through universities and government research institutions, vaccines remain a private investment—a role defined clearly by the polio-fighting NFIP and more recently by groups like the Bill and Melinda Gates Foundation, which drives global vaccine markets and outreach programs. If vaccines were a public good, they would be free, as they are in many parts of the world. As the single largest purchaser of vaccines, the government could more aggressively negotiate prices for vaccines, but does not. Yet healthcare providers have accused public health agencies of interfering with profits and have sabotaged efforts to expand free vaccine programs for all children, not just those unable to pay private fees. This private fee schema supports a view of vaccines as a technology for individual benefit. Parents question a for-profit, publicly mandated intervention for which they will be expected to pay. This profit motive undermines a collective understanding of vaccines as a community-produced technology and public good.

Fourth, the shielding of vaccine makers from tort liability for a potentially dangerous product also underscores these conflicting understandings of vaccines. Threats to cease manufacturing have resulted in legal protection—both in 1976 against the swine flu program and later in the no-fault, no-liability vaccine compensation system. These historical trends inarguably shape perceptions of vaccines today.

2

Parents as Experts

I knew at home millions of mothers had been waiting years for what was coming in the segment after the commercial break. Mothers who have been silenced, mothers whose child's own pediatrician had called them stupid or ignorant, mothers who had been accused of causing their child's autism with their own negligence, mothers who had waited years for one person to break through in the media and say what they have been screaming for a whole decade. This wasn't my moment in the spotlight coming up. It was theirs. I was their voice and ready to speak on behalf of these amazing women. . . . "The statistics are one in one-fifty. I'd like to know what number does it have to be for everyone to start listening to what the mothers of children who have autism have been saying for years, which is, . . . We vaccinated our baby and SOMETHING happened. SOMETHING happened. Why won't anyone believe us?" . . .

I continued to speak about how the Centers for Disease Control (CDC) acts as if vaccines are one-size-fits-all, as if they should be administered at the same rate for all children without regard to the individual child's needs and biological makeup, and I felt something even more profound. I felt the collective energy of moms everywhere. I felt them jumping up and down on their couches. I felt them calling their own moms on the phone screaming, "Are you hearing this? She said it!"

Oprah finished the segment with a statement from the CDC, which said there was no science to support the connection between vaccine and autism. I couldn't help but think, "Who needs science when I'm witnessing it every day in my own home? I watched it happen." I replied with all the love that I could muster in my heart. "At home, Evan is my science."

—Jenny McCarthy, *Mother Warriors*[1]

Parents try to consider the possible risks and benefits for their individual children. They make what they understand to be the best choices they can for their children's health, with the information they have. They assess the risk of exposure to the disease and feared adverse reactions. They weigh those against the potential benefits of vaccines, as they understand them. This process of evaluating risk and benefit is an example of what the sociologist Deborah Lupton calls "lifestyle risk discourse," which places responsibility on the individual "to avoid health risks for the sake of his or her own health as well as the greater good of society."[2] The discourse of health promotion and illness avoidance, that is, managing risk to avoid sickness, frames health as an individual pursuit. This focus on the individual undermines the collective nature of vaccine policy, where individuals might absorb some small amount of risk for the good of others. It also reminds consumers, as illustrated in Jenny McCarthy's remarks in the passage above, that they—and not their physicians or vaccine researchers—are the experts on their own needs, their own risks, and their own children. By closely examining parents' perceptions of risks and benefits, we can better understand their insistence that they hold unique expertise that makes them best qualified to make vaccine choices for their children.

Parents' views of themselves as experts are not surprising. Parents make decisions for their children based on their own assessment of their children's needs, desires, abilities, and ambitions daily. In an expanding number of spheres—schools, media, extracurricular activities—parents generally, and mothers specifically, are expected to be experts on their own children. As parents are increasingly expected—and expect—to cultivate children into adulthood, it is not surprising that this culture of individualism and demands for parental expertise extend into areas of healthcare, including childhood vaccine choices.[3] Parents who opt out of vaccines are often portrayed as either ignorant or armed with "internet educations."[4] This dismissive view of the small number of parents who intentionally refuse vaccines underestimates the labor and intent these parents bring to their vaccine choices and to claiming their expertise.

Decisions about vaccines can be said to embody the rational choice framework, in which all individuals are presumed to be informed consumers out to maximize the benefits and minimize the costs for themselves and their own children. The public health system asks parents to consent to vaccines based on the general recommendations of scientists and public health practitioners at the same time that most of the healthcare landscape is increasingly individualizing risk and customizing choice. Vaccine decision makers—that is, those choosing whether to consent to consume vaccines for their children and sometimes themselves—view the vaccine choice through this individualized lens, with disease prevention a process of personal risk assessment, lifestyle adjustment, and individual choice. We see an ethos that disease is largely preventable through personal responsibility. This shift of responsibility from the state to the individual shapes how parents approach their choice about whether to vaccinate.

The precepts of informed consent, a bedrock concept in American medicine, reinforce this individualism. Healthcare must honor the individual, a concept that infuses the mandate for informed consent, which requires individuals to be informed of the personal costs or risks and potential benefits to themselves before receiving a medical intervention; they must have access to this information in a manner that does not require them to have advanced medical training. The concept of informed consent draws on an ethical principle of patient autonomy and human rights. The root premise is the concept, fundamental in American jurisprudence, that "every human being of adult years and sound mind has a right to determine what shall be done with his own body." As stated by the U.S. Circuit Court of Appeals in the 1972 case of *Canterbury v. Spence*, a decision that shaped expectations that patients should be informed of risks and benefits so they may voluntarily consent,

> True consent to what happens to one's self is the informed exercise of a choice, and that entails an opportunity to evaluate knowledgeably the options available and the risks attendant upon each. The average patient has little or no understanding of the medical arts, and ordinarily has only his physician to whom he can look for enlightenment with which to reach an intelligent decision. From these almost axiomatic considerations springs the need, and in turn the requirement, of a reasonable divulgence by physician to patient to make such a decision possible.[5]

This case makes clear that patients have the freedom to decide what should happen to their bodies, without coercion, and that physicians are to act as facilitators to patients' efforts to reach these decisions. How to provide informed consent for vaccines, as we saw in the last chapter, has been perplexing. On one hand, vaccines are compelled, making refusal difficult. On the other, they are a medical intervention into the body that carries benefits and risks, which should be fully understood and accepted before individuals receive them. Yet parents are asked to make these choices on behalf of their children, despite the fact that they are juggling unknown risks and partial knowledge. How they do so animates the next two chapters.

Parental Expertise and Informed Consumers

Parents view themselves as best able to decide whether consent to a vaccine is warranted because they most intimately know their own children, understand their unique health statuses and vulnerabilities, and believe that they can most accurately estimate risk. They also engage in a process of empowering themselves, usually through self-education, to make informed decisions, with information coming from books, websites, physicians or other health providers, peers, family members, advocacy organizations, or publications committed to natural living. Critically, mothers also weigh their information alongside what they often see as their trump card: a sense of intuition about what they feel their children need. The constellations of sources parents seek out, alongside their intuition, represent their intent to make good decisions for their children and become more credible than advice or recommendations provided by scientific advisory panels. Illustrating this, Jenny McCarthy explains above, "Who needs science when I'm witnessing it every day in my own home?" This form of expertise is both specific and irrefutable. Science, which studies patterns and trends—sometimes from thousands of participants—seems less able to speak to parental concerns for their child. As parental experts, parents see themselves as best able to conduct "research" to become informed decision makers on the best possible care for their children.

One online exchange between parents opposing vaccines illuminates what parents mean when they talk about research. One mother introduced herself as a "vaccine researcher" for more than a dozen years. As I read her commentary, it became clear that her definition of research—

like that of all the parents I spoke with—is not research as those who produce expert knowledge define it, which would usually be defined as the *systematic* process of evaluating phenomena to establish facts that are generalizable and verifiable. Just as consumers are encouraged to conduct their own "research" on products before purchase and patients are told to "research" their options, parents conduct research by gathering information for personal use, which they see as central to their role as good, informed experts on their own children. In calling herself a "vaccine researcher," a term usually referring to immunologists or microbiologists who spend decades in laboratories after years of postgraduate training, she challenges the very meaning of expertise and considers her qualification as a vigilant parent to be equivalent. The role of research played out dramatically in my conversations with parents. Heather's story illustrates this.

Heather Moss, a thirty-two-year-old mother of two, works part-time as a childbirth coach and educator. She consented to fully vaccinate her first son on the schedule recommended by her pediatrician. Over time, she began to feel uneasy about having followed that advice without question. As a result, she committed to educating herself before her second son was born. She describes the change between her two children: "I had gotten a lot more educated about things and the process and had gone to a seminar on vaccinations taught by a naturopath in the area and learned a lot more about it so that I decided—we wanted to delay some of those early vaccinations."

In explaining her rejection of the interventions offered at birth and shortly after, she confidently accounts for her decision: "I researched that and I just felt like the risk factors for him were very low." Many of these interventions would be automatic shortly after delivery. Heather describes conducting her own research to equip herself with information she could use to challenge the medical recommendations she would be offered (often with some insistence on the part of healthcare providers). She weighed her perception of benefit against risk of illness, and opted out.

Shortly after her second child's birth, she began training to become a childbirth educator. She describes her subsequent transformation, going from a hospital birth with her first and fully vaccinated son to a home birth with her second son, who has had only select vaccines. "Becoming a childbirth teacher, you're just exposed to a lot more information about that. That's why I think the change from [my first son's] to [my second son's] birth was different." She explains how she now works to empower other mothers:

> I teach moms about vaccinations. And when I say "teach," what I do is I inform—I inform prospective parents of the facts of vaccinations and I try not to get into what you should do or what you shouldn't do, but I just try to say, "This is what this is. This is what it's for. This is— potential risk, potential benefit kinda thing," and let them really make their own decision on that. I try not to be an influencer as far as trying to talk them out of it, you know, because I mean, I've gotten my kids vaccinated, too.

Throughout my study, parents describe the importance of conducting their own research, considering their own children's needs, and making independent decisions, based on their own knowledge and intuition. Katie Reynolds, a mother of two partially vaccinated children, recommends this for other parents:

> First of all, I think everybody's gotta do what works for them and their family and their own individual situation and their own individual belief system. . . . I guess the only thing I would say is just educate yourself and try to know the plusses and minuses of any decision you make and then be okay with the decision that you've made, but, you know, just be conscious of making the decision and don't do it if you feel like it's a decision you're being forced into.

Elizabeth Nowak, a mother of two unvaccinated children, similarly advises, "My only piece of . . . advice would be just to do as much reading and research and then make an individual decision. I don't think that our experience is ever gonna be the same as somebody else's experience." As these stories illustrate, demands that parents conduct their own research and make individual decisions are central to how parents describe the vaccine decision. As they identify these practices as belonging to good parents, they communicate their belief that all good parents should engage in this process. In thinking about her interactions with friends who fully vaccinate their children, Janine Bouche, a mother of an unvaccinated toddler, recalls,

> I think that the people who do it, there is just as much tension as there is in anything, any kind of life choice like that. Like, I really think that the people, our friends, that did vaccinate think that we are picky, that it was just like that weird choice to [not vaccinate]. And then there are those on the flip side that say that they only did it because their doctor said. I have a judgment about that too. . . . It is just, like, making any uninformed decision that feels important is just kind of dumb to me. I would certainly say that I have some judgment about that.

Janine elaborates that she respects parents who choose vaccination so long as they do so after weighing the choice for themselves. "But people that make unconscious choices, I don't. It is the people that are saying, 'Oh, the doctor told me to' [I don't respect]." As parents construct themselves as experts on their own children, they highlight the importance of information, the process of education, and intuition. With intrinsically imperfect knowledge of possible future outcomes—both of adverse reactions and disease exposure—parents highlight their role as the best able to make these important decisions and communicate the value of claiming that expertise.

The logic that everyone must do what is right for them and their children underscores gendered meanings of parenting. Overwhelmingly, vaccine choices are mothers' choices, a pattern that is not surprising, as childhood outcomes reflect most heavily on mothers. Culturally, mothers are responsible for the physical, emotional, and psychological health of their children; healthy children symbolically represent good mothering and, inversely, mother-blame proliferates when children are sick.[6] Embracing cultural expectations that they invest heavily in their children (but not necessarily all children), mitigate risk, and protect their children's bodies, mothers work hard to support their children and in doing so, aim to define themselves as good parents.

This view is predicated on the belief that each child is unique and as such, institutions should be malleable to the needs and desires of each child and her or his family. This can be observed in discussions of school choice or charter schools, particularly as parents may choose to separate children from the same family into different schools to accommodate each child's talents, interests, or learning styles. This strategy is but one example of parents' willingness to expend considerable parental resources—in terms of time, emotion, and money—prioritizing each child's individuality. In the vaccine case this is no less true. Parents might craft different vaccine schedules for different children and prioritize vaccines differently based on perceptions of need, as parents define themselves as best able to make these decisions.

Parents' belief in the individuality of each child and each family makes population data—from which disease morbidity and mortality as well as vaccine safety are calculated—relatively uncompelling. Paula Parenti, for example, faces criticism from close friends who are physicians for not vaccinating her children. Her response to them is informative:

> I understand from your perspective, you know, in treating disease, that
> it's better to err on the side of caution, but that's not my perspective and,
> while I can appreciate that you have that data worldwide or whatever,
> . . . if you look at the statistics from a parent's perspective, there's not
> enough data to support in our culture—in my lifestyle—that my children
> would be at risk.

In viewing her family as unique, Paula renders public health data, including claims that unvaccinated children are at increased risk for disease, irrelevant. Parents like Paula receive support for this view. This rhetoric is also promoted by organizations that oppose vaccine mandates and position themselves as advocates of informed choice. For example, the American National Vaccine Information Center's website insists, "Your Family. Your Health. Your Choice. Know the risks for you and your child." Similarly, the Canadian Vaccination Risk Awareness Network touts on its website, "Your Child. Your Future. Your Choice."[7]

The ethos that parents should conduct their own research rather than rely on the advice of their pediatricians or the prepackaged advice from public health agencies serves as a way for parents to feel that they are ensuring the best outcomes for their children. It bears noting that parents who choose to vaccinate, even if only partially or on a delayed schedule, engage the same process of making choices based on their own research, evaluation of risk, and consideration of their own child's needs—assessments they feel uniquely qualified to make.

Evaluating Potential Benefits of Vaccines

The sociologist Jacob Heller usefully describes what he calls the "vaccine narrative" in the United States. Noting that a master narrative is "an overarching storyline or sequence of events that anticipates and therefore reinforces our established expectations," Heller explains that, regarding vaccines, Americans have little experience with the diseases vaccines work to prevent and few have technical knowledge to understand how vaccines work, but support for vaccines remains high nonetheless.[8] He argues that the reason for "vaccines' continued public support is that vaccination works; the technical knowledge has been transformed into lay knowledge, something people can grasp without the baggage of scientific jargon and data."[9] Most parents accept that vaccines are necessary, with U.S. vaccine rates remaining around 90 percent for most childhood diseases. These parents most often trust their health provider or have a parent or grandparent or other trusted source that successfully communicates the horrors of infectious disease before vaccines.

For parents who reject vaccine recommendations, the process of considering necessity is more complex and draws on cultural information that challenges the vaccine narrative that vaccines are always intrinsically good. Anyone who questions that narrative by calling vaccine safety, necessity, or beneficence into question, Heller notes, is seen as a "crackpot."[10]

We know from other contexts that for individuals to be motivated to seek health interventions for their own benefit, they must believe that they are susceptible to a particular health problem, that it is serious, that a treatment or medication will reduce the harm of that condition, and that there must be few barriers to accessing the treatment.[11] Those who would seek out health interventions must also find ways that the prescribed treatment fits their lives and matches their goals, and they must also fear a negative outcome should they refuse that intervention.[12] In deciding whether to consent to vaccines, parents engage in a process of evaluating the benefits of vaccines. First, parents consider the likelihood that their children will encounter disease. Second, they assess how badly the children would be affected if they were to become sick. These assessments drive their decisions.

Likelihood and Severity of Disease

In this cost-benefit analysis, parents weigh minute risks of vaccines against the small risks of infection of diseases that are rarely seen in the United States. For example, parents are often aware that wild-virus polio has not been seen in the United States since 1979 and in the Western Hemisphere since 1991.[13] Citing this information, they suggest that public policy's insistence on subjecting young children to a vaccine against a disease they are unlikely to encounter is unreasonable and introduces potential harm to their children unnecessarily.

Parents also understand the relative benefit of vaccination in terms of the seriousness of the disease the vaccine prevents. They often dismiss vaccines for diseases that they understand to be minor. Anna Chase, a mother of two, spends a great deal of time considering vaccines. She is a former public health worker and now a part-time acupuncturist, and as such, she considers the meanings of health deeply. Several times in our interview, Anna makes clear that she agrees with "the theory and concept of vaccines" but challenges their relevance. Although she has consented to allow only one of her sons to receive the tetanus vaccine, unavoidably bundled with diphtheria, she does not doubt that vaccines work. But as mortality from infectious diseases—and even the diseases themselves—have become less common, she sees vaccines as less necessary. In sorting through the perceived risks and benefits of each vaccine, Anna considers potential benefit in terms of the vaccine's efficacy, seriousness of the disease it protects against, and relevance. "I think that vaccines were, for example, polio—you get a polio vaccine, you don't get polio. You know, I believe in that and I'm not like, 'Oh, it doesn't work.' But I don't believe that's true for all immune diseases."

Anna laboriously parses out the logic of different vaccines. She considers how severe infection would be for her children should they become ill, and how that would vary depending on her children's age and gender. With confidence in her own research, she defines specific strategies for her children, rather than the approach to disease prevention universally recommended by the healthcare community. She explains,

The vaccines that I think make sense are tetanus. Diphtheria is kind of a nasty thing to get; totally believe in polio. I think that for boys it's probably better that they, you know, either get the mumps when they're little or if they don't get it when they're little then they have it before they're a teenager, because if they get it then they're at risk of sterilization. German measles, don't really care about. Regular measles for boys, I don't care about. Girls, if I had a girl, I'd want her to have the measles when she's little, or if not, to have the vaccine by the time she's a teen, because if she got it when she was pregnant, it'd be very sort of life-threatening to her fetus. So measles I think for girls makes sense.[14]

By managing vaccine choices in a "cafeteria" fashion, Anna articulates a strategy that illustrates parents' efforts to separate out the risk of disease and potential benefit of vaccines as they vary depending on the individual child and include the variable long-term effects of exposure, perceived probability of exposure, and severity of the disease. In this way, risk and benefit remain situated in the individual, and might shift as her children grow. Because risk lies in the body, boys don't need to be vaccinated against diseases that can cause, for example, fetal demise, even as they may choose to be involved with women who could be pregnant or might encounter women in their neighborhoods or communities as they grow. Rather, Anna's children are the center of her assessment. She considers the reproductive capabilities of her children, but not others they may encounter.

Anna is not unique in this process of evaluation. She is articulate in accounting for the process, even as others engage in a similar method of decision making. This can be seen most clearly in discussions of the vaccine against tetanus, which was often sought out, even by parents who reject all other vaccines.

Considering the Benefits: Tetanus

Tetanus is a bacterium ubiquitous in soil but not communicated between people. It infects individuals most commonly through deep puncture wounds, like those caused by stepping on a nail, but can also enter the bloodstream in more benign ways. Worldwide, neonatal tetanus, where the bacteria enter the umbilical stump after birth, remains a significant public health problem. This is possible in the United States, but less likely since newborns rarely encounter dirt. Once in the body, the spores from tetanus release a neurotoxin that interferes with neurological function and causes muscle spasms, including lockjaw, spinal contraction and curvature, and even death. Tetanus, which is not infectious, is one of the few compulsory vaccinations that carry no capacity for collective benefit; the benefits are only to the person receiving inoculation and there is no herd immunity against tetanus. Yet, because of the high use of vaccines against tetanus, there are fewer than fifty reported cases annually in the United States.[15]

Many of the parents in this study who rejected all vaccines consented only to the tetanus vaccine, suggesting that despite distrust of vaccines generally, risks of tetanus seemed compelling, particularly as there is no community protection. Marlene Bryant, who rejects virtually all vaccines for her three children, consented to tetanus since her sons were active in the Boy Scouts, which requires tetanus vaccination because of their increased time outdoors and accompanying increased risk of exposure. She explains, "Well, the boys have all been in Scouts, so now they've all had tetanus [vaccines], and that's the main thing [the Boy Scouts organizers] look at." Anna, who rejected all vaccines for her sons, opted to vaccinate the oldest against tetanus at the age of four years (tetanus is typically given in a series in the first two years of life with pertussis and diphtheria[16]). Although she does not believe that children's bodies are most able to safely absorb vaccines and mount a strong immune response, and thus prefers to wait as long as possible, she explains why this vaccine was compelling to her: "It was a tough decision. I was weighing in between wanting him to get it as much toward his immune system being fully formed as possible so that he could handle the vaccine. I was weighing that in between that and like, 'Okay, he's a boy and at what point is he going to be exposed to tetanus?'"

For some, the severity of the disease and challenges treating it swayed their decision. For example, Lauren Tate's knowledge of the primitive nature of tetanus treatment—which requires large quantities of antitoxin to counteract the toxins the bacteria release—inspired her to seek out the vaccine. She elaborates, "Tetanus is the only one that they haven't made modern medical advances to treat. There's really not a good treatment for it, whereas, like, whooping cough, they can intubate you now, whereas before they didn't used to be able to do that." Lauren's evaluation of whether vaccines are necessary reflects consideration of the options should her child become sick. In fact, tetanus infection requires hospitalization and treatment with "either human tetanus immune globulin (or equine antitoxin if human immune globulin is not available), a tetanus toxoid booster, agents to control muscle spasm, and aggressive wound care and antibiotics."[17] If immunoglobulin is not available, tetanus antitoxin (the original treatment, derived from horse blood serum) should be used in a single large dose, although some with allergies are not good candidates. In my interviews with pediatricians who work in hospitals, I found that few medical centers stock adequate supplies of antitoxin and often rely on interstate collaboration to acquire enough, making treatment even more challenging. Even with modern intensive care, tetanus is associated with death rates of 10–20 percent.

Lauren's choice to reject most vaccines does not mean that she rejects medical advice or expertise; rather, she sees technological innovation in medicine as facilitating her ability to reject vaccines. "You know, as far as, like, a lot of the infections and secondary infections, the treatments, the drugs, and everything that we have now are much better than they were back when these sicknesses were sweeping across the country and killing children." She believes that medical technology will manage acute illness should her children become infected; hence vaccines are less important and diseases less feared.

Evaluating Risk of Vaccines

Parents often fear that their child will react badly to a vaccine and will suffer an adverse reaction that will affect their health immediately or in the future, setting them up for health problems. Although much attention (spurred by activists like Jenny McCarthy) has focused on autism as an underlying fear, in fact parents fear a broader array of conditions, including a long-term autoimmune disorder, cognitive challenge, cancer, or other chronic health conditions that might not appear until adulthood. According to medical research, adverse reactions to vaccines that physicians tend to view as not serious and not a reason not to vaccinate include fever, redness, swelling, or soreness at the injection site, fainting, headache, fussiness, poor appetite, tiredness, vomiting, itching, wheezing, rash, or chills. More serious, albeit rare, adverse reactions include soreness in the shoulder with limiting range of motion, seizure, nonstop crying for more than three hours, long-term brain damage, serious allergic reaction, or hives. One vaccine (MMR) carries about a one in a million risk of very serious complication, including long-lasting seizures, deafness, temporary low platelet count, which can lead to a bleeding disorder, intussusception of the intestines, pneumonia, or Guillain-Barré syndrome.[18] Although the CDC is quick to point out that the risk of disease complication is significantly higher than the risk of adverse reaction, parents are not certain the risk of exposure to these diseases is reasonably high compared to adverse reactions. There is no well-established relationship between childhood vaccines and chronic autoimmune diseases, cancers, sudden infant death syndrome, or autism, but the impossibility of disproving such a causal relationship makes it difficult to reassure parents.

It is difficult to predict which children are likely to suffer an adverse outcome, in part because they are so exquisitely rare, but assumptions are that some children may carry an unknown genetic predisposition to an adverse reaction. In my discussions with attorneys who represent individuals in the Vaccine Injury Compensation Program, the federal court that compensates those harmed by vaccines, the probability of an unknown predisposition came up often. One attorney explains, "There's still a tremendous amount of research that's being done that is getting closer to understanding the ways in which certain kids, because of genetic predisposition, might have developed or regressed following vaccines in a way that resulted in their being on the autistic spectrum." Another argues that more research is needed to understand why some people experience complications from flu vaccine, insisting, "They need to keep better data on the people who get sick" to better understand what kind of predisposition may make someone vulnerable to an adverse reaction.

Serious adverse reactions are exceedingly rare, but also hard to predict, leading to the view that something in the child places them at risk. Without knowing what kinds of traits would mark vulnerability, parents search for signs of whether their children are possibly at risk in making the decision to vaccinate them. In considering whether to consent to vaccines, parents evaluate each of their children as individuals and sometimes create vaccine strategies for each child in the family, based on perceptions of risk. Thus, as parents file a personal belief (or religious) exemption claiming their objections to vaccines, the state imagines that the family philosophically and uniformly objects to vaccines for all children in the family. In fact, many parents perform an individualized risk-benefit calculus for each child and decide accordingly, often coming to different conclusions. Parents consider vaccine risk in many ways, including family history of adverse reactions, particular vulnerabilities a child might have that they see extending to their capacity to "handle" vaccines, and whether there are too many vaccines given when children are very young, which they imagine are not likely to be safely absorbed.

Family History as Risk

As parents search for information with which to estimate their children's risks of an adverse reaction, they often report looking to family history for indications of whether their children might be vulnerable. Some noted family members who had responded badly to vaccines, which they interpreted as a sign that their children might also react poorly. Anna, for example, describes this process:

> Oh, during pregnancy I knew I wasn't gonna vaccinate. I actually have a niece who was having really horrible, horrible health problems, she's still not totally okay. But at the time, her health problems all started up, like, mysterious disease, like, no one could figure out what was wrong with her kind of thing, right after she got a hepatitis B vaccine at age twelve. I mean, she went from being totally normal to, like, skin and bones, missed a year of school.

Anna relates that her family searched for explanations.

> My mom, being a nurse, helped them do a lot of research and that's when we started learning about the whole vaccine thing and—that was my brother's daughter. . . . And then my sister's boy, her boy almost died when he had the pertussis vaccine, he had such a reaction, . . . super super high fever, I think he might have convulsed; just a horrible, horrible reaction.

Anna acknowledges that she herself was vaccinated without incident, but sees the current schedule, which includes many more vaccines, to be qualitatively different from the one she received and thus sees her niece's and nephew's experiences as a better predictor of adverse outcomes than her own history.

Billy Folsom is a father whose teenaged son developed a seizure disorder as an infant. Although no one can tell him for certain whether the vaccines caused the seizures, he feels that it is likely they did, a theory first introduced by his son's neurologist, who was concerned that his son had received the now-discontinued DPT vaccine.[19] After years of unbreakable seizures, which seemed to begin between six and nine months of age, his son became permanently disabled, devolving into a vegetative state. It took nearly a decade for Billy and his wife—who is a nurse—to have another child, in part because they wanted to be certain that the seizure disorder was not a genetic condition that another child could also develop. After having a baby girl, and convinced the vaccines had triggered their son's seizures, they decided they would not vaccinate her. In discussing their choice with a pediatrician, Billy recalls one doctor telling him, "Off the record, if it were me, I would not have vaccinated her either." Later, his son's neurologist expressed his concerns more strongly: He recalls the doctor telling him, "No. Under no circumstances—do not vaccinate her. And also under no circumstances don't— don't get [your son] flu shots." Billy also recalls that he and his wife were advised not to receive the flu vaccine, in case they could shed the virus and risk infecting their medically fragile son. "We were told not to do flu shots or anything because of the fact that we could give it to him. So if we did anything like that we would have to be away from him for forty-eight hours and then we may or may not be contagious to him." Billy's story illustrates both the risk of vaccine and the inability to predict how one might react. They collectively avoid vaccines for fear their daughter could share the same vulnerability as their son, even though that DPT shot is no longer given.

Parents also adjust their approaches to vaccines based on how older children fared, even with less dramatic consequences than Billy's son. For example, Heather believes that her oldest son, Daniel, "had damage from his vaccinations in his body." As she sees it, Daniel has respiratory problems that may have been caused by the vaccines, and she believes that the vaccines more generally have "compromised his immune system." She also recalls that at the age of five years, he "did have a serious reaction to polio [vaccine]." She recalls, "We had to take him to the ER. He couldn't breathe and his throat and tongue was swelling up." In the emergency room, she remembers the physician's resistance to seeing this reaction as vaccine-related:

> I took him to the ER and the strangest thing was they would not entertain the idea that this could possibly be a vaccine reaction. They were searching for some other explanation for all this and they never did identify it as a vaccine reaction, although he'd had the vaccine that afternoon. He came home and started blowing up. . . . I kept saying, "He had a vaccine this afternoon." Like, "Oh, well. Never mind that, but look at this." And so they ended up just giving us, like, Zyrtec for an allergy reaction.

Because that injection completed the polio series, the issue of future vaccines against polio was moot. Yet Heather recalls that an allergist with whom they followed up advised her that if he had needed more vaccines, he should not receive them. This information informs Heather's vaccine decisions for her son, as well as her decision to delay vaccines for her younger child.

Fear of genetic predisposition overwhelmingly shapes vaccine refusal. Across the board, those who question vaccines argue that there is not enough research devoted to understanding these predispositions. Jake Kalman, a chiropractor and parent who opposes the use of vaccines, argues that healthcare, as it is practiced, is intrinsically flawed in its lack of attention to individual predispositions. Drawing on the goals of his own practice, he explains,

> What we're trying to do is create a new normal for healthcare, but we have to unthink the old healthcare first, you know, and at least to have somebody understand the mechanisms of disease, how somebody becomes autistic, and say, "Okay, does my child have any of these markers already?" You know? "Has anybody—has any of their brothers or sisters ever had a reaction? Has a mom or dad ever had a reaction?" . . . You know, simple things.

For some parents, the belief in a preexisting vulnerability makes vaccines unacceptable, but also can raise concerns about infection as well. Patricia Etter, a mother of eight, notes that when she was homeschooling her children, "we were less exposed to the community. It was a little easier." Yet as some of her children have entered school, disease prevention has become more complicated. "Now that I have kids coming in, you know, they have to wash their hands when they come into the house. Well, we've always had that rule, but there's just—there's two ways to look at it." She explains that although she does not have reason to believe that her children have a compromised immune system that would not be able to handle vaccines, she fears it nonetheless. This same weakness, however, might also mean that they would not handle infectious disease well either:

> If their immune systems hereditarily are compromised at all, then I don't want to be giving them vaccinations. But I also really don't need them to be exposed to stuff either. So it's both ways. It's like, you know, I don't want them doing harm from the vaccines, so we have to be careful. It's a constant battle to try and keep people healthy and I think that's the best thing to do is kind of teach them healthy lifestyles and to keep their immunes boosted. It's not easy, though.

The Vulnerable Child

Parents who distrust vaccine safety fear unknown predispositions that might make a child vulnerable to an adverse outcome. They evaluate each child to assess their risk and feel compelled to remain vigilant for possible vulnerabilities that could suggest a predisposition to an adverse reaction. They consider whether their child seems less resilient and would therefore seem like someone who would handle vaccines less well, an assessment they believe that as parents, they are uniquely qualified to make. Concerns about genetic predisposition were not always separate from a perception of particular vulnerability. Margaret Spencer, whose children—now young adults—were never vaccinated, explains, "You know, there's so many individual situations where there's a predisposition—genetic or otherwise—to having problems. Boys are four times more likely to have autism, for example, and ADHD, because testosterone does not protect as well as estrogen." As such, she suggests that boys might be more vulnerable to a reaction.

Lauren's process of coming to reject vaccines illustrates the process of evaluating each child's resilience and vulnerability. Lauren, like others, considers her family history in opting to delay vaccines indefinitely. Even without a history of vaccine reactions, she sees other health risks that might make her son vulnerable, including food allergies, which, she insists, "are very serious in my family" and which make some vaccines, particularly those made from eggs (like the seasonal flu vaccine) seem more risky.[20]

Lauren's fears of food allergies were confirmed when her son developed them. In addition to food allergies, her son seemed to face other health challenges. She recalls that when he was an infant, a pediatrician told her that "they thought he was brain-damaged at the time. He just had his eyes tightly shut all the time and he screamed and screamed and he didn't roll over until he was over eight months old," months after he would be expected to hit that developmental milestone.

Her son has caught up developmentally, but Lauren says that he continues to face health challenges. He has participated in early interventions through public agencies designed to work with children who are developing more slowly than expected. He has mostly caught up in terms of speech and motor skills, but she believes she must remain vigilant. Rather than start him in preschool or other interventions, Lauren chose to work with him at home and then transitioned as he became school-aged to homeschooling him. She jokes, "I basically just went from therapy to school and now he's so far advanced that it's kind of funny." Lauren is proud that her son is thriving, yet still views his body as potentially vulnerable. As the person who brought her son from developmental delay to academic achievement, Lauren describes herself as his greatest advocate and the one most able to assess what he can handle.

Too Much Too Soon

Parents focus their efforts to identify whether their children are vulnerable by considering their particular needs. Many parents in my study voiced concerns that the federally recommended vaccine schedule has too many shots, as most childhood vaccines are given in two- to four-shot series, spaced over time, which could overwhelm children's bodies. For example, the inactivated polio vaccine (IPV) is to be administered in four separate doses by the age of six years, while the measles-mumps-rubella vaccine (MMR) vaccinates against three diseases simultaneously at two points in time. As they consider the safety and necessity for their children who are small or seem vulnerable, the quantity of vaccines presents a different risk. Parents voice concern that children get too many at once, too many before the age of two, and too many over time. As Heather, who fully vaccinated her first child before conducting her own research and opting out for her second, recalls of her decision, "There was enough that I'd learned that made me feel like, you know, there's no rush to do all of them all at once and so I—my main goal when I had [him] was just, I don't want to give him a bunch of vaccines at a time. Try to do one at a time or, just, you know, one or two at a time, and not do them so early." Sharing this view, Marlene, whose four children have not received any vaccines, explains, "Wouldn't it be nice to be able to immunize the kids and not overwhelm their systems? I can't believe the numbers they—things they want to stick into little people nowadays, with very immature immune systems. And they don't know the long-term things."

Intuitively, the vaccine schedule may feel overwhelming to many parents. Studies have found that parents fear "immune-overload" from combination vaccines, where multiple antigens are given in a single injection, and believe that children receive vaccines too early.[21] These feelings may be widely shared; research suggests that even among parents who fully vaccinate their children, more than 20 percent believe that delaying vaccines is safer than following the recommended schedule.[22]

Likening vaccines to other challenges that could overwhelm the immune system, Leanne explains,

> You know, you get somebody in the hospital with pneumonia and a leg infection and earache. You're trying to deal with all different kinds of things in the body system, and I felt the same way with the shot. They're trying to deal with all these different chemicals and just an overload on their system.

Leanne's common-sense approach may resonate with other parents, but it is not supported by practitioners, who know that individuals encounter and manage exponentially more pathogens each day than are in vaccines.[23] Yet as parents see themselves as experts based on what feels true for their families, they reject the recommended vaccine schedule, which seems overwhelming, in support of individual children's needs.

Developing Unique Plans for the Unique Child

In all my discussions, it was clear that parents who reject mainstream vaccine schedules view each child's immune system as unique. Parents assess each child's age, gender, health status, and perceived predispositions that would make them more vulnerable to an adverse reaction. Leanne's description of how she manages vaccine decisions for her four children illustrates the proactive efforts parents take to manage risk, often laboriously parsing out different schedules for different children, each of whom they see as having separate and distinct needs. Leanne's first child was given vitamin K, but she declined the infant hepatitis B vaccine. She did consent to other infant vaccines, except MMR, which made her uncomfortable. At about nine months old, her oldest developed eczema and was identified as suffering food allergies, including an allergy to eggs. When she had her second son, two years later, she noticed very quickly that if she ate nuts, he showed a reaction after nursing. She recalls becoming cautious. After seeing small cuts or cracks along his mouth that emerged after nursing, she "really went hard-core on avoiding all dairy products, all nuts, all eggs, and so my diet was very restricted."

Leanne had become cautious about food during her pregnancy with her daughter a few years later, "as well as once she was first born, really watching what kinds of things were introduced to her." The process of remaining vigilant about food motivated her to think about vaccines. "It made me question the whole shot regimen, thinking, you know, because I read somewhere that that can have a link to immune reactions, since the eczema and allergies are an immuno-response. It made me question that. And so we did a delayed schedule with her."

Her daughter did not develop allergies and Leanne loosened her vigilance. She is the only one of Leanne's children to receive the MMR vaccine, which seemed safe since, she explains, "She doesn't have any of the allergies. She's just fine." Her fourth child was born two years ago and has not yet received vaccines. Leanne wants to see him protected, but believes that she should delay vaccines as long as possible. She also believes that he is at reduced risk for infection. "Our feeling has been, he will need those, he still has a chance of needing to build up those immunities to those kinds of diseases, but without traveling, without having a whole lot of exposure, it hasn't been pressing." Since the youngest does not show signs of allergies, Leanne imagines she will consent to have him vaccinated in the coming year.

Like most of the parents in this study, Leanne conducts her own research but also relies on her intuition about her children. She describes this process: "I weigh it out in my mind. I obviously ponder it and try and sense if . . . [intervention] seems appropriate. And I do feel, like, in a way I'm either comfortable or uncomfortable with it. And whenever I'm uncomfortable I won't move forward." Reflecting on how she and her husband reference the sense of intuition, she continues, "We call it guiding of the spirit, but yeah, that confirmation of peace and comfort or an unsettled feeling. It's walking into that dark alley and saying I don't feel comfortable, that's something telling you this is not a comfortable situation."

Paula also considered vaccines differently with each child. Her first daughter, now a young adult, received all recommended vaccines, in large part because it hadn't occurred to Paula to question it. She explains, "She had, I think, all of the normal vaccinations. She went through the series." Her daughter began having seizures at about one year of age. Paula believes that this was related to an excessive use of antibiotics rather than vaccines. "She had a lot of respiratory problems and colds, and the pharmacist that filled her last prescription at eighteen months said that she was being poisoned by too strong of—too many antibiotics and that that was causing them." Although she became critical of prescription medications, she did not question vaccines. "At the time I don't think there was any awareness that, you know, I mean, everybody had their kids vaccinated."

By the time she had her second child, two years later, Paula began questioning a range of interventions, including vaccines. Her second child did not receive any vaccines until she was hospitalized at the age of ten years and was given a tetanus vaccine, which, Paula recalls, was part of the hospital regimen. She remembers thinking that her kids were "growing up barefoot" and probably would benefit from protection against tetanus, and as such, she didn't object.

More than a decade later, Paula gave birth to a son with Down's syndrome. He was sick frequently with respiratory infections, and a pediatrician convinced her she should consent to give him the vaccine against Hib. As she recalls, the physician advised her that the infection "he might be exposed to the most and be the most vulnerable to would be that one. She said, 'If there's only one you're gonna get, that is gonna be the most important for him, this is gonna be it.'"[24]

In thinking about her different approaches to each child's vaccines, she explains that in part, she consented to that vaccine for her son "just because he had more vulnerability." It is also clear that Paula sees the changes in her family life as also transforming her approaches to health:

Life's just different. It's a different planet. . . . I mean, I was a single mom with two girls at home for a long time and I think it's just being, you know, what I call guerrilla parenting. You just have to be so on all the time.

As Paula became older and focused on a child with a disability, her strategies changed. "I think everything needs balance." She manages her son's care differently. "We keep him off junk food, we keep him off dairy. He doesn't get food colorings, he doesn't get sugar because he has a susceptibility to having allergies or food sensitivities. And I, you know, I just fell in love with great vitamins and [chiropractic] adjustments and the things that are gonna boost up his immune system so he doesn't get sick." Drawing on these resources, Paula feels she can make different choices in terms of his health generally and vaccines specifically.

Landscapes of Risk and Choice: Katie Reynolds

Thus far, I have shown how parents weigh risk and benefits of disease and vaccines and make individual decisions about vaccines for each of their children. Often, critics of those who opt out of vaccines portray parents as either wholly disapproving of vaccines or as underestimating the risks of diseases. The choice not to vaccinate is seen in isolation from the other strategies parents adopt. I find instead that the vaccine choice is one choice among a broad landscape of other choices parents make: about schools, religion, nutrition, neighborhood, youth sports, or discipline in the broader context of their children's lives. In the following section, I take one parent's explanation of her anxiety about vaccines to illustrate the many factors at play as parents strategize vaccine choices.

Katie is a forty-one-year-old mother of two. Her son, Julian, is five years old and in kindergarten and her daughter, Maya, is two years old and home with her full-time. Katie has a master's degree in economics and when she could not find a job in her field, became a freelance financial writer. Katie recalls questioning vaccines when her son was due for his first round:

> I'm one of those people who researches everything to death, and reads every book I can read, so it was like the night before he was getting his first round of immunizations and I [felt like] I made the decision to give him—I mean, I just felt like I had made a lot of decisions without really researching them.

It is worth noting that Katie regrets many of what she now sees as uninformed parenting decisions. For example, she regrets consenting to having her son circumcised without conducting research first. She also regrets allowing her physician to give her a booster against measles, mumps, and rubella (MMR) during her hospital delivery of Julian. This latter intervention is common, as physicians routinely check the levels of immunity in soon-to-be mothers and boost their immunity if needed in an effort to protect them against infections that could lead to birth defects in future pregnancies or to infections their babies might suffer. Aiming to do her best as a parent, the night before the well-child appointment at which vaccines would be offered, Katie began her research. She recalls,

> I was reading *Mothering* [magazine] and I went to the *Mothering* website and I started doing research and one of the things that came up was—and I was always really worried about autism to begin with. That there was some study that was done where children whose mothers had received

the MMR vaccine while they were nursing, the child went on to develop autism in, like, twenty out of twenty-five cases in some study in England. And it was actually in a testimony before Congress but it was kind of hushed up. So I was freaking out about that, you know, because I thought, here I am worrying about his vaccines and I totally agreed to do that and didn't think twice about it. You know, and here I won't take an aspirin while I'm nursing, but I did that.

Her understanding of this research pushed her to fear that her nursing son could develop autism because of her own MMR booster. It is worth noting that this study she cites does not represent mainstream knowledge and links to a broader debunked study linking MMR to autism.[25] Yet, based on her research, this felt like a significant risk and informed her choices. At the time she found this study, she had only started her research and did not feel certain of her views or able to articulate her concerns well. At this appointment, Katie felt pressured by the pediatrician she saw that day and by her mother, who accompanied her on the visit; she reluctantly consented to infant vaccines, including Hib and DTaP. Julian tolerated the vaccines well and Katie convinced herself that she was "freaking out about nothing." However, several friends she considered knowledgeable continued passing on their research about the risks of vaccines to her. Katie describes that time period:

> Now around this time one of my friends who was sort of into all these questions too told me she had read something, and I guess the crucial thing with this study with the MMR booster and the mother was the child developed autism after receiving their own MMR booster. So that was sort of like the trigger. And it doesn't necessarily have anything to do with the shot, it has to do with—I'm totally gonna screw this up, because I don't really know if I quite understand the science, but certain people are born with a resistance to the MMR vaccine and that has something to do with yeast in their gut. . . . So for some reason, this is more a marker of people that for some reason the vaccine triggered something—some intestinal thing.

Fear of the vaccine and possible susceptibility to developing autism drove Katie's choices, which she claims full control over making. "At that point I said to my husband, 'If I get hit by a bus tomorrow, the one thing you have to remember is do not give Julian the MMR booster,' because you know, I kept thinking, to me that was gonna be, that would be the trigger."

Katie admits that her son never had a fever or showed any signs of adverse reaction to the vaccines he received. However, by the age of two years, she remembers, "he still wasn't talking hardly at all," which frightened her. He was also a child who "has had a lot of allergies, eczema, immune-deficit, immune system issues." Believing he was vulnerable and that her own MMR vaccine while breastfeeding placed him at increased risk of developing autism, Katie continued to refuse the MMR vaccine. "Maybe if it hadn't been for me getting the MMR [while breastfeeding], I would have done all of them and not question it, [but] that was always in the back of my mind."

Katie seems to know her son's strengths and weaknesses well. She notes that "he's probably ahead for his age intellectually or cognitively, but, you know, his language skills, his motor skills and other things are a little, you know, behind." She notes, though, that it was not until entering preschool that the ways her child was different from other children were pointed out to her. "He's never been a really social child; you know, he liked to play by himself in the corner and wouldn't join in with the group and everything." As she remembers it, the teacher told her, "You know there's something—something's off with him." Katie remembers feeling resentful of the teacher and her feedback, thinking, "My child's perfect. It's you who doesn't know what you are doing." But she had his hearing and vision evaluated anyway; both tests came back normal. Next, several people recommended they look into whether he suffers from a sensory processing disorder, so they "had him evaluated for that and he did have that."

At his small private school, Katie recalls, "he had a definite problem; he doesn't always get social cues with other kids, and some of the kids were, like, a year older and were sort of pushing him and he was pushing back and getting into scuffles with them, and he just didn't seem to get what was going on." After he was switched to another class, he began to do better, as the class had more kids his age and a teacher who "runs a much tighter ship." Nonetheless, the new teacher encouraged Katie and her husband to seek out a full developmental workup at the local children's hospital. Instead, Katie sought out an evaluation through her local public school district's office charged with accommodating students with disabilities. The district explained that Julian did not have any disabilities that would qualify him for special accommodations, because "they don't accept sensory processing as a thing." Katie adds, "But they did say, you know, if you want to pursue an autism diagnosis then we could, you know, talk." Katie briefly considered this, but declined, explaining, "I just don't want to have him labeled that."

Notably, Katie has refused to enter the pediatric world of autism assessment and diagnosis, even as she describes herself as desperately searching for answers. "It really bothers me when people who look at him are like, 'He's got this wrong with him,' or 'He's not doing this for his age level,' but then [don't] see, like, all the really great things about him." This view changes how she approaches healthcare systems.

> So to me it's like looking at it in a very holistic way and not trying to change him or fit him into a box or label and—when I'm talking to a medical practitioner, they don't address him as a whole person, you know, or maybe only as, like, a diagnosis or potential diagnosis.

As her son's advocate and the person who knows him best, she rejects medical definitions of her child in hopes that he will be viewed as the more complex person he is who will best thrive without diagnoses.

Despite her view of healthcare providers as reductionist in their approach, Katie has developed a relationship with a pediatrician she trusts. She describes him as "probably the most alternative" in a group known for embracing alternative and complementary medical practices. While she feels supported in her effort to identify her son's challenges, she refuses vaccines, without the same support. Her son's doctor reminds her at each appointment that Julian is due for five boosters, but she refuses. "I don't even want to go there. I don't want to do anything that's gonna throw off his system." Katie continues to seek advice from people around her about the challenges she faces in advocating for her son and receives support for rejecting vaccines. "I've had a number of different practitioners we've seen [including a homeopath, cranio-sacral practitioners, and naturopathic allergists] who have said to me, 'Don't, whatever you do, don't do the MMR.'"

Katie also considers whether her own mental health at the time Julian was born contributed to his deficits.

> One of the things I wonder with my son too is he was born a month after 9/11 and I was just a basket case the whole month before he was born. Because I tend to be a little neurotic anyway. . . . So I was pretty tense.

Much of her search for her culpability is informed by questions various providers ask her—about her family, their diet, and even her pregnancy.

> People are always asking you questions about it all too. Like, "Okay, tell us again about his birth, tell us again about your pregnancy." And you start thinking, "Well, maybe I—I thought I had a really easy pregnancy, but maybe I didn't. You know, let me think. You know, maybe I ate a lot of tuna at the beginning of the pregnancy. Maybe that was it." I think about the mercury in the tuna, you know.

Katie considers the possibility that her son has autism, which she refuses to have diagnosed, and feels possibly responsible. "The ironic thing is I feel like I attracted, I was so fixated on being afraid that he had autism [that I might have brought it on]."

Woven through all these possible explanations is the recurrence of her belief that the MMR vaccine she received at his birth contributed. "There's part of me who thinks, 'Gosh! Was it that shot? Was it because I did that? Or would it have been worse if I had gotten [him] some more of the shots, specifically the MMR?'"

Katie's story illustrates several crucial points for understanding the choice to opt out of or modify vaccine schedules. First, research and advocacy are central to her parenting. With schools, disabilities, and vaccines, Katie sees her role as requiring her to read everything and become as pushy as needed to get what she believes her children need. On occasions when she did not conduct research or do her due diligence, she expresses regret for what she sees as negative outcomes, even when they are uneventful (like the lack of complication for her son's circumcision). Second, Katie feels a sense of responsibility as a mother and consumer for failing her children. Her conviction that her own MMR vaccine or her distraction post-9/11 in the months after her son was born might have led to her son's cognitive delays demonstrates her beliefs that as a mother she should be able to manage risk and that children's challenges represent her failures. As an active consumer, she should be able to make choices to optimize her children's health. Poor health, then, suggests she missed the mark.

Being Good Parents

Much of the culture of individualist parenting demands that parents maintain vigilance in considering their children's needs and advocating for them with institutions. This has in many ways become the cornerstone of concerted cultivation, where investing in children's well-being demands intense resources to ensure that children have optimal outcomes. The parents in this study take these duties to heart. They conduct research, share information on listservs and in online forums with other parents, discuss their children's care with friends and providers, and consider the ways their children are unique.

As parents weigh risk and make vaccine choices, they do so in ways that illustrate how the mandates of public health and informed consent lie in tension. The narrative that vaccines are beneficent and should be accepted without question undermines the tenets of informed consent, which require providers to communicate potential risk and benefit so patients can decide whether and when they want an intervention. Although public health officials who develop vaccine schedules would disagree with the process that leads these parents to opt out, it is clear that parents thoughtfully consider the meanings of each vaccine, even if their understandings of science, risk, and benefit are different from expert views. In understanding risk and benefit, parents must believe that the risk of illness is significant and that vaccinating will mitigate that risk. Healthcare providers and policy makers might identify the statistical likelihood of infection, or of a significant injury from vaccination, but in order to choose to vaccinate, parents must perceive that those risks apply to their own children and that the vaccine will prevent those specific and identifiable risks while not causing other harm to their vulnerable children.

Some of these parents believe that vaccines work in general but believe that they are unnecessary or too risky; others do not accept that they are necessary and effective for their children at all. What is common to all of the parents in this study is the view of their children as individuals with unique bodies, immune systems, vulnerabilities, and lifestyles that predict different vaccine needs for their own health. In contrast to public health, which looks at immunity and efficacy at a population level, these parents evaluate their own children's lifestyle, diet, nutrition, social networks, and health to evaluate vaccines and then reject or accept them accordingly.

3

Vaccines as Unnatural Intervention

One thing that completely confounds me is that there are no studies comparing the health of unvaccinated children to the health of vaccinated children. This seems like such an obvious study and it should have been conducted decades ago. Why hasn't it been done yet? My guess is because the health of the nonvaccinated children would so totally blow away the health of the vaccinated children that the discussion about the dangers of vaccines could finally be put to bed and the case would be closed emphatically in favor of those that accuse shots of causing chronic illness and auto immune disease. . . . Take an informal poll of the folks in your circle and see for yourself. Observation is a powerful tool, so put it to use. The kids with the most problems—allergies, asthma, ADHD, autism, coordination and other gross motor issues, etc. sure seem to be the ones that are right on track with their vaccination schedule, don't you think?
—Sarah Pope, The Healthy Home Economist[1]

For many parents, there is nothing more natural than their newborn baby. Almost all referred to newborns as perfect. Ruby Caine, a mother of two, says of her son, "He's not circumcised, and he has no vaccines, because I was like, 'Look, you came out perfect. We're leaving you alone.'" This view of children's bodies as naturally perfect is a sharp contrast to perceptions of vaccines as artificial. I find that parents overwhelmingly identify prenatal and neonatal interventions, especially vaccines, as corrupting this natural state. Illustrating the subjective meanings of "natural," some mothers describe using Clomid or other medications to assist them in becoming pregnant, even as they felt protective of natural birth. Some describe accepting other interventions around delivery but valorize the lack of medical technology in their children's bodies.

For example, when Tracy was twenty weeks into her pregnancy, she experienced preeclampsia, a potentially serious complication. As she thinks about the experience, she recalls with relief how her daughter did not require technological interventions after birth. "She came out, she weighed exactly five pounds; she was breathing on her own. Never required being in an incubator or anything. She was perfect." Gabriela Luce, who refused additional prenatal testing after a screen for birth defects came back positive, remembers just knowing that the fetus was fine and that her pregnancy would go well. "It was perfect. I knew it was. Yeah, I felt more intuitive when he was born than at any other time in my life." These women, like most in this study, recall the newborn period and their children's early days as magical, as a natural and thus ultimately superior state. Newborn interventions, in contrast, are seen as undermining that natural state, which as the scholar Chris Bobel explains, is powerful, pure, and superior, embodying a logic beyond the control of the individual and beyond human reason.[2] For example, Patricia, a mother of eight, explains her concern over the early use of vaccines and other interventions as unnatural:

> Like, we didn't come into this world, you know, requiring a shot. . . .
> We have a God-given immune system and it's sad that the medical field
> doesn't recognize that. It's like, you don't have to shoot things into the
> body. . . . Let's support what we already have.

Patricia's view, like those of virtually all the parents in this study, valorizes the natural body. These views are in many ways driven by timing, as many vaccines are offered in the first days and months of life, when parents see their babies as the epitome of innocence and purity. It is an image in stark contrast with lurking needles and the perceived toxins within them. The medical rationale is that since infants have naïve immune systems, are the most vulnerable to infection, and are also likely to suffer the worst complications from many vaccine-preventable infections, early vaccines will help protect them. As a result, public health policy aims to vaccinate those babies at the time they are most vulnerable. In contrast, parents focus heavily on the age, weight, and maturity of babies when explaining their reasons for rejecting or delaying vaccination. Carolyn Kalman, a mother of three, recalls, "We went for a well-baby checkup, and all they did was hassle me, . . . and I said, 'You know, I'm making a choice, and who are you? And why is it that I have to do this in this time with a little infant?' And I said no way."

Similarly, Elizabeth, a mother of two children who have not received any vaccines, describes her concern that vaccines could overwhelm them, physically and emotionally. She explains that vaccines make sense with older children, who have "most importantly just better-developed immune systems. More able to handle it, I think, from a social-emotional perspective." Anna explains, "You know a child's immune system really isn't fully formed—it's better at two, but . . . it's not really formed until about seven."

Physicians do not dispute that infant immune systems are underdeveloped. Yet *how* that underdevelopment matters is where the parents in this study diverge from generally held public health principles. The parents see infants as too young to handle vaccines. Vaccine proponents argue that, in fact, infants are capable of building an immune response within hours of birth, and that vaccines actually help that process. The vaccine researcher Paul Offit and colleagues in a frequently cited medical journal article explain,

> The development of active humoral and cellular immune responses in the newborn is necessary to meet the tremendous number of environmental challenges encountered from the moment of birth. When children are born, they emerge from the relatively sterile environment of the uterus into a world teeming with bacteria and other microorganisms. Beginning with the birth process, the newborn is exposed to microbes from the mother's cervix and birth canal, then the surrounding environment. Within a matter of hours, the gastrointestinal tract of the newborn, initially relatively free of microbes, is heavily colonized with bacteria.[3]

Parents are unlikely to view birth as an experience "teeming with microorganisms." Instead, most describe birth in romantic terms that reflect the view of it as beautiful, miraculous, and natural. These fundamentally different, yet by no means mutually exclusive, views of birth underscore how parents envision neonatal interventions as invasive. In many ways, the timing of initial vaccines—after birth—highlights the sense of vaccines as an artificial intervention on the heels of what many parents see as one of the more natural moments in life, but one they spent a great deal of energy planning: birth.

Natural Birth and Newborn Interventions

Parents invest birth with great significance. More than half of the parents in this study had at least one child born at home, and almost all conducted extensive research and planning for their births. Despite these efforts to control it, women were quick to refer to birth as the most natural of experiences, often characterizing it as empowering. Molly Jones's description of her son's birth illustrates this: "I felt like I was in charge of my body. . . . I felt like I could do anything. If I could go through that experience and, you know, push out this baby, I could take on the world, basically." She continues, "I think it was three hours before I gave him up to anybody. Just held him and said, 'I did that. I pushed you out.'" Women in this study offered stories of birth as a way of explaining their commitment to a more natural, and thus superior, state as women. As Marlene, a mother of four, explains, "Well, birth is such a defining event for women. . . . There are some things we can't intellectualize away, and giving birth gets you way out of your mind and back into your body."

The Newborn, Vitamin K, and the Underdeveloped Immune System

Birth was inscribed with symbolic meanings as a natural and often enchanted state, which led many mothers to question why anyone would disrupt it with chemical interventions, like vaccines or other newborn interventions. In fact, parents are asked to make medical decisions in the first moments of becoming a parent. Newborns are often given antibiotic eye ointment to protect against possible exposure to syphilis during delivery, which could cause blindness; vitamin K to address a serious but rare risk of spontaneous bleeding due to a vitamin K deficiency; and the first vaccines against hepatitis B, intended in large part to prevent transmission from mother to newborn during delivery. For many parents, medical justifications for these interventions are unconvincing, particularly as they see their babies as naturally perfect. For example, Janine explains her choice to decline newborn interventions: "Like the eye ointment that they put in if the mom has syphilis. Well, she doesn't, so that is just dumb to do that. So, we didn't do that. And then the vitamin K for blood clotting felt irrelevant too. She is going to be at our house, . . . why would she bleed out?"

Because medical interventions are offered immediately after birth, mothers in this study recall being aware that they needed to be prepared to make these decisions, or in some cases, voiced regret that they were not better prepared to give truly informed consent (or refusal) at birth. In all cases, parents described self-education as key to their strategic efforts to make an informed decision for their baby. Heather, a mother of two young boys who later received some vaccines, attended seminars on vaccines taught by a local naturopath and researched newborn interventions. She explains, "I knew I didn't have any infections, so I didn't want to give him antibiotics or the vitamin K. . . . I researched that and I just felt like the risk factors for him were very low." Considering her own health during pregnancy, Heather continues, "I had been taking alfalfa and vitamin K, things to increase my vitamin K in my blood, so that he would be, you know, less likely to have problems, and we didn't circumcise him." Many women, like Heather, identify how their management of their prenatal bodies could protect their babies, and that prenatal health predicts child health.[4] Heather's explanation presents a common misunderstanding of how vitamin K deficiencies actually present, not from openings to the body, but with internal bleeding, including but not limited to life-threatening bleeding in babies' brains or digestive systems.

Vitamin K deficiency bleeding is rare—affecting only about 4 to 8 babies per 100,000.[5] Intramuscular injections of vitamin K have been used since the early 1960s and are completely effective in preventing deficiency bleeding. Some babies will show signs of vitamin K deficiency bleeding shortly after birth, but it is much more common and much more dangerous for babies to develop it between two weeks and two months after birth. Since breastfeeding confers less vitamin K than formula, exclusively breastfed babies are at higher risk for bleeding disorders, which seems counterintuitive, as the more natural practice of breastfeeding is widely understood to be superior.

Rates of rejection of vitamin K have increased recently, with few parents communicating that they understand the possibly life-threatening outcomes of doing so.[6] Reasons vary, but generally show parents' beliefs that vitamin K injections are unnecessary, unnatural, and potentially toxic. Some websites aiming to inform parents of the risks of vaccines and vitamin K, for example, argue that while vitamin K is necessary, synthetic vitamin K is not well-absorbed, compared to that derived from natural plant-based sources.[7] Others suggest that injections are unnatural, even as some research indicates that oral doses are less effective for newborns. A widely discredited 1992 study in a midwifery journal linked vitamin K injections to leukemia, which is still discussed in the blogosphere. More generally, parents who prioritize natural living, aim to have good nutrition for themselves and their families, and voice a commitment to protecting the natural state of the body don't see the vitamin K injection as necessary or relevant for newborns, envisioned as naturally perfect. Rather, these interventions seem unnecessary, unnatural, and even dangerous.

Hepatitis B

Parents reject the vaccine against hepatitis B, a virus that causes chronic liver disease, for several reasons, some similar and others quite different from the reasons they reject vitamin K. Parents also see the vaccine and its timing as unnatural—both as an intervention on newborns' perfect bodies and as a vaccine against risks in a different phase of life. In these ways, the newborn vaccine against hepatitis B represents a disruption of the life course of illness risk and behavior, which makes it unacceptable. Katie's story illustrates both these dynamics.

Katie's first child was born in a hospital, and she did not question the newborn interventions that were offered. By the time she was pregnant with a second child, her toddler son suffered chronic ear infections, allergies, and eczema. Fearful that medical interventions in his first days led to these health issues, Katie explains, "So with [my daughter] I decided I wanted to do my birth completely differently, the way I wanted to do it." This included using a midwife, practicing yoga all through her pregnancy, and being "very holistic." Although she delivered her daughter at the hospital because she wanted to ensure she would have access to medical care should anything go wrong, she describes her labor as easy and natural.

After she delivered her daughter "naturally" in the hospital, she remembers that a nurse came in and asked whether she would consent to a hepatitis B vaccine for the baby. She recalls responding with a sense of dismay. "She'd just been born and I was like, 'What?' And I was like, 'Why?' And they're like, 'Well, in case she's sexually active when she's a teenager.'" Katie was unconvinced and declined. She recalls, "They kind of hassled me a little bit in the hospital about it, but I was so—I was pretty firm in my convictions by this point in time and I was just like, 'No, I'm not doing it.'"

Hepatitis B is a virus that causes inflammation of the liver. It is the leading cause of liver cancer and contributes to cirrhosis as well. It is contagious and spread through contact with the blood, semen, vaginal fluids, and other bodily fluids of someone who already has a hepatitis B infection. Common routes to transmission include blood transfusions, direct contact with blood in healthcare settings, sexual contact with an infected person, tattoo or acupuncture with unclean needles or instruments, shared needles during drug use, sharing personal items (such as toothbrushes, razors, and nail clippers) with an infected person, or being born to someone who is infected.[8]

The virus for hepatitis B was discovered in 1965 by Baruch Blumberg, who was awarded a Nobel Prize for this discovery. By 1971, he and the microbiologist Irving Millman had helped to develop a test for the virus, which made it possible to screen blood. A hepatitis B vaccine was first licensed in 1981, and a more sophisticated recombinant vaccine, one that does not use blood products and therefore carries no risk of accidental infection, was licensed in 1986. In 1991 three doses of the vaccine against hepatitis B were added to the schedule of recommended vaccinations.[9] Initially, the hepatitis B vaccine was recommended only for people identified as being at risk for infection, which included those who are sexually active or use intravenous drugs. However, this strategy proved ineffective for limiting transmission, in large part because those at greatest risk do not regularly access healthcare systems. Recommendations changed to universally vaccinate all infants.

This policy is driven by three general concerns. First, babies born to mothers who carry hepatitis B are at significant risk of infection. Babies who are infected are most likely to develop chronic hepatitis, which makes them always contagious with recurring symptoms, and for which there is no cure. Children infected before the age of five years face a 15–25 percent increased chance of premature death from liver disease and are 50–90 percent more likely to develop chronic liver disease (depending in part on the age of infection).[10] Second, children can be infected by family members, childcare or healthcare providers, or others near them. Our vocabulary of harm reduction communicates that through behavior modification and deliberate efforts, we can identify and reduce risk. Yet approximately 35 percent of people who get hepatitis B do not have any identified risk factors, and do not know where they contracted the virus.[11] Third, infants represent a captive audience for healthcare delivery. When individuals face the greatest risk of infection—in adolescence and young adulthood—they are least likely to be seen by doctors. Thus, vaccinating them before they face risk is seen as the best way to prevent future infection. As a CDC brochure for parents explains, "Hepatitis B vaccine is your baby's 'insurance policy' against being infected with the hepatitis B virus."[12]

This third rationale for vaccination is the most controversial and is the focus of most parental objections: babies are vaccinated to protect them and those around them from infection in adolescence and adulthood should they participate in behaviors that risk exposure, like those involving the exchange of bodily fluids or intravenous drugs. Lauren's objections to this vaccine best illustrate this:

> I don't even remember if I read it in a book or if I went to, like, my Lamaze class at [the] hospital and they said that they were gonna give the hep B shot to the babies . . . and I was just outraged. . . . And so I started looking into it and they're like, "Well, you know, vaccinating the adult population has been a total failure; they're not gonna comply. So now we're gonna do it with newborns."

Lauren, a mother of four unvaccinated children, understands that the reason for the vaccine is to reach adults who are difficult to find later. She finds this objectionable in large part because she understands the vaccine to be dangerous to babies. Lauren recounts her understanding that an equal number of adults die of hepatitis B infection as children die from complications of vaccination. This understanding informs her views, but is statistically unlikely. The World Health Organization (WHO) estimates that about 780,000 people die yearly of hepatitis B disease, with the CDC estimating about 1,800 hepatitis B–related deaths in 2011 in the United States.[13] It is difficult to account for deaths caused from vaccines, since most vaccines are given between two and four months, which is considered the peak age for sudden infant death syndrome as well. Most of what is known of vaccine injury comes from the Vaccine Adverse Event Reporting System (VAERS), a federal database of adverse reactions from vaccines to which healthcare providers, patients, or families can *voluntarily* report, though it is admittedly not an exhaustive system for vaccine safety surveillance. According to VAERS data, there were fifteen reported deaths from hepatitis B vaccine in 2010 in the United States.

For parents like Lauren, the perception that an equal number of children die from the vaccine as adults from the disease, and the accompanying horror that public health officials seemingly accept that this exchange is justified, shape their objection to the vaccine and fuel distrust of public health systems. Lauren explains her outrage:

> Their whole reasoning that I could find was there's so many adults that died of what was basically, it's transmitted like an STD [sexually transmitted disease]—not that that's not the only way you get it, obviously—versus this many babies die if we give the vaccine, so therefore that equals it out. Well, I don't consider a newborn baby to be the same as an adult.

Newborns, as Lauren sees it, are vulnerable and innocent, facing unknown risks of vaccines, which may be "changing them or altering them." She stacks that perception against the less sympathetic adult who engages in risk behaviors, including drug use or sex, after which she imagines him saying, "Oh gee, I have all these problems now." Disgusted, she explains her resulting distrust of medical systems: "That is the number one thing that has totally eroded my trust in the medical system, and they'll never get it back, because I think that their values and my values are different, because if they don't see the difference between a newborn and an adult, then there's not much to talk about."

As the earliest vaccine offered, hepatitis B is the focal point of parents' concerns. The controversy around it illustrates constructs of risk, need, health, and nature. One pediatrician who rarely recommends vaccinating newborns against hepatitis B explains, "You know, we vaccinate every newborn for hepatitis B, but what's the true statistical chance of them getting it in a place like Boulder? It's very close to zero." In contrast to this wealthy and predominantly white university town, he clarifies how he weighs risk and necessity: "If I lived in sub-Saharan Africa, ... I'd be for using hepatitis B vaccine on every newborn." In this explanation, the social location of the parents—both geographical but also in terms of race and class—supports a view of them as low-risk and exempt from the assumptions of public health policy.

These views also reflect a commitment to therapeutic nihilism. This perspective, originating in medicine in the nineteenth century, holds that the body is powerful enough to heal itself and also that medical intervention or treatment is generally useless or even harmful—that when it comes to medicine, less is indeed more and better. In this view, vaccines are at best a necessary evil to be avoided when possible. Parents continue to weigh risk and benefit, but they do so from the starting point that risk of disease exposure is identifiable (particularly in their own communities, where they feel safe), while risk of vaccines is not. In part, what their calculus rests on is the view that the natural body can manage disease, but vaccines are an unnatural intervention containing dangerous chemicals, which introduce new unknown risks to young bodies. As they question the safety and necessity of vaccines, they also doubt whether vaccines actually save lives and build strong immune systems over time.

Vaccines as Unnatural Immunity

Another way that the division between natural and artificial is articulated by parents is in discussions of the differences between immunity generated by exposure to a wild virus and that which comes from a vaccine. Joseph Mercola, an osteopathic doctor and health product salesman with one of the most-visited natural living websites in the world, advises parents, "There is a major difference between natural acquired immunity and vaccine-induced immunity. Obtaining natural immunity has far greater benefits, but this fact seems to be completely overlooked in the United States."[14] The view that natural immunity is better, and vaccines are inferior, shapes many parents' sense of why vaccines should be avoided.

Unnaturally Entering the Body

In part, parents view the mode by which vaccines enter the body—mostly through injection—to be unnatural. Parents often describe how natural infection—from one infected person to another—would enter the mouth, nose, or throat and gradually work its way into the body, through the mucosal, digestive, or lymphatic systems, where, they imagine, the virus or bacteria are more successfully defeated or at least significantly weakened before entering the bloodstream. Tara Milon, a mother of one unvaccinated toddler, explains, "We have issues with the shots. Because when you go through the first two layers of the immune system and then the immune system goes, 'Oh, God, what is this thing in my body?' The immune system says, 'I'm not working,' and the immune system starts to shut down." Similarly, Gabriela explains, "I would love it if they would put more research into edible vaccinations so that it goes through the digestive system rather than directly—bang!—into the bloodstream."

Jake, a chiropractor and father of three unvaccinated children, has a similar concern about vaccines. "When you inject something into a person, you're bypassing up to nine major organ systems that are supposed to protect you from getting sick. So you can't call the vaccination or immunization a natural immunity. It's not." Citing something he read, he explains his understanding of how the immune system processes pathogens and how vaccines interfere with this process by using a football metaphor of better "first-string" players and backup, "second-stringers":

> When you get an artificial immunization, then the rest of your life now your immune response will be basically, like, sending in the second string. Your body will not have the natural immune response, or its best immune response. It has a weakened immune response. When you—if someone sneezes on me or I let my child get chickenpox by itself, or mumps, rubella, whatever these things are, even polio, now my body says, "Oh, that's already gone through the lymph channels. It's already gone through the mucus channels. It's already gone—so by the time it hits the bloodstream, the immune system says, "Hey, we've already weakened this germ to the point where now we can kick its butt and send in the first string." Okay?

And now once your body defeats that bug naturally, through the first string, that first string now—anytime anything else comes at the immune system, that first string gets released immediately, and now you have lifetime immunity. You don't need boosters. You don't need anything, because you've got it.

Highlighting the ways he perceives the natural immune system as different from immunity from vaccines, which drives his decision to reject vaccines, he continues, "I don't care what you call it, that vaccine—that vaccine's never gonna do better than [what] my body can produce if my body's healthy enough to produce, so that's what we went with." Jake is articulate in his view of how the natural immune system is superior. He does not acknowledge how many diseases that cause natural immunity can also lead to serious illness, disability, or death. Rather, he communicates his strong faith in the body to heal and protect itself.

Since the natural state of the body includes becoming sick and recovering, some see vaccines as causing long-term weaknesses in the immune system. Margaret explains, "When you basically inject a concoction into the bloodstream and you set up a permanent antibody response to where these antibodies are—they're like little soldiers in there; they basically are committed to keeping the immune system strong. But then [a vaccine] compromises the immune system. I mean, the body just doesn't have all the resources necessary to offset other things coming in." From this perspective, vaccines, which some parents see as the antithesis of nature, can also be understood as obstructing the natural immune response.

Many parents cite the need for boosters as a sign of vaccine failure. For example, one mother offers advice to another mother on a parenting listserv about whether to consent to the mumps vaccine for her teenage son, who is at heightened risk of sterility should he become infected. On the heels of a measles outbreak in the United States, the mother of the teen boy felt newly vulnerable and turned to a parent listserv for advice. The reply from another mother shows how perceptions of disease as natural and vaccines as inferior justify vaccine refusal:

I read something recently about how, if we think about the first, probably, ten or fifteen years of the MMR vaccine push, no one got boosters. Pretty

much all those people NEVER got boosters and we're talking about millions of people who, according to today's standards of boosters every few
years, are potentially susceptible to getting measles, mumps and rubella,
yet there haven't been any mass outbreaks. If you listen to current wisdom, that measles is just a plane ride away, you would think all those millions of people would be coming down with measles right now. Keep in
mind that "they" are freaking out about 159 measles cases in a population
of over 300 million. Mind boggling. Mumps isn't even on the radar. . . .
I know the whole vaccine thing can be scary if we get caught up in scare
tactics, but really, look at your family tree—you and your husband might
be the first of your family to even get the MMR, and yet you made it
onto this Earth. No one in your family (prior to your birth) went sterile
because they had mumps and they all likely had mumps at one point or
another!

In this explanation, the ability of one's ancestors to procreate after
mumps exposure illustrates that the vaccine is not necessary. The writer
does not consider that risks of sterility increase with age, so individuals
might have encountered mumps as younger children before vaccination. Further, it downplays the reality that some number of children
who experienced infectious disease may not have survived to become
adults who procreate, or may not have procreated to have progeny to
participate in online forums. Rather, the narrative claims the powers of
the natural immune system over vaccination and the lack of necessity of
vaccines, demonstrated by continued human existence.

Vaccines are designed to inspire the immune system to respond as
though it were infected with a particular pathogen without the risk of
the illness. This can mean that a virus is weakened so it may replicate
but not cause illness (as in the case of measles, mumps, rubella, rotavirus, varicella); that a virus is inactivated or killed so it cannot reproduce but can be recognized by the immune system (polio, hepatitis A,
influenza); or that part of the virus or bacteria—like a surface protein
or sugar—is used in the vaccine so the immune system will recognize it
and launch an immune response (as with diphtheria, tetanus, pertussis,
Hib, hepatitis B, HPV, pneumococcal, and meningococcal).[15]

Both immunity inspired by vaccines and immunity inspired by
infection can be seen as *natural immunity*. In both cases, the body's

own immune system is launching an immunological response. These responses, however, are not identical. The capacity for the body to remember and recognize that pathogen over time is sometimes lower with vaccine-inspired response than from becoming sick and recovering. Although a handful of vaccines seem to work better than immunity from the virus or bacteria (this appears to be the case for tetanus, HPV, Hib, and pneumococcal), much of the time, immunity is better and longer-lasting after illness than after vaccine.[16] However, the cost of that immunity is sickness and the potential complications that may accompany it, which may be serious and even life-threatening. Parental resistance to varicella (chickenpox) vaccine illustrates the perception that the weaker immunity resulting from vaccines is reason to avoid them.

Varicella

The varicella vaccine, which immunizes against chickenpox, is broadly viewed by parents—many of whom consent to other vaccines—to be inferior and unnecessary. In contrast, wild-virus varicella, which parents often seek out in hopes that their children will catch it and develop natural immunity, is seen as natural and superior. It is also largely seen as risk-free.

Before the varicella vaccine was introduced in 1995, there were about four million cases of chickenpox annually.[17] Most of the parents in this study recall having chickenpox as children. As the National Network for Immunization Information, a clearinghouse of medical vaccine research, describes it,

> Varicella (chickenpox) is an infection caused by the varicella-zoster virus (VZV). The infection usually starts as a rash on the face that spreads to the rest of the body. The rash begins as red bumps that eventually become blisters. A child will often get 300 to 500 blisters during the infection, which crust over and fall off in one to two weeks. The virus can be spread in the fluid from the blisters or droplets from an infected person's nose or throat.[18]

Because many of us remember having chickenpox and recall the pain of infection as well as the social aspects of classmates, neighbors, or sib-

lings also suffering in solidarity, we seldom think of varicella as dangerous. Parents' resistance to the varicella vaccine stems from both their
lack of firsthand experience with negative outcomes and a sense that the
disease itself is not very serious. As Steph O'Neill explains, "I know I'm
just one person, but I don't know of anyone who's had severe complications, let alone died, from chickenpox." Steph, a mother of one, considers the risk of the disease, but rejects the vaccine, explaining that she
derives "some comfort in knowing" that neither she nor her husband experienced any severe effects from the disease. She notes, "I survived it."

Outside personal experience, the story of chickenpox is more complex. According to public health researchers,

> Varicella is generally a mild disease, but it is highly contagious and can
> be severe and even fatal in otherwise healthy children (less than 1 out of
> every 10,000 cases). Chickenpox can cause pneumonia (23 out of every
> 10,000 cases), and is an important risk factor for developing severe in-
> vasive "strep" (group A streptococcal disease), commonly referred to as
> "flesh-eating disease." Treatment of this deep infection requires antibiot-
> ics and surgery to remove the infected tissue. Complications of varicella
> include bacterial infections (up to 5 percent of cases), decreased platelets,
> arthritis, hepatitis, and brain inflammation (1 in 10,000 cases), which
> may cause a failure of muscular coordination. Complications are more
> common among adolescents and adults, and in immunocompromised
> persons of all ages, than in children.[19]

Like measles and rubella, chickenpox holds additional risks for pregnant women; a woman infected early in pregnancy carries a 2 percent
chance of having a fetus with abnormalities, potentially including scar-
ring of the skin, limb deformities, eye damage, or mental retardation.
Infection can also lead to spontaneous abortion and increased risk of
death in infancy. Age also matters. Of the four million cases per year in
the United States before the vaccine, about ten thousand people were
hospitalized with complications, and approximately a hundred people
died. Although only 5 percent of reported cases of varicella are in adults,
adults account for 35 percent of the deaths from the disease.

Researchers invented the varicella vaccine in Japan in 1974, but it
was not licensed in the United States until 1995. In 1999 the Advisory

Committee on Immunization Practices (ACIP) began recommending varicella as part of the routine immunization schedule. Those recommendations have been twice updated and now include recommendations for a booster, as evidence showed that immunity may wane after inoculation.[20] As of November 2012, all states except Montana require either one or two doses of varicella vaccine for school entry. Evidence of two doses is required in all but nine states for children in childcare settings, schools, or both.[21]

Because of high rates of vaccination, it is becoming increasingly difficult for parents to find wild-virus varicella. Parents like Steph insist, "I think I would be more inclined to stick [my daughter] in a room with a kid I know who has chickenpox than I would be for her to get the vaccine between now and when she starts school." Katie, too, would like her son to contract varicella in childhood, when risks of complications are lower. In thinking about the possibilities of finding wild-virus exposure, she explains her strategy: "Actually, there are lots of nonvaccinated kids, I believe, at [our private school], and there was a huge outbreak of chickenpox—and I was like, "Can I bring my kids over?" . . . [but] they didn't get sick, which I was bummed out about."

The lack of easy opportunity for exposure has led to innovative efforts by parents. Many phone doctors' offices to ask whether they have any patients with active infection with whom they could be put in contact. Others set up online forums for parents to share information about chickenpox outbreaks. Some have even attempted to acquire it through unusual means. In one notable example, Wendy Werkit, a Nashville mother, offered a "fresh batch of pox" that she would ship on suckers that her infected child had sucked, or with spit-on Q-tips for fifty dollars. As she explained of her efforts, "They can't get [chickenpox] the normal way anymore of just naturally catching and just naturally getting the immunity for life."[22] Infectious disease doctors warn that infection on sucked lollipops that had been mailed would be unlikely to successfully communicate varicella, but could carry other diseases, including hepatitis, bacteria, or strep. Sending biological material through the postal system is also illegal. It does demonstrate the lengths parents will go to obtain "natural immunity" from wild-virus infection over vaccination.

Ironically, even the failure to become infected can underscore the success of natural living as a way of promoting wellness. For example, one mother posts in a parent forum, "If anecdotal stories help, both my children are unvaccinated and we have not had any issues. In fact, their immune systems seem to be so strong that they avoided contracting chickenpox on three different exposures (the last one even involved shared toothbrushes and clothing)."

The immunity conferred by the varicella vaccine does indeed wane over time, usually over twenty years, though there is variation.[23] As such, recommendations for boosters have increased. Before the vaccine, varicella, which is highly contagious, was nearly ubiquitous. So when those who had the disease cared for their own children who were infected, their immune system responded to the re-exposure to varicella, which essentially boosted their immunity to it. As varicella becomes increasingly rare with vaccination, there is a generational gap. Those who were infected with wild-virus varicella carry the virus in their nerves. Yet, without reinoculation from exposure to what would be the next generation of infected children if not for vaccines, they will likely require boosters to keep it in check.

The outcome of this may be increasing rates of shingles, although several studies show that rates of shingles were also increasing prior to the introduction of the vaccine, suggesting that something else is leading to the increase.[24] Shingles, a painful rash often accompanied by nerve pain, results from the reactivation of the varicella zoster virus that causes chickenpox and also lies dormant in the nerves of someone who ever was infected. One in three adults will get shingles during their lifetime, and at least half of all people eighty-five and older have had it.[25] In the United States, there are about one million cases of shingles each year, which is most often brought on by stress, immune-compromise, illness, or age. Getting the chickenpox vaccine does not erase the possibility of developing shingles. However, the frequency and severity of shingles is much less in those who were vaccinated against varicella than that following natural infection. The result of all of this has been the development and marketing of a vaccine for adults against shingles.

The natural health website proprietor Joseph Mercola writes of this development, "The FDA approved Merck's shingles vaccine (Zostavax) for use in people age 60 and older in May of 2006. So they have come out with a vaccine (shingles) to reverse the damages to your health caused by their earlier vaccine (chickenpox). Sound familiar?" From this perspective, vaccines and medications are seen as actively undermining health and removing the body's natural ability to heal. Connecting this to the larger view of chemicals and medications for chronic illnesses promoted by for-profit pharmaceutical companies who manufacture vaccines, Mercola writes,

> It is very much like the polypharmacy used to "treat" chronic disease. You get a drug to supposedly make you better, but it causes adverse side effects, so you are given another drug to treat those side effects. Then, THAT drug creates more problems, and pretty soon, no one can tell what's causing what, and down the drain of poor health you go. Meanwhile, you are taking a long list of drugs, and the only people truly benefiting are the pharmaceutical companies who make money each step of the way. In the case of varicella vaccines, they are profiting from the cause of an epidemic, as well as the supposed cure. But is it REALLY a cure? Will a shingles vaccine prevent a shingles epidemic?[26]

Because varicella is very rarely life-threatening, the vaccine for it triggers more questioning from parents than those for more dreaded diseases. In those cases, the natural history of disease, which includes disability and death, is harder to ignore. Chickenpox, in contrast, can seem a rite of passage that was a natural part of the life course that has artificially been removed from children's lives.

The Natural Body as Naturally Immune

Parents often cite their lifestyle, informed by a commitment to what they define as natural living, as rendering vaccines unnecessary. As they support their children's general health, they imagine their children naturally immune to infection. Tom Sanders, a father of four, points to the reality that some people are vaccinated and still contract illness, while others who are not vaccinated never contract illness. Rather than considering differences in patterns of infection, Tom insists that this latter group proves that health is complex, and that immunity to infection can come from many sources other than vaccines. "There's too many parameters. Was it nutrition? Was it exercise? Was it obesity? Was it diet alone? Was it the sugar consumption of the U.S.? It's outrageous, from a health standpoint."

Tom's insistence that diet, nutrition, and lifestyle are more important factors in protecting against infection than vaccines was shared by
many parents in this study. For example, Margaret explains of her family's health, despite lack of vaccination: "It's like we're using the body's
natural immunity and promoting . . . natural supplements or herbs or
whatever, that are attuned with nature." For Margaret and others, weakness in immune response, which she defines as becoming sick when infected, ties back to failures to live naturally. "We compromise ourselves
through not eating correctly or taking care of ourselves, and that's a hard
pill for a lot of people to swallow, because a lot of people don't want to
give up their vices. . . . So most people are gonna be prone to cancer and
other problems."

This framing infuses the ways many parents describe their choice
to opt out. Melissa Pallamore, a mother of one, for example, expresses
similar concerns, explaining that she and her husband came to endorse
"the whole natural family planning philosophy and the whole not putting artificial things into your body and listening to our bodies." With
the goal of protecting the natural state of her child's body, Melissa questioned vaccines, but also worried about how to protect his health. "For
the people who don't vaccinate, what do you do? Do you give them
supplements, or do you just give them extra fruits and veggies?" Melissa joined "a small mommy group" where women with new babies get
together, walk, and share parenting stories and experiences. She recalls
that one woman in the group who hadn't vaccinated her two-year-old
recommended vitamin or immune-promoting drops instead of vaccines, and touted the importance of taking her child to a chiropractor
once a month for well-care because, she explained, "that affects everything in their body." Looking for alternatives to vaccines, Melissa seriously considers these suggestions for the future, but thus far has opted to
consent to some vaccines for her son. Yet, even as she evaluates alternatives, she accepts that vaccines are separate from the natural body and
can potentially undermine it. Parents like her then search for ways to
promote their children's health through means they see as more natural
that might allow them to opt out while also believing that their children
are safe from infection.

In addition to individual decisions about lifestyle, parents also look
to regions with high rates of infectious disease and point to the living

conditions that they believe promote disease, like lack of sanitation. In these explanations, sanitation and clean drinking water are constructed as natural, despite being technological innovations built by public health systems, and diseases and pollution are unnatural. These explanations ignore how communities with high rates of infectious disease also often have weak healthcare delivery systems, poor access to nutrition, unclean water supplies, and low vaccination rates. Rather, parents take these patterns and extrapolate to feel assured that their lifestyle (facilitated by resources) is protective against infectious disease, that their children's bodies can resist infection, and that vaccines are unnecessary and unnatural.

Reconnecting Vaccines to the Natural

Clearly, the dichotomy between "natural" and "artificial" is constructed, maintained, and deployed in these parents' vaccine decisions. As they voice strong preference for natural health over what they see as chemical or technologically mediated health, agencies and providers are reconsidering how they communicate with parents about vaccines. In many visible ways, the public conversations around vaccines are shifting to better engage these concerns. The Colorado Children's Immunization Coalition takes these issues on directly. On the website for the statewide campaign, "Immunize for Good," the coalition explains,

> In the past decade we've seen a shift toward green, eco-friendly and natural living. Many of us have worked to reduce our personal waste, preserve nature's gifts, and keep toxins and anything labeled "artificial" out of our homes and our bodies. Some parents want to "green our vaccines" by calling out chemicals and seemingly scary-sounding ingredients. The truth is, all vaccine ingredients are tested together to be safe, and each ingredient is there to produce a stronger response in your baby's body to immunity toward a specific disease. Some of the ingredients in vaccines have raised concern among parents and have increased the appeal of natural immunity, but the only way to get natural immunity to a disease is to acquire it through actual infection. This means that you have to get sick—sometimes very sick—to develop resistance. Vaccines, on the other hand,

induce a natural immune response in the body without the suffering of getting sick with disease.[27]

Pediatricians are also considering how to best approach these concerns with parents. As they aim to reassure parents about the safety and necessity of vaccines, they also adopt the vocabulary they feel best addresses their concerns. For example, Carrie Mathers, a pediatrician who advocates for universal vaccination, describes her approach:

> I say, "You're introducing a very mild or, you know, inactive form of this illness to your body, allowing your body's natural immune response to create protections for you for the next time you encounter this virus, or this illness. So your body is producing its *natural* reaction, so it allows you to protect yourself without actually getting the illness."

The Immunization Coalition statement directly addresses the slogan "green our vaccines" and the parental concerns it embodies. Yet, as this chapter shows, this discourse is unlikely to be adequate in addressing parental concern as those issues remain more diffuse. They also fail to address a broader chemical-filled environment in which families live. Children are indeed growing up in environments with unavoidable exposure to plastics, chemicals, and toxins. Vaccines, in contrast, require consent. This allows parents to control one kind of intervention into their children's health. Pediatricians and websites that aim to convince parents that vaccines are also natural and also elicit a *natural immune response* aim to address these concerns.

4

The Limits of Trust in Big Pharma

I am sitting at a long table in a huge ballroom in an expansive hotel in Reston, Virginia. There are about 700 people sitting at similarly long tables, organized in rows with a long center aisle that serves as a wide walkway, with many large cameras placed strategically. In the front are panelists on a huge stage. Their faces and PowerPoint presentations project onto big screens on either side of the stage. Occasionally, these screens show pictures from the organization's memorial for vaccine victims, "those who are casualties of mass vaccination policies." There are also two microphones on stands that will later host audience comments and questions.

Two seats from the outer edge of the table midway back, I sit next to a woman, frantically typing notes from each presentation into her laptop. The cord stretches to an outlet on the outer wall and on occasion, she flinches as sometimes someone walks by and trips on it. She listens, types, and occasionally sighs or shakes her head in disbelief. This is the meeting of the National Vaccine Information Center, the largest organization that advocates against mandatory vaccines. Throughout the room, activists, alternative health providers, chiropractors earning continuing medical education credits, and concerned parents wanting to make good choices for their children take notes.

During a break in the morning session, I ask her what she will do with her notes. She explains that she is a former high school teacher who now runs a preschool parent co-op. She is collecting information for her own benefit and explains her concerns and priorities as a mother and educator. Then, a smile crosses her face. She turns and lifts an empty Starbucks cup. "This belonged to Andrew Wakefield." Starstruck, she announces that he "just threw it away" in front of her. Andrew Wakefield, a speaker the day before and the

recipient of the organization's Humanitarian Award at the reception the night before, is most famous for his claims in Great Britain that the measles-mumps-rubella (MMR) vaccine might cause autism. The British journal, *Lancet*, later rescinded Wakefield's article making that claim, and the General Medical Council of the U.K. revoked his medical license. Among U.S. and U.K. doctors, researchers, and public health officials, Wakefield is a pariah. Here, where he presents his new research on the suckling patterns of infant monkeys after vaccinations, he is, as the organization's leaders introduce him, a doctor of "conscience and courage" who stands "up for truth and freedom in science" and suffers the consequences.[1] Although discredited by mainstream science, he is a trustworthy expert here, and deserving of fandom.
—Fieldnotes, 2009

Parents who reject vaccine recommendations see vaccines as composed of toxins that can harm children. They doubt claims that vaccines are safe, question the ingredients in vaccines, and distrust the systems of scientific testing and regulation that are supposed to ensure vaccine safety. In this chapter, I parse out parents' logic that vaccines represent chemicals that are dangerous to children's bodies and should be avoided. I examine the views of vaccines as toxic and how this toxicity narrative justifies parents' refusal of vaccines.

The Toxicity Narrative: Fear of Vaccine Ingredients

Currently, federal agencies recommend vaccination against fourteen vaccine-preventable diseases, which can result in as many as twenty-six shots by the time a child is two years of age and as many as six shots in one visit.[2] Parents who distrust that vaccines are safe question what the combined toxicity of vaccines might be, what chemicals are contained in them, and what risks they might present.

Those who promote vaccine safety argue that vaccines are cleaner today and contain fewer unintended proteins—less contamination—as technologies for isolating proteins and mimicking viral DNA have improved. The pediatrician and vaccine researcher Paul Offit and colleagues explain, "Although we now give children more vaccines, the actual number of antigens they receive has declined. Whereas previously one vaccine, smallpox, contained about 200 proteins, now the eleven routinely recommended vaccines contain fewer than 130 proteins in total." In explaining the improvements in vaccine technology, they note, "Advances in protein chemistry have resulted in vaccines containing fewer antigens."[3] Although intended to reassure parents that vaccines are better refined to include only the desired antigens, these highly technical ways of manufacturing vaccines underscore the unnatural basis of vaccines themselves and do little to reassure parents.

Virtually every parent in this study cited concerns about ingredients as a reason they view vaccines as dangerous. Many feel that doctors and vaccine manufacturers are deliberately vague about the necessity of many chemicals and preservatives in vaccines. Margaret is a mother of two college-aged unvaccinated children. She describes her concerns about the number of chemicals in vaccines, which she learned from a friend who was a nurse and shared with her the vaccine package inserts:

> I wanted to make an informed decision. And so she said, "Do you want to look at an insert label?" I said sure. . . . She said, "Okay, here's what's in a vaccine." . . . All these chemical names, and she said basically that formaldehyde, aluminum, thimerosal, which is approximately 50 percent in weight, ethyl mercury, ethylene glycol, which is antifreeze, MSG, squalene, carbolic acid, neomycin, streptomycin, foreign viruses, dead animal parts, all this crap. And I said, why would I put this in my baby? I mean, it was just such a logical decision for me.

Other parents relay similar stories. They often describe the process of finding out about ingredients—from package inserts included in the vaccine boxes, friends, online forums, or websites—from sources other than those provided by doctors or CDC informational handouts. This perceived lack of official disclosure fuels suspicion. For example, Barb Schoenhorn, a mother of two, describes her frustration:

The fact that they don't tell us the truth anymore is really criminal. It's criminal to me. That they are allowed to say there's a trace of mercury when in fact that is not the truth. The fact that they are saying there is no mercury, that's not the truth. The fact that they don't tell you there is aluminum or formaldehyde, or the equivalent of antifreeze and aborted human fetus cells and portions of immunizations that's being incubated on monkey innards.[4]

Discussions of vaccine ingredients as harmful are plentiful in parent forums. In one online exchange, a pregnant woman asks other women in a discussion forum for advice to convince her husband that vaccines are dangerous. She receives dozens of suggestions for places to look for information. In one poignant example, another mother directs her to the FDA.gov website, where, she is told, she can look at each vaccine ingredient and at package inserts. The woman offering advice acknowledges, "Sometimes it's hard to understand what exactly an ingredient is because of the name, but the FDA explains some of them as well." By unveiling the toxic ingredients, she imagines the concerned woman's husband will also see the risks: "This alone can help your husband begin to understand your concern. The ingredients listed even at the lowest levels have been known to be harmful and even cumulative when you combine more than one vaccine." As the advice-giver provides her understanding of the risks of chemicals, she also includes advice to stay healthy naturally, breastfeed for as long as possible, and to seek out naturopathic remedies instead of vaccines.

Sometimes those who support vaccination programs challenge the perception that all chemicals are intrinsically harmful. For example, a supporter of vaccination posted online that there is more formaldehyde in a pear than in a vaccine, along with a list of other formaldehyde-producing fruits and vegetables. Some supportive followers agreed, adding additional information like, "Every single cell in the human body produces formaldehyde. It is a byproduct of normal cellular respiration. The body is well capable of removing formaldehyde." However, more responders disagreed, arguing instead that naturally produced formaldehyde must be less dangerous than that produced in laboratories, that chemicals consumed in the digestive system must be less dangerous than those injected, or that only older children can eat a pear, making

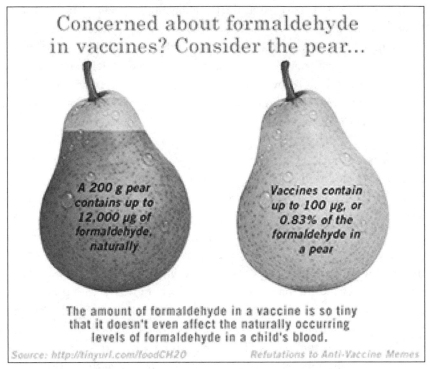

"Concerned about formaldehyde? Consider the pear . . ." Posted on "Refutations to Anti-Vaccine Memes's Page" March 20, 2013. https://www.facebook.com/RtAVM/photos/a.414675905269091.96547.414643305272351/484442114959136.

them better able to process the chemical, highlighting why infant vaccination is a mistake.[5]

These arguments reveal different understandings of chemistry. For some people, chemical compounds are meaningful outside their context, so for example, formaldehyde is always formaldehyde. For others, toxicity depends on the mode of production, the path of consumption, and the social context in which it is encountered. In these ways, beliefs about toxicity are deeply engrained in parental distrust and inform vaccine decisions.

Green Our Vaccines

This notion that vaccines are toxic received the greatest attention in 2008, when the celebrities Jenny McCarthy and Jim Carrey, in collaboration with several autism advocacy organizations, including Talk About Curing Autism (TACA), Generation Rescue, HEAL Foundation, and Moms Against Mercury, protested in Washington, D.C.[6] The June 4 march culminated in a rally and a call to reassess mandatory childhood vaccine schedules, which protesters insisted are too toxic. Jenny McCarthy spoke passionately at that rally:

> This is not an anti-vaccine rally. This is not an anti-vaccine group. We are an intelligent group of parents that acknowledge the vaccines have saved many lives. What we are saying is that the number of vaccines given and the ingredients, like the freaking mercury, the ether, the aluminum, the antifreeze, need to be removed immediately after we saw the devastating effects it took on our children.

As McCarthy continued her speech, she focused on the dangers of toxins beyond vaccines, as a call to make vaccines less toxic. Highlighting both the responsibility of individual parents to protect their own children's bodies and the role she sees autistic children playing in families' lives, she called for the prioritization of natural living as a means to protecting children:

> I want to empower parents to educate themselves and take safety back into their own hands. Everyone, not just parents of kids with autism, need to seriously pay attention to the warnings. These children are trying so hard, you guys, trying so hard to show us how to live in a cleaner world. These kids are here for a reason, to teach us to eat better, clean up the air, get rid of toxins because they can't survive.[7]

The "Green Our Vaccines" rally was among the most public protests against vaccines in the United States in recent history. With environmental activists like Robert Kennedy Jr. as a speaker, the campaign marries environmentalism, natural living, and children's health in ways that make vaccines suspect. Protesters also want agencies to develop a new schedule they imagine would be safer, arguing that until that happens, parents should reject *recommended* vaccines (which they note are not required, even if they are presented as such).

Managing Toxic Exposure

The fear that vaccines present a risk of toxic exposure stems from the broader context: children live in polluted environments and are exposed to chemicals each day. Some are manageable or more easily eliminated, like plastic storage containers or BPA-containing water bottles, while others are perceived to be more perniciously, even invisibly, poisoning children's bodies. The sociologist Norah MacKendrick suggests that this new form of "precautionary consumption" represents additional work mothers must perform to ensure the well-being of their children.[8] Parents' fears are shaped by their perceptions of widespread proliferation of chemicals, lack of environmental regulation, and corporate practices that lead to development of new artificial and questionably safe products and increased pollution. Anna describes her fears of chemicals generally, and how they impact vaccines:

> Somebody told me once that . . . there's something like two thousand new chemicals made every single year, and I just think about that and, like, all the shit that I think that's going on with our world, and I just wonder about, like, what's in the vaccines now, you know?

Some parents identify some chemical exposure as inevitable and dangerous, but also potentially necessary, like that from prescribed medications. Vaccines, in contrast, become additional exposures that might be optional. For example, Steph rejects interventions in her daughter's body, in large part because she feels that her daughter has already had too many, including those given to support her after birth when she was in the neonatal intensive care unit. "We felt she had had so many interventions, like, on day two of her life, that we started to really question whether or not—how we wanted this to go in her life, you know?"

Steph's daughter was prescribed Prevacid in her first months of life. Prevacid and other proton pump inhibitors (PPIs) are a class of acid blockers that includes Nexium, Prevacid, and Prilosec. They are not approved for babies and are not proven to be more effective than placebos for them.[9] Yet they are commonly prescribed for infants who spit up often, cry frequently, or have colic. They also cost approximately $120 per child each month. Steph recalls receiving the prescription:

> That was not something I wanted to do, but I felt like, you know, as an exhausted new parent at that point you've exhausted all other ideas that anyone has given you—I mean we were avid at swaddling, we were big on putting her halfway upright to nurse her—I mean everything that we could do nonmedically, . . . [even] gripe water, which is an all-natural colic remedy.

When none of these natural remedies worked, Steph agreed when her pediatrician suggested this drug. Having accepted a prescription for a pharmaceutical product for her young infant—and then regretting it—she became uncomfortable with other pharmaceutical products, including vaccines.

Steph brought her partially vaccinated daughter to her one-year checkup, which is when she "started to realize what this vaccination schedule would be." Steph and her husband attended the appointment together and were shocked that the physician wanted to give her baby six vaccines that day. She recalls, "I was like, 'My child is eighteen pounds and you're gonna give her six shots today?' I said, 'No. No. We're not doing that.'"

After discussion with the physician, Steph reluctantly agreed to three vaccines. Leaving the appointment, she remembers her daughter "passed out to a point where she was like—like a sack of potatoes." Noting the difference in her child, she recalls, "Quite honestly, [it] scared the heck out of me. . . . She was just dead weight in my arms, and it really scared me and I thought that was even more proof to me that I was so glad she only did three." In identifying her primary concerns about vaccines, Steph returns to fear of chemicals. She explains, "She's eighteen pounds. I just think that that's a lot of fluid to put into such a little body. It's a lot of chemicals. It's a lot of unnatural things to put into such a tiny little person." Steph sees the value vaccines can provide in protecting her daughter but is only willing to consent to some, "because it's still that many more chemicals, you know? . . . It's the number, but I think the number, to me, is synonymous with the chemical level."

Many parents echo what I heard from Steph. Parents fear they are being asked to deliberately expose their children to those toxins, and see opting out as a chance to mitigate chemical exposure, rather than taking on the more challenging task of addressing broader issues of environmental regulation or exposure. One mother, posting online, illustrates this fear:

Sometimes, I wish I hadn't breastfed, though—keep thinking that was not good for my son. I'm sure I was pretty toxic. I'm sure I still am very toxic. . . . Ever notice how some children/babies really sweat during sleep? I think some of that is not just that they are hot, but their bodies are working hard to purge toxins from their system—their bodies use their skin to get rid of things.

Similarly, Carolyn remembers testing her own levels of heavy metal accumulation in her body and discovering it was high, which she attributes to mercury amalgam fillings in her teeth since childhood as well as possible environmental exposure. She explains how she seeks to limit further exposure for her and her family. "My children have never been vaccinated. They've never had a mercury filling in their mouth. There has been no area where they've had mercury." As part of her efforts to control exposure, Carolyn had her children tested for heavy metal accumulation, only to discover that despite her hard work to avoid contamination, their tests showed high levels, equal to her own. Rather than suggesting that vaccines do not contain heavy metals that accumulate in the body, this surprising information instead confirms her belief that toxin and heavy metal exposure is unavoidable, but vaccines are. Since some vaccines contain or have in the past contained preservatives derived from mercury or aluminum, vaccines are a potential exposure she can and should avoid. Of all chemicals mentioned, heavy metals generally and thimerosal specifically were of greatest concern to parents.

Thimerosal and Vaccines as Poison

Thimerosal is an organic compound used as a preservative in vaccines since the 1930s. As a preservative, it prevents microbes from developing in vials that contain multiple doses of vaccines, a risk that arises as multiple unused hypodermic needles enter the vial over time, which can lead to accidental contamination. Among the most often cited examples of the importance of a preservative for vaccines are a 1916 incident in which a tainted bottle of typhoid vaccine led to sixty-eight reactions, twenty-six abscesses, and four deaths, as well as a tragic 1928 incident in Queensland, Australia, where twelve of twenty-one children inoculated against diphtheria died after becoming infected with staphylococcus, a bacterial infection.[10] Since 1968, federal regulations have required that all multi-dose vials contain a preservative, with only a few exceptions. The law requires that preservatives be "non-toxic so that the amount present in the recommended dose of the product will not be toxic to the recipient," and that when used in combination, will not change the vaccine or its potency.[11] These regulations arose in part in response to past tragic episodes of infection from contaminated vials.

Thimerosal, which is approximately 50 percent ethyl mercury (not the more toxic methylmercury) by weight, has been one of the most widely used preservatives in vaccines. Mercury is a naturally occurring element, often found in water, soil, plants, and animals. It accumulates in the aquatic food chain, primarily in the form of methylmercury. Humans are exposed to methylmercury primarily from consuming seafood, although industrial exposure increases risk.[12] Methylmercury is a neurotoxin when consumed or absorbed in high doses. According to the FDA, the toxicity of methylmercury was first recognized during the late 1950s and early 1960s, when industrial contamination of mercury in Minimata Bay, Japan, led to the widespread consumption of mercury-contaminated fish.[13] Epidemics of methylmercury poisoning also occurred in Iraq during the 1970s, when seed grain treated with a methylmercury fungicide was accidentally used to make bread.[14] We also know a great deal from studies of island populations with high levels of seafood intake from the top of the aquatic food chain, including pilot whale meat in the Faroe Islands.[15] These epidemics and patterns of exposure reveal that fetuses are more sensitive to the effects of methylmercury than adults and that pregnant women who are exposed often give birth to newborns with high mercury levels, which can cause neurological damage.[16]

Because of the known risks of methylmercury exposure, several agencies in the U.S. government have issued advisories about how much

seafood to consume or how to limit exposure to mercury. These guidelines have historically varied between agencies, so Congress asked the
National Academy of Sciences to study methylmercury exposure and
provide recommendations.[17] This request was made in late 1997, as an
addition to a larger bill, the FDA Modernization Act, which aimed to
streamline pharmaceutical distribution and licensing and allow more
experimental drugs to get to patients faster. During discussion of the
bill, New Jersey Representative Frank Pallone, concerned about mercury
exposure from seafood, amended the bill to give the FDA two years to
compile a list of drugs and foods that contain intentionally introduced
mercury compounds and to provide a quantitative and qualitative analysis of the mercury compounds on the list. This process was complex,
with study of dose-response, levels of toxicity and exposure, and organ
processes.

Methylmercury is absorbed easily in the gut and then accumulates
in the body, where it slowly converts to inorganic mercury.[18] Yet individuals who receive the same exposure may be affected quite differently, depending on a wide array of variables, including but not limited
to genetics, age, sex, health status, nutrition, the time and intensity of
methylmercury exposure during critical periods of brain development,
and variability in how individual bodies process the chemical. Although
not the original goal, these explorations led agencies to also question
whether the quantity in vaccines.

The Mercurial Rise of Autism

Mercury in vaccines became a flashpoint issue in the late 1990s, coin-
ciding with a growing awareness of autism. Autism spectrum disorder
is a developmental disability that generally describes individuals with
different degrees of difficulties in social interaction, challenges in verbal
and nonverbal communication, and a propensity for repetitive behaviors. Although autism has been described in medical literature since the
1940s, it was not until 1994 that the Diagnostic and Statistical Manual,
the handbook of psychiatry, clarified autism as manifesting in five disorders, which exist along a spectrum.[19]

It is clear that autism rates have increased dramatically, from 1 in
5,000 in 1975 to about 1 in 68 in 2014; the reasons for the increase are

not clear.[20] Although better diagnosis likely accounts for a portion of the increase, it cannot account for the entire increase. Instead, some combination of genetic predisposition and environment, including but not limited to parental age, neighborhood, social influence, nutrition, prenatal health, or toxic exposure, is likely at work.[21]

As rates of autism rose, social institutions were ill-equipped to provide care. Schools were often unable to meet the special needs of their children; doctors who were not familiar with the disease could not provide adequate care; and researchers offered few answers of cause or effective treatment. As a result, parents had to become activists who shared information and resources. Parents of autistic children formed multiple groups and organizations that are sometimes allies and sometimes opponents. Although they all want to see better resources and more research on autism, much of the disagreement between them stems from whether they believe that infant vaccines cause autism.[22]

Autism activists had been focused on diet as a possible strategy for improving autistic children's behaviors for some time, but the late 1990s brought evidence of an alleged link between the gut, autism, and vaccines. In 1998, the British gastroenterologist Andrew Wakefield—along with a dozen collaborators—published a report in the *Lancet*, one of the premier medical journals in Great Britain, suggesting that in their study of twelve children with bowel disease, nine were autistic and eight had experienced diarrhea after receiving the MMR (measles-mumps-rubella) vaccine. On the eve of the publication, Wakefield held a press conference to announce the findings. Passionately, he cautioned against the use of the MMR vaccine, and recommended that the combined MMR vaccine should be administered separately rather than in combination until the full relationship between the vaccine, autism, and the gut could be understood.

In Great Britain, parents took Wakefield's warning to heart. Vaccine rates dropped precipitously, from 92 percent to 80 percent, below the level of herd immunity. In the United States, the Wakefield study was met with great interest, and when U.S. Senator Dan Burton heard the news, he held a series of congressional hearings to discuss the possible relationship between vaccines and autism, a particularly significant issue to him personally as his grandson was diagnosed with autism at the age of twelve months.[23] Despite the strength of existing national organizations committed to challenging vaccine mandates, it was in fact parents of autistic children who raised concerns about thimerosal.[24] Publicity surrounding the Wakefield study, rising rates of autism without explanation of cause, and parents' frustration with the lack of information they were provided about their children's condition collectively drew attention to the possibility that vaccines contributed to what was now referred to as the "autism epidemic."

Wakefield's study and accompanying concerns about vaccine safety and the possible connections to autism dovetailed with the U.S. government's newfound interest in examining levels of mercury exposure with the goal of standardizing recommendations across agencies. Since the infant vaccine schedule had expanded over the prior decade, it became clear that an infant could theoretically be exposed—depending on the frequency in which vaccines were administered—to high levels of ethyl mercury. Not knowing safe levels of ethyl mercury, the Center for Biologics Evaluation and Research (CBER) pointed out that this level would likely exceed EPA standards on methylmercury.

Thimerosal is chemically different from methylmercury. Unlike methylmercury, which converts to inorganic mercury, thimerosal converts to organic ethyl mercury, a different chemical compound, which generally has a shorter blood half-life, does not accumulate in the body in the same ways methylmercury does, and is more easily eliminated from the body.[25] However, since there were until recently virtually no studies on the effects of ethyl mercury exposure, agencies extrapolated from the toxicity profile of methylmercury, which had a known risk threshold.

In 1999 the U.S. Public Health Service, which comprises the FDA, the National Institutes of Health (NIH), the Centers for Disease Control and Prevention (CDC), and the Health Resources and Services Administration (HRSA), joined the American Academy of Pediatrics to issue a statement urging vaccine manufacturers to reduce or eliminate thimerosal in vaccines as soon as possible.[26] Although they insisted that thimerosal was not damaging to babies, they also insisted that removing it would be the best way to exercise precaution. The statement explained,

> The recognition that some children could be exposed to a cumulative
> level of mercury over the first six months of life that exceeds one of the

federal guidelines on methylmercury now requires a weighing of two different types of risks when vaccinating infants. On the one hand, there is the known serious risk of diseases and deaths caused by failure to immunize our infants against vaccine-preventable infectious diseases; on the other, there is the unknown and probably much smaller risk, if any, of neuro-developmental effects posed by exposure to thimerosal. The large risks of not vaccinating children far outweigh the unknown and probably much smaller risk, if any, of cumulative exposure to thimerosal-containing vaccines over the first six months of life. Nevertheless, because any potential risk is of concern, the Public Health Service, the American Academy of Pediatrics, and vaccine manufacturers agree that thimerosal-containing vaccines should be removed as soon as possible.

Announced as a precaution against a hypothetical risk, the statement reiterated the collective faith in vaccine safety and aimed to increase faith in vaccination. In 2001 the CDC and NIH asked the Institute of Medicine, "an independent nonprofit organization that works outside of government to provide unbiased authoritative advice to decision makers and the public,"[27] to assess the scientific plausibility and broader societal implications of the thimerosal question. The IOM convened to evaluate all data that could speak to the possible relationship between autism and mercury. In providing an overview of the research on mercury exposure in the infant vaccine schedule that led to the joint statement, the IOM aimed to be reassuring. The report notes, "The methylmercury exposure limits calculated by these agencies are not limits above which injury is certain to occur. Rather, they should be interpreted as general levels of exposure below which there is confidence that adverse effects will be absent."[28]

On October 1, 2001, the IOM's Immunization Safety Review Committee's report concluded that the evidence was inadequate to either accept or reject a causal relationship between thimerosal exposure from childhood vaccines and autism, attention-deficit/hyperactivity disorder (ADHD), and speech or language delay. The committee called for future research in order to establish or reject a causal relationship. However, the report also indicated that the hypothesis that exposure to thimerosal-containing vaccines could be associated with neurodevelopmental disorders was biologically plausible. As a result, the committee supported the voluntary removal of thimerosal from "any biological product to which infants, children, and pregnant women are exposed." In explaining the rationale, its members characterized the removal as "a prudent measure in support of the public health goal to reduce mercury exposure of infants and children as much as possible."

The IOM continued its work and in 2004 issued a new report, which reviewed new epidemiological evidence from the United States, Denmark, Sweden, and the United Kingdom, and studies of biologic mechanisms related to vaccine absorption. The report concluded that this new body of research supports rejecting the hypothesis that vaccines, particularly the MMR vaccines singled out by Wakefield and the vaccines containing thimerosal, are causally associated with autism. Further, the committee stated that the benefits of vaccination were proven, in contrast to the hypothesis of susceptible populations, which they saw as "presently speculative." Widespread rejection of vaccines, the IOM cautioned, would lead to increases in incidences of serious infectious diseases like measles, whooping cough, and Hib bacterial meningitis.

Simultaneously to the government's work to identify mercury risks, several researchers aimed to reproduce Wakefield's study on a larger scale. Although some identified gastrointestinal issues in children with autism, none claim a vaccine link and several argued against the biological plausibility of a causal relationship.[29] In fact, studies consistently pointed to the safety of vaccines. These studies, along with the IOM report, were meant to create clarity and certainty that, with great scientific evidence, there is no causal relationship between vaccines and autism. Medical experts, policy makers, and government health officials imagined that this now voluminous body of research showing that vaccines are safe would reassure parents.

Notwithstanding, many parents remain distrustful of vaccines, and their resistance has actually increased rather than decreased. This in many ways reflects the importance parents assign to their own expertise and that of other parents over that claimed by institutions. This is illustrated in part by the continuing story of Andrew Wakefield. Discredited in Great Britain, he moved to the United States, finding support for his continued research and efforts at Thoughtful House, a research center in Austin, Texas. In 2010, after losing his British medical license for academic misconduct, which included a previously undisclosed effort to patent single-dose vaccines of measles, mumps, and rubella (to be administered separately rather than in combination like the MMR he cautioned against), he left Thoughtful House, which subsequently renamed and rebranded itself. Nonetheless, parents of autistic children and those concerned about vaccine safety continue to see him as a champion for their cause. Many see him as a martyr. One post on the Age of Autism website, an autism advocacy organization that strongly supports the continued belief in a causal relationship between vaccines and autism, writes to Wakefield, "To Andy, your continual concern for our children while you must deal with professional and personal injustice is nothing short of heroic. Thank you for never giving up."[30] Wakefield's widespread discrediting among professional organizations alongside the continued tribute he receives from parents who believe that vaccines are dangerous succinctly illustrates the different meanings of expertise, knowledge, and trust.

Distrust of Safety Claims

Parents are aware of much of the debate about the safety of vaccines, the controversies about mercury, and the arguments about the cumulative effects of multiple vaccines. They understand that there is a lack of scientific clarity, but also understand that the schedule of vaccines might potentially create toxic levels of exposure. Professional organizations and government agencies argue that these issues have been resolved and the scientific questions have been adequately answered, but parents don't agree.

Parents search package inserts or ask providers about ingredients, but often they distrust the information provided, particularly about thimerosal. They question the veracity of claims that thimerosal was removed. For example, Anna, who had rejected vaccines for her sons, decided that she wanted her older child to get a tetanus vaccine, decoupled from diphtheria and pertussis, with which it is usually distributed. Yet she felt compelled to verify information about the vaccine's ingredients, especially the claims that the vaccine is thimerosal-free. She recalls, "I had tried to get him a tetanus shot earlier and a doctor was like, 'Oh, they don't use thimerosal anymore, blah blah and it's totally fine.' And I said,

'Well, let me just—I just want to read the box. You need to show it to me,' and there on the box was thimerosal.'"

Pediatricians are aware of parental distrust and encounter questions about mercury quite a bit in their practices. Kevin Sato explains of his pediatric practice, "People still ask about that. 'Is there mercury in these vaccines?' I still get that question, even from people who have done some research." He describes these encounters: "Some of the parents, moms and dads, who are pretty informed, say, 'Yeah, I'm still worried about that autism controversy. I know all the medical studies have shown there's no link'—they'll even offer that up, the ones who have been following these things."

Kevin aims to reassure the parents with data and reports of medical studies. Rather than evaluating the science, he observes, parents are instead more comfortable drawing on their own sense of expertise, which is often informed more by intuition than science. Parents frequently counter discussions of science, he notes, by explaining, "But it just doesn't feel right to me." Many pediatricians describe similar interactions, in which their reports of science are unconvincing when stacked against parents' faith in their own intuition. As Kevin reflects, "People who have a basic distrust of the pharmaceutical industry have a basic distrust of the mainstream medical literature." Distrust of science, providers, and claims of vaccine safety are informed, as Kevin suggests, by parents' larger sense of distrust of the known profit motives of pharmaceutical companies. They also more generally distrust the process that creates scientific knowledge about health, illness, and immunization.

Doubting Knowledge Production and Vaccine Regulation

For a drug to come to market in the United States, it must undergo several stages of study. A company must identify an illness or condition a drug addresses and isolate the cause of the disease. Increasingly, vaccines are developed using isolated proteins, rather than the entire disease-causing organism. Developers demonstrate a vaccine's safety using animal models. After the clinical trial is licensed, the tested medication or vaccine must be shown to be safe and able to generate an immune response on healthy volunteers. In the second phase, researchers determine the appropriate dose of a vaccine by enrolling hundreds of healthy participants. In the third phase, thousands of individuals are usually enrolled so that both safety and effectiveness can be better documented. The FDA notes that "at any stage of the clinical or animal studies, if data raise significant concerns about either safety or effectiveness, FDA may request additional information or studies, or may halt ongoing clinical studies."[31] If each phase is successful, the vaccine will be submitted for licensing, at which time a multidisciplinary FDA review team will examine the efficacy and safety record, calculate the risks and benefits of the new vaccine, and review proposed product labeling and directions to practitioners who will administer the vaccine, including what they should tell patients and their families. If licensed, the manufacturing plants will also be inspected and licensed. After licensing, the FDA will continue to oversee the vaccine production, manufacturing, and ongoing safety, which often draws on reports from VAERS. The FDA explains, "Until a vaccine is given to the general population, all potential adverse events cannot be anticipated. Thus, many vaccines undergo Phase 4 studies—formal studies on a vaccine once it is on the market."[32] These multiple phases and ongoing monitoring aim to examine not just the safety and efficacy of the product as designed, but also challenges that may emerge as it is used.

Despite assurances that these procedures are rigorous and ensure public safety, many parents do not trust these processes. In part, the structure of the FDA's budget encourages distrust. Beginning in 1992 and reauthorized several times since, the Prescription Drug User Fee Act (PDUFA), approved by Congress, allows the FDA to collect funds from those who manufacture drugs, devices, and vaccines. These funds are intended to expedite drug approval, since delays cost companies money and presumably harm patients who may need new remedies for serious health conditions. The law seems to have worked, cutting review times on new drugs by about half.[33] User fees constitute about a quarter of the FDA's budget, a portion that may go up as Congress continues to cut funding to the FDA and shifts more burden onto manufacturers. Many consumer groups worry that if pharmaceutical funds are paying to monitor their own products, conflicts of interest may arise that will not support rigorous monitoring.[34]

The 2002 reauthorization of PDUFA was closely linked to the Bioterrorism Act, which included new limitations on what kinds of materials and biologics could be accessed and by whom. It also created new funds to develop new vaccines against possible bioterrorist attacks and to stockpile them along with other pharmaceutical products.[35] Among the continuing linkages between bioterrorism and vaccine regulation, the 2009 H1N1 flu vaccine is not eligible for compensation under the Vaccine Injury Compensation Program, but instead falls under the Countermeasures Injury Compensation Program, which most specifically compensates injuries related to "a declared pandemic, epidemic or security threat."[36] This program and its ties to governmental claims of bioterrorism also fuel distrust.

Barb, a mother who stopped vaccinating her children when her oldest developed autism as a toddler, explains her distrust of pharmaceutical research on vaccines:

> Pharmaceutical companies make about $80 billion a year off of immunizations. This new H1N1 hasn't even been tested except on all the lab rats that have died, and they hid that. Did you know that? The first round of H1N1 testing was all done on lab rats and they all died. So they adjusted it a little bit and they refused to divulge all of the ingredients. But yet they put together a removing themselves from all liability clause, so if you die from the H1N1 [vaccine], they would not be held responsible.

The connections between federal regulation, the pharmaceutical industry's "pay-to-play" funding of the FDA, increasing emphasis on expedited review, which inevitably limits certainty of safety, and corporate profit motives that are enhanced as the government commits greater resources to developing and stockpiling drugs and vaccines all undermine parents' trust in the systems designed to protect their children's health. Illustrating this, Jake describes his view of biomedical research as largely untrustworthy, identifying the influence of pharmaceutical funding of research specifically. "Well, first of all, it's biased because it was paid-for studies. They'll take—they'll take the numbers and twist them. . . . You can make the numbers come out and say pretty much what you want and you'll have somebody who is unbiased do the exact same research and it's night and day."

Jake has a broad view of the dangers of vaccines and refuses them for his own children. He conducts his own research from sources he trusts, and brings in speakers and hosts community educational events about the dangers of vaccines. In explaining his position and willingness to find experts he trusts more than those in medical or regulatory systems, he highlights the conflicts of interest pharmaceutical companies create: "This is not conspiracy theory stuff, this is just credible science that has no financial ties to Merck or Pfizer or Novartis, you know?"

Similarly, Marlene describes her distrust of safety claims: "They're not doing much new research, and anything I read tends to be saying that vaccines can have a negative impact." As she and others see it, vaccine manufacturers and the FDA they fund have little incentive to continue researching adverse reactions since it can only be to their economic detriment.

The distrust of medical providers and vaccine ingredients represents a larger distrust of pharmaceutical companies, which exist to make a financial profit. Parents frequently explain how the goals of vaccine safety are incompatible with for-profit pharmaceutical companies, particularly as they are shielded from liability claims by the National Vaccine Injury Compensation Fund. Illustrating these concerns, Katie explains, "I think that the drug companies push vaccines that they don't know are 100 percent safe. I think trying to put fifteen vaccines—you know, six doses of vaccine—in one shot is crazy. And I don't know if we know the whole health ramifications of giving so many vaccines to children." As parents believe that pharmaceutical companies' primary goal is to promote vaccines rather than ensure safety, they reiterate their role as uniquely qualified to protect their children's bodies by limiting exposure to vaccines.

Concerns about vaccine safety come from broader distrust of vaccine production and regulation, which take a toxic product to market with, as parents see it, limited oversight. Parents make their vaccine decisions based on the degree to which they trust the systems responsible for vaccines. The parents in this study make it clear that they especially do not trust the pharmaceutical industry and its government regulators.

Vaccine Failures and the Meanings of Regulatory Systems

Vaccines are indeed imperfect, and in fact there have always been problems with them. As with any scientific endeavor, there have been failures, where clinical trials sometimes show no success from the vaccine and at other times cause the harm that the vaccine was intended to prevent.[37] Some are made incorrectly, as was the case in an early smallpox vaccine or during the Cutter Incident, when 120,000 doses of polio vaccine were not fully inactivated, infecting more than 40,000 children, killing 10 people, and paralyzing 169.[38] At other times, vaccines become contaminated during manufacture, as was the case in 2010 when a rotavirus vaccine was found to be contaminated with material from a pig virus,[39] or in 2013 when Merck recalled 743,360 vials of Gardasil because they may have contained particles of glass from a breakage during manufacturing.[40] Manufacturing shortcomings sometimes appear during inspections, raising additional concerns. Illustrating this latter point, a 2012 warning letter issued by the FDA to Sanofi Pasteur, a major vaccine manufacturer, cited more than twenty-five concerns about safety and quality in its plants. Among these, the company failed "to assure an adequate system for cleaning and disinfecting aseptic processing areas and equipment," to "establish and follow appropriate written procedures designed to prevent microbiological contamination of drug products purporting to be sterile," and "to establish laboratory controls that include scientifically sound and appropriate specifications, standards, sampling plans, and test procedures designed to assure that components, inprocess materials, and drug products conform to appropriate standards of identity, strength, quality, and purity."[41] Given the few manufacturers of vaccines, most production problems lead to shortages of required vaccines, which in turn require federal advisory bodies to issue substitutive recommendations of how providers should modify schedules to ration vaccines or minimally vaccinate those most at risk.

Those who advocate for vaccine use and trust their safety point out that each of these is a *known* failure precisely because it was rapidly detected in the systems set up to monitor vaccine safety. When we experience a shortage of influenza vaccine, as we did in 2004 because of mold contamination in manufacturing that was detected before any was distributed, vaccine proponents suggest we should feel *more* secure that inspectors identify breakdowns in vaccine safety before anyone is harmed, not *less*. Those on the other side wonder how many risks are undetected or unknown.

Vaccines can also be produced perfectly and still cause rare but serious bad outcomes. Some adverse effects—particularly those that are statistically uncommon—are identified only when hundreds of thousands of doses are consumed, as was the case with the oral polio vaccine, which could cause polio. A more recent example lies in the Rotashield vaccine and its complicated history, which shows the challenges in addressing the potential dangers of vaccines, particularly those that can be manufactured perfectly and still harm people. Rotashield provides an excellent opportunity to more fully consider vaccine risk alongside regulatory success to consider the potential dangers of a manufactured pharmaceutical product.

The Case of Rotashield

Rotavirus is, globally, the leading cause of vomiting and severe diarrhea. Rotavirus infection is responsible for about 600,000 deaths per year in children, which translates to about 5 percent of deaths worldwide to children less than five years.[42] Eighty percent of those deaths are to children in resource-poor countries in sub-Saharan Africa and south Asia. Without a vaccine, rotavirus worldwide causes approximately 114 million episodes of gastroenteritis requiring home care only, 24 million clinic visits, and 2.4 million hospitalizations in children five years of age or younger. By age five years, nearly every child in the world, irrespective of nation or access to sanitation, will have an episode of rotavirus gastroenteritis. One in every five of those children will visit a clinic, one in fifty will be hospitalized, and approximately one in 205 will die.[43]

Although the impact is felt greatest in the global south, the impact in the United States before vaccine was also significant. According to the CDC, before the vaccine, rotavirus was responsible for more than 400,000 doctor visits, 200,000 emergency room visits, 55,000–70,000 hospitalizations, and 20–60 deaths in the United States each year.[44] The creation of a vaccine held great promise for both saving lives worldwide and reducing healthcare costs in the United States and abroad. Rotashield was supposed to be that vaccine.

As a live oral vaccine to be taken in three doses, Rotashield immunized children against the four most common strains of rotavirus. According to one of the researchers involved in testing this vaccine, clinical trials lasted more than fifteen years, cost "hundreds of millions of dollars, involved multiple government agencies, industry, and dozens of clinical investigators. It was given to more than 10,000 infants in 27 clinical trials conducted in nine different countries."[45] After this lengthy process, results were submitted to the U.S. FDA, while a rotavirus working group at the Advisory Committee on Immunization Practices (ACIP—the same group that sets vaccine schedules) simultaneously reviewed reports of adverse effects and efficacy, and considered recommendations for use. The data showed that among 10,054 vaccinated babies, there were five cases of intussusception, a painful condition where the intestine folds or telescopes on itself, requiring medical intervention and sometimes surgical correction. There was also one case among the 4,633 members of the placebo group. After much analysis, the group determined that the intussusception was unlikely to have been caused by the vaccine, although it was mentioned as a possible side effect on package inserts.

The vaccine was licensed in August 1998 and the ACIP issued its recommendation that infants receive it in three doses at two, four, and six months of age. After ten months and 1.5 million doses of Rotashield had been given to approximately 600,000 infants, information about a possible increased risk of intussusception appeared from two sources: reports made to the Vaccine Adverse Event Reporting System (VAERS), a passive surveillance system where individuals and physicians can voluntarily report possible adverse reactions, and in studies conducted in closed managed healthcare systems (like Kaiser Permanente, where patient care is more closely tracked because their prescriptions, visits, and other records are all centralized). After some debate, experts agreed that Rotashield increased risk of intestinal intussusception at a rate of about one for every ten thousand vaccinated infants, twenty to thirty times their base level of risk.[46] The ACIP immediately rescinded its recommendation for the routine use of Rotashield. Fourteen months after licensing, Wyeth, the manufacturer of the vaccine, voluntarily withdrew it from the market.[47]

Those concerned about vaccine safety see the Rotashield failure as an example of why parents cannot fully trust vaccine manufacturers or those charged with overseeing vaccine safety. The vaccine was licensed and recommended, even as it was unsafe. Yet those who promote vaccines can look at the same information about Rotashield and see assurances that, in fact, our systems are working. As an information sheet from the CDC about Rotashield explains,

A primary goal of CDC is to protect the health and safety of the general public in the United States. One of the most effective ways to prevent disease is through vaccination. However, when a vaccine is discovered to have a serious side effect, a recommendation to continue using the vaccine will be reconsidered and the vaccine may be withdrawn, in spite of the beneficial effect of the vaccine to prevent disease. The vaccine safety monitoring systems worked to detect an uncommon side effect. Rotavirus vaccination was promptly suspended and new cases of intussusception were prevented.[48]

How one views the success of the vaccine monitoring processes, as illustrated in the Rotashield experience, likely reflects how one views those charged with public safety. If, for example, you are someone who trusts public systems to regulate corporations and trusts the peer review process of science to ensure good outcomes, the quick withdrawal of Rotashield after a small number of adverse outcomes were identified is reassuring. However, for many parents, the people and processes responsible for vaccine decision making feel distant from the people consuming those vaccines, and that raises anxiety. They do not feel connected to the ACIP and the CDC and do not believe that the members of these groups understand them or their children. And while most ACIP members are parents or healthcare providers themselves, they are not generally perceived as sharing the concerns of parents. Further, media coverage of events like the Rotashield withdrawal or of manufacturing problems potentially heightens parents' sense that vaccines are dangerous and informs their choice to reject vaccines, which they believe may have unknown adverse outcomes.[49]

Whether parents see vaccine regulation as imperfect but the best way to monitor vaccine safety or whether they view the bodies charged with monitoring vaccines to be unreliable or corrupt depends on their views of government, corporate responsibility and, even more fundamentally, research and the scientific method used to produce biomedical knowledge.

From Toxic Product to Promises of Green Vaccines

Parents frequently assert that the profit motives of companies drive biomedical research. Which questions are researched, how the terms of health are defined, and what findings are released are guided, parents believe, by pharmaceutical profit motive. There is a well-established critique that pharmaceutical corporations do not research diseases with the highest morbidity or mortality because they are unlikely to be profitable.[50] As parents raise questions about the range of diseases against which children are vaccinated, they echo some of this complaint.

Many focus their critique on the ways companies charged with illness prevention profit from illness management. More hardline rejecters trust that the body can better heal itself than be protected by immunization. Some point to children they personally know who are frequently sick and attribute their illnesses (and the weakened state that invites illness) to the vaccines themselves. As they trust that their children's unvaccinated bodies are stronger and their deliberate efforts to maximize their families' health are superior, they question why pharmaceutical companies or medical researchers don't study health promotion. Illustrating this, Margaret, a mother of two unvaccinated children, argues that profit motives of companies drive science: "Nobody's doing the studies to find out why the people that aren't getting vaccinated or aren't doing the drugs or the statins or whatever are staying healthy. Because there's no money there for the drug companies. Because they're not controlling the market. They don't control supplements. They don't control broccoli. They don't control sunlight."

Parents like Margaret frequently define their unvaccinated children as healthy, a state they refuse to risk with vaccines. Yet their critique calls into question the way scientific research is conducted and research questions are identified, funded, and pursued. Some parents believe that these issues could be better understood if researchers conducted comparative studies of children who have and have not received vaccines. Marlene, a mother of unvaccinated children, explains, "It would be really interesting to see what they'd find if someone did do a study [comparing vaccinated and unvaccinated children]." Recognizing the likely objections to doing so, she adds, "But then you'd have to leave some kids out and they would consider that a public danger to the child so they're not gonna do it." Parents regularly mention that a comparative study of children of different vaccine statuses would be a good way for federal agencies to convincingly establish that vaccines are indeed safe.

This kind of study, which parents believe will never be carried out by those responsible for vaccine safety, is so often called for that the National Vaccine Information Center at its 2009 conference launched an effort to fundraise for such a program. All morning, panelists came on stage in the packed Virginia ballroom and called for a comparative study. By midday, the organization's founder, Barbara Loe Fisher, rose and announced that they would start collecting for a research fund. Throughout the afternoon, individuals would contribute sums of money to the new research fund. Ally, alternative medicine proponent, and osteopathic physician Joseph Mercola announced he would match funds. According to the NVIC's press release, the organization raised more than $100,000 to launch its own research program. Fisher explained this success:

> The people are taking back vaccine science from the institutions which have failed us. . . . We are not going to wait any longer for government and industry to answer the big question of whether one-size-fits-all vaccine policies using multiple vaccines during the past quarter century have contributed to the unexplained chronic disease and disability epidemic among our children. It is critical that independent researchers from multiple scientific disciplines act now to evaluate and protect the biological integrity of our children.[51]

The NVIC research program, which, as of 2014, has not yet released any research findings, speaks to the broader distrust of science, which is largely funded by pharmaceutical companies, and the broad-based belief that it can and should be democratized. As parents question what is known about vaccine safety and what remains uncertain, they raise questions about the kinds of inquiry that lead to vaccines, which they see as consistently furthering profit motives and narrow investigations by regulatory bodies.

These parents and their organizations might initially appear to be simply anti-science or ignorant of research. As such, they are easily dismissed. In contrast, those who trust the current scientific methods for evaluating vaccine safety and accept the claims of companies and regulatory agencies perceive themselves to be drawing upon superior knowledge. Carrie Mathers is a pediatrician who supports vaccination and aims to fully vaccinate all of her patients. Her explanation for why she adopts this position illustrates how her view of science and knowledge production is different from those of the parents who question or refuse vaccines. Carrie explains, "I feel like I am a truster of research that goes into vaccines and so, you know, would I say that I read every single piece of data that goes into this new vaccine? No. But I do have a lot of faith in the CDC and the FDA and the process that a vaccine needs to go through before it's approved."

Carrie ponders what kinds of concerns would inspire her to question vaccine safety or to adopt a more cautious approach. In thinking about reasons to approach vaccine recommendations more cautiously, she considers the levels of reports of adverse outcomes she would need to see before she would stop recommending a vaccine and repeats her faith in vaccine safety monitoring: "I need to have data that says, 'Oh, it's greatly increased the rate of something or other' before I'll really back off."

Carrie believes that parents who trust anecdotes or intuition over systematically collected data are misguided, a position she says many of her colleagues share:

> You'll be hard-pressed to find a resident here [at the children's hospital] that doesn't get their fire lit when the family says, "No thank you, vaccines." I mean, that just fires everyone up—because, it just is illogical to us. We're like, "You have the AAP and the CDC recommending these things, so you're gonna listen to Jenny McCarthy?" That doesn't make any sense to us. It's just totally illogical.

Yet Jenny McCarthy and others address crowds as concerned parents who do not appear to have a motive other than the care of their children. This makes their claims that vaccines are dangerous, toxic, and unsafe easier to trust than the organizational, bureaucratic, or corporate expertise provided in impersonal encounters with those who might simply identify as "trusters of research." Those who question vaccine safety seem invested in individual children, which from the perspective of individualist parenting, is more trustworthy than claims in support of public health.

5

Who Calls the Shots?

"He was one of those kids that everybody liked instantly," Regina Booth recalls of her son Austin. He was a seventeen year old honors student who played every sport he could, including varsity football and varsity baseball and basketball. "When he got sick the first day, he didn't feel good. We knew it was flu season. A couple of other kids on the basketball team had come down with flu so we knew that was going on." But Austin didn't want to miss school, which would have meant missing that night's game. "He was strong, healthy. We assumed he had an awesome immune system, so we didn't worry." He felt well enough to go to school the next day, although the basketball coach sent Austin home from practice when he didn't seem up to it.

Regina kept her son home the next day. "By about 10 a.m. that Thursday he had coughed up some blood," she said. She rushed him to the emergency room, and they airlifted him to the nearest big hospital in Grand Junction, Colo. But even then it didn't seem dire.

Doctors used sedatives to put Austin into a medical coma and dosed him with more antibiotics than Regina could remember. A ventilator was helping him breathe. He had the B strain of influenza, which developed into pneumonia, and an infection called methicillin resistant Staphylococcus aureus, or MRSA. Despite treatment, his organs started to shut down. Austin died on Monday, Jan. 17, 2011.

Although the CDC says everyone over the age of six months should get a flu shot, most still don't, with only about half of children aged 6 months to 17 years vaccinated. Just under 75 percent of babies aged up to 2 were vaccinated. A third of kids in Austin's age group, 13 to 17, got vaccinated. "I was one of those people who didn't think they needed it," Regina says. "I was one of those people who thought if you get the shot, you are going to get sick."
—NBC News and FamiliesFightingFlu.org[1]

Flu vaccine is different from most other vaccines in that immunity is fleeting. The influenza virus mutates easily and often, and since the vaccine targets surface proteins that change (a process known as antigenic drift), vaccine manufacturers must develop new vaccines to address these changes and better target the virus. In the United States, flu vaccines are developed based on the strains that are common in the Southern Hemisphere in the six months prior. Some years, this extrapolation goes better than others, leading to a more or less effective protection. (For those who contract flu, they too experience limited protection, since that same antigenic drift limits the relevance of their naturally gained immunity, which is why individuals can suffer flu multiple times.) Protection from flu requires vaccination every year.

From parents' perspectives, flu vaccines represent short-term and imperfect protection against an illness that does not seem serious, but which may carry unknowable serious long-term risks. From this view, avoiding vaccines is logical, especially if parents remain focused on their own children. The stakes for vaccines and vaccine-preventable illnesses are high, as the Booth family's story above illustrates. They are also largely unknown and unknowable, and often rare, rendering parent decision making imperfect, even as parents assert themselves as experts.

Throughout medical training, physicians learn science and practice standards, but vary on what parts of their work they see as most pressing.[2] Pediatricians are not monolithic administrators of uniform advice, but make decisions on how to practice medicine, how to advise parents, and how to communicate about risk, health, and illness. As they develop their primary care practices, they develop their own strategies for managing patient interactions around these questions of disease risk, performing emotion work, in which they manage parental anxiety, and supporting or challenging parents' choices for their children.[3] Doctors do so within boundaries set by insurance requirements, billing schemas, time limits with patients, and varying patient needs. To what extent healthcare providers support parents' insistence that they are experts on their children and how the institutional structures of medical practice respond to parents significantly shapes parents' vaccine decisions and experience of primary care.

The parents with whom I spoke communicate their confidence in their own expertise and the importance of a provider who considers their child as an individual. From this perspective, they search for physicians for their children to serve as consultants, rather than as experts to whom they might be expected to defer. Yet pediatricians, who have at a minimum completed four years of medical school and no less than three years of pediatric residency, have different kinds of knowledge and varying willingness to assume the role of consultant. In this chapter, I examine variation in physicians' approaches to parents who reject expert recommendations on vaccines by profiling three pediatricians who organize their practices differently. In doing so, I elucidate the challenges pediatricians face in balancing the competing priorities they and parents may have and how these negotiations are bound by institutional forces that structure patient interactions, including time, rules, and payment. I then return to the different understandings of influenza to examine how pediatricians and parents view vaccine necessity and disease risk in these interactions.

Doctors as Consultants

Pediatrics as a specialty of medicine is many jobs in one. Parents expect pediatricians to respond when their children are sick and to provide treatment for illnesses or injury. Most of pediatrics, though, involves health supervision, or well-child care, which includes screening for risk of illness, monitoring growth and development and checking for delays, consulting on psychosocial challenges, providing education on safety to parents (known as anticipatory guidance), and providing consistent preventative care, of which vaccines are a key component.[4] Although care is provided to children, parents and/or caregivers are intermediaries, creating additional interpersonal challenges to the patient-provider relationship.

Complicating this multifaceted job, professional organizations advise pediatricians in ways that are complex and sometimes contradictory. For example, pediatricians are advised to build strong relationships with families and make each patient a priority. They are advised that their work includes "listening to and respecting each child and his or her family," and "honoring racial, ethnic, cultural, and socioeconomic background and patient and family experiences and incorporating them in accordance with patient and family preference into the planning and delivery of health care." Care should be individualized, which requires them to maintain "flexibility in organizational policies, procedures, and provider practices so services can be tailored to the needs, beliefs, and cultural values of each child and family" and to facilitate "choice for the child and family about approaches to care." Pediatricians are to share "complete, honest, and unbiased information with patients and their families on an ongoing basis and in ways they find useful and affirming, so that they may effectively participate in care and decision-making to the level they choose." They also are advised to recognize and build "on the strengths of individual children and families and empower them to discover their own strengths, build confidence, and participate in making choices and decisions about their health care."[5]

Simultaneously, pediatricians are also encouraged to assume responsibility for community health more generally. According to the American Academy of Pediatrics, the community-based pediatrician's work should, in part, include "a perspective that enlarges the pediatrician's focus from one child to all children in the community." Pediatricians are encouraged to synthesize "clinical practice and public health principles directed toward providing health care to a given child and promoting the health of all children within the context of the family, school, and community" and to advocate for all children, "especially for those who lack access to care because of social, cultural, geographic, or economic conditions or special health care needs."[6]

These sets of professional obligations are important, but contain internal contradictions as they are realized in daily practice. Most of these goals speak to an obligation to advocate for children who lack care and to work toward the health of all children in the community, with an eye on the unique experiences of individual children within one's care. Most physicians also want to empower patients and their parents to participate in decision making, even as those decisions might undermine the other goals of working toward public health. Vaccination is a clear example where the tension between individual choice and the well-being of all children manifests. Although empowering patients to make independent decisions around a host of other health conditions may have effects on the individual, efforts to prevent infectious disease squarely straddle the line between the individual and the community. The following sections illustrate three models for providing pediatric care around this tension.

Ben Kirkland: The Individualized Vaccine Schedule Practice

Ben Kirkland has been both a hospital-based pediatrician and a primary care provider in a large practice; ultimately, Ben opted to open his own practice. He operates a boutique practice and like other providers with similar setups, rejects insurance payments and requires patients to pay for services directly instead. Ben explains that choice: "Well, if you take insurance, you basically are working for the insurance company, so then they dictate how much you can charge and how much you get paid." Ben charges three hundred dollars per hour, which he likens to attorneys or therapists, who also charge by the hour. This is in sharp contrast to how most physicians bill—by the procedure or diagnostic category. Ben explains why he rejects that model: "You can see a patient for ten minutes or sixty minutes for a regular doctor, it's all based on a diagnosis. And I don't understand why somebody would make fifty dollars for a runny nose and seventy dollars for doing stitches. Like, to me, it's really my expertise and my time that you're paying for."

Doctors who take insurance—public or private—are bound to the payment schedule set forth by the insurance or Medicaid reimbursement systems and spend however long necessary to see their patients. They cannot afford to support a practice by seeing only nine patients a day at the contracted payment rate. In contrast, Ben often schedules patients for one-hour appointments; because he charges per hour, he can afford to spend as much time as he and his patients want and see fewer patients each day. Ben believes he can more effectively meet each individual patient's needs and make them feel heard in ways more challenging for other pediatricians.

> We're able to provide a level of service, I think, beyond medical expertise and all of that. I mean, just availability and, you know, being able to be likeable and all those things. I think it's so much easier for us in a way because we don't have the constraints of the finances like they do.

Ben recognizes the elitism of a cash-only practice, and will see patients "for free for a while until they end up getting back on their feet"; he says he would like to eventually find a way to accept Medicaid.

Patients also have the option of submitting their bills to their own insurance companies for reimbursement, which some are able to do successfully.

Ben admits that his unusual style of care has led to an unusual practice that includes on one extreme, "the total hippie mom who is not married, has a kid and is just, you know, has almost no money but basically has made [her child's health] a huge priority" and on the other, fairly wealthy parents for whom payments are not a burden. He does not collect information about his patients' family incomes or finances, but believes that the majority are "just looking for something better for their money, basically." He continues, "You know, they just want—they want better attention. They have been dissatisfied with the kind of care they've gotten somewhere else." He notes that the common denominator in his practice is parental anxiety about medical care, with some patients as old as twelve years having never been to a doctor until they come to his office. In many ways, Ben's practice is the answer for parents who feel that no one understands their unique family's healthcare needs. His entire practice is built on individualization. Not surprisingly, vaccines feature prominently.

Ben frequently explains—both in our interview and in his community educational events I have observed—that although he is often asked whether he believes in vaccines, vaccines are not "like the tooth fairy." It is not a question of whether he believes; he is certain vaccines work. Yet, he explains, *none* of the children in his practice—with the exception of older children who have come from other practices—are fully vaccinated.

> I encourage people not to fully vaccinate. It depends. It's totally like everything else in a practice based on a per-person, individualized schedule. There's no one schedule that works for anybody, but some of the things just don't make sense. . . . Some of the vaccines are really important at certain times in life and not in others, and some of them are really important in later life, which I'll recommend doing.

Ben sees his approach as not necessarily individualistic, so much as holistic. He views his process of assessing risk as requiring him to consider the whole family and others they might encounter.

It needs to be individualized within the whole, and that's why it's holistic medicine. . . . What's really going on in the child's larger picture? . . . It's the child in their own personal environment, their house, so what kind of bed are they sleeping in? What kind of toxins are in the home? What are the families like? What are their personalities like? What town do they live in? What are their high-risk behaviors? You know, whatever it might be.

Ben's efforts to customize risk assessment and tailor vaccines accordingly operate with assumptions that risk is measurable and identifiable. His favorite example of his tailored risk assessment—one I heard him offer in several different venues—points to the ways that the child of a school bus driver likely faces more risk of infection than does the child whose parents are home full-time. As a result, that child is more likely to receive vaccines.

Most of Ben's descriptions of risk assessment focus on the child as the center of the family and of possible infection. Unlike other health-care providers, Ben does not articulate a meaningful difference between making choices for one's own child and making choices for the community. He admits that vaccines do affect those around the child, but conceptualizes the importance of vaccinating children to protect others as more limited. Rather than communicating a sense of shared responsibility in communities for disease prevention, Ben sees a much narrower view of "community": vaccines protect those you know and for whom you care. This extends to families where "you have multiple kids in the family and there's a really young child" or for adults who work with very young children.

Ben is a proponent of natural immunity over vaccine-generated immunity and does not recommend some vaccines against diseases like chickenpox (varicella) that he sees as minor, unless a child lives with or is close to someone who is immune-compromised. Arguably, those same children present risk to others—at the grocery store, in schools or parks, in community interaction—but broader risk is not a reason he would encourage vaccination against more illnesses. He clarifies his position: "I'm certainly not anti-vaccine by any sense of the imagination. We order a lot of vaccines and we give them every single day in our practice, but we just try to be more judicious about how we do them."

Ben is one of several pediatricians I interviewed who aim to provide high-quality, individualized, appropriate, and intentional care—and who feel they must rescript how medicine is delivered. In many ways, these doctors represent the greatest ambitions of the women's health movement, to empower patients to manage their own care on their own terms. Yet they also require strategies that are out of touch with or even directly challenge the core tenets of public health and a willingness to serve only those with the resources to buy their services.

The structure of Ben's practice allows time to develop a strong relationship with families and communicate about their fears, concerns, and needs. Parents expend significant personal resources to bring their children to his practice. Other physicians with whom I spoke questioned the ethics of practices like Ben's, where profit motives and parental fears mix. As one pediatrician explained, "I can talk to you for an hour. I can fill an hour. But is it a benefit to you? Maybe not. . . . I could ask you a lot of extra questions, right? I mean it just, that doesn't feel good to me." Despite ethical questions that arise in cash-only practices, some research suggests that patients are more likely to perceive physicians as working for them or more trustworthy when not paid by a health plan that may alter their priorities.[7] It strikes me that, in contrast to doctors who maintain a wider payer mix of patients—some who are publicly insured, some who are privately insured but cannot afford cash-pricing for each child's care—a pediatric practice that focuses on monetary exchange risks tipping too far away from pediatric mandates to serve as an advocate for all children.

Kevin Sato: Balancing Patient Preference with Public Health

Kevin Sato is a pediatrician and parent who passionately wants to serve as a resource to families. He works in a large pediatric group in which no more than 20 percent of their patients receive Medicaid. Compared with the hour-long visits provided by doctors like Ben, Kevin's patients are scheduled throughout the day in twenty-minute visits.

Kevin believes that his role is to give parents all the information about vaccines and then allow them to choose what they want for their children. In doing so, he feels he balances the tension between individual choice and community health, though he strongly encourages parents to follow the routine schedule. In recommending vaccines, he draws in part on his experience in residency with seeing children ravaged by vaccine-preventable diseases.

I think there's a gut reaction amongst pediatricians who have been in an academic children's hospital because you've seen all the diseases. For example, in the vaccine talk, we all come from our own biases, and I had a child who was devastated by pertussis who was unvaccinated, neurologically devastated. So I always tell people that that's a bias that I'm carrying with me. That's a child that I saw in my own individual experience. It would be very difficult for me not to recommend that vaccine and not to give it to my own kids. So as long as you know that that's a bias that I'm coming from, plus the training that I've had, and you make your own decision about that pertussis vaccine, I'm totally comfortable with that.

Kevin is driven by his own experience and extensive training, but insists that doctors are not any more equipped to decide about vaccines than are parents. He recognizes that he has more training and experience, but also sees the importance of honoring parents' expertise on their own children so that they feel secure with their choice. He explains his strategy:

My overall approach in all of medicine, not just for vaccines, is that the people I value the most in healthcare are the people who come to a discussion with a sense of humility. And that doesn't mean that you don't acknowledge the training that you have, but it means that you understand that there are limitations to your training, limitations to science. So sometimes I have a lengthy discussion with parents where I explain why I think it probably is a good idea, it's important, and then I do use that kind of wording where I say, "You are the expert on your child." So I wouldn't turn that around the other way. I don't even talk about my training. People don't need to hear that. If I was on the other end, I wouldn't want to hear about that. If you want to know about my training, you can look in my bio.

This approach, of recognizing parents as the experts on their children, is important to parents. Yet it also runs the risk, Kevin feels, of failing to communicate that there are facts we do know from science, including disease risk and vaccine safety. "That's something that I'm conflicted about at times, because sometimes—I'm not sure if I'm advocating strongly enough for the vaccines, because I want to make sure I'm honoring where they're coming from."

As Kevin considers his role in families' lives, he sees his approach as one where he both supports parents' choices and encourages them to continually revisit them.

> So what I tell them is, "If you've come to the point where you've done all the research that you can and I've given you what I know and then you come to that point where you've made the decision one way or the other, then my job is to support you through that, keep checking in," I bring it up at every visit, but not in a pressure way. So for a family who's decided not to vaccinate, I'll say, "Where are you at with the vaccines today?" and leave it open-ended.

One challenge is the wide variation in what parents understand about science and how they approach vaccines. He explains, "I try to find out where they're at. I don't want to use a cookie-cutter approach." Yet, he notes, while some parents "have done tons of research and know exactly what their science is," other parents are far less informed. Kevin aims to assess these differences. "I try to ask them where they're coming from. 'What are you concerns about the vaccine?' Leave that open-ended."

Kevin acknowledges that he likely gets more patients who question vaccines because he has developed a reputation as a physician who is "okay having that conversation." Rather than announcing which vaccine he will give, he sees his role as starting a conversation at the newborn visit and then returning to it at the two-month well-child appointment, when vaccines would be routinely given. He encourages parents to conduct their own research and invites them to call him with questions. Although few parents actually do call, he believes that this offer communicates his willingness to discuss their concerns. He would like to see all children in his practice fully vaccinated, but does not feel that this is his only role as their provider. "So you've cultivated that relationship and you've given your recommendation and you feel like you've communicated it, then people are on their own path." He sees myriad other health concerns beyond vaccines he can address to help his patients, so long as he can maintain a relationship of trust. "People have to not only trust you, but feel like you're on their side."

There are limitations built in to his practice. He notes that it is often difficult to raise questions of vaccines during the short twenty-minute appointment "and not have people feel like they're being made to feel guilty about something, which, I just think [is] part of the doctor-patient relationship." He also finds that his low-income, Medicaid-enrolled patients are more likely to defer to him as the expert and ask what vaccines he recommends, without a long discussion. He explains,

> They have an acceptance of conventional medicine, and they're not—I don't know that it's that they don't have time to question it, they're not coming from a place of questioning. You get the sense right when you bring up that question, "What are your thoughts about vaccines today?" That's how I bring it up. . . . And most people say, "Whatever the routine." Or I'll offer that up. "Are you going to do the routine schedule?" And you get a very quick sense. Like some people right away know exactly the answer to that question, which is, "Yes, we're going to do the routine schedule. Yes, of course."

In thinking through which parents come from "a place of questioning," we see how class shapes perceptions of expertise. Privileged parents committed to individualistic values more commonly perceive their parental work as actively cultivating their children into successful adults. They are more likely to demand individualization of vaccines—and feel entitled to get it. Although Kevin wants parents to feel empowered, he also sees limits in individualizing all care. As a physician he feels a tension between his duty to treat his patients and his duty to be mindful of the well-being of all the children in the community, not just those in his practice: "We have to be the individual doctor and we have to also think about public health." As a result, he feels comfortable administering the routine vaccination schedule and opted to do so for his own children.

Carrie Mathers: Public Health and Time Limits

Carrie Mathers is a pediatrician who works in a clinic where over 90 percent of her patients are publicly insured or have no insurance. In a typical clinical day, she sees between fourteen and twenty children in appointment slots that are fifteen or thirty minutes long. She is fluent in Spanish, which is helpful for many of her patients. She actively chose this patient population, explaining,

> I feel like our patient population for the most part really responds to medical advice and follows physician's recommendations and really appreciates things. Also, I feel like they are underserved and not necessarily understanding, a lot of times, the services that medicine can provide and [the benefits of] health supervision visits.

Identifying how patients who have fewer resources may not see the ways pediatric well-care can optimize their children's health, Carrie aims to educate and empower these parents. "I feel like I'm doing them a lot more of a service than I am for people who get on the Internet and look up stuff on their own."

Vaccines, she says, are a significant portion of her practice. Because her clinic trains pediatric residents, she has help with much of her work, and therefore has more time "to have longer conversations with parents about vaccines." She explains, "I feel like a lot of pediatricians are limited in their time so they're not able to engage in a longer debate or discussion about vaccine safety and the importance of vaccines. So I'm at an advantage that I can take that time. And I always do when it comes up."

In Carrie's practice, vaccine decisions arise in the context of larger discussions of care for infants. For example, each of her patients' parents is given a booklet at the first well-child visit, usually at two weeks of age. The government-funded booklet, which is made available to practices with a significant portion of low-income families, provides advice on how to feed infants or safely position them for sleep, as well as information on how long they likely sleep at each age, and which vaccines are recommended at each age. Carrie explains,

> So when I talk about the packet, I always pull that out, and I say, "Here's information for you about how to feed your baby"; that's everyone's priority, feeding and sleeping at that age, right? But then I say, "You know, this is the vaccine schedule as it stands now, so it kind of gives you an introduction as to when vaccines are given. And it's not hugely detailed

but it just says, at two months, at four months, at six months." So parents kind of know when to expect them, if not what to expect.

Unlike many other pediatricians, Carrie meets few of her patients' parents before birth. Although she acknowledges that it would be preferable to discuss vaccines with expectant parents, it is not feasible, since few attend childbirth classes where it could be raised. She notes, "It's harder to know when the exact appropriate time is. I try to bring it up at least for them to start thinking about it at the newborn or two-week visit, but a lot of moms are just exhausted and if it's a new baby, they're just emotionally [tired]." For many of Carrie's patients, vaccines are not their most pressing concern.

In well-child visits in her clinic, Carrie explains that in the majority of cases,

> I come in and I say, "Hey, today is two months, we're doing the vaccines today. Do you have any questions about vaccines? Have your other children been vaccinated in the past?" And then I say, "You know severe side effects are rare, and sometimes there is local pain, swelling, or fevers that can be caused. If your baby seems fussy or in pain, give a little bit of Tylenol; you can repeat it in four hours if they're still fussy. And then if the next day there's big swelling, come call us." You know, and that's the end of the discussion.

Carrie says that her patients rarely ask about specifics of vaccines, a pattern that matches those of all the pediatricians I interviewed who treat low-income patients. When they do, she starts with the more familiar diseases and aims to educate parents about health more generally.

> I talk a lot about the bacteria, because I think not all families understand what a virus is and what bacteria are and why they're treated differently. But lots of people understand the ideas of germs and bacteria. So if you focus on severe bacterial meningitis in an infant, I think that's really scary for a lot of families, and that can help, I think, promote interest in preventing that. So I do do that.

In Carrie's view, her patients have limited knowledge of science, limited time to research each vaccine, and would struggle should their children become ill. She also recognizes that for her patient population, vaccines are mostly trusted and not often questioned. Thus, she spends little time reassuring her patients' parents about why they are necessary and safe.

Carrie has a toddler-aged child herself, whose pediatrician primarily serves privately insured patients. This experience with another practice reveals to her the differences between how her daughter's pediatrician approaches vaccine discussions and how she herself does with her patients. She explains, "They have such a different patient population that their attitude as clinicians towards it is different, . . . but I was surprised." Most notably, Carrie recalls how differently influenza vaccine was treated in her practice and in her daughter's doctor's office. At that private practice, Carrie was asked whether she wanted thimerosal-containing flu or thimerosal-free flu vaccine. (Recall that because thimerosal is a mercury-based preservative, it was the source of great controversy and was removed from all childhood vaccinations, but not all flu vaccines.) She recounts the experience: "It was just such an interesting question. And I said, 'Wow! That must come up quite a bit in your area?' and it does." In contrast, Carrie's clinic until recently offered only one flu vaccine, which was the last vaccine to contain thimerosal; parents seldom asked about it.[8] This difference illustrates the varied demands patients of different backgrounds make on clinical encounters and how pediatricians respond accordingly.

Vaccine Choice, Pediatric Advice, and the Flu Vaccine

The vaccine against influenza occupies an unusual place in the landscape of childhood vaccines. As the Booth family's story at the beginning of the chapter illustrates, it is the most likely to be refused by parents at all income levels and also is capable of killing otherwise healthy children. Children can also carry infection to seniors they encounter, who are most vulnerable to complications.[9] The influenza vaccine illustrates many of the tensions of physician practice—the line between public health and individual preference—and the different ways parents understand necessity and risk. In its worst forms, we see strains like the one in 1918 that killed millions of people worldwide and, according to world almanacs, lowered the average life expectancy that year by ten years.[10]

In other years, the strain is less lethal. Influenza in the most general of terms is a virus that attacks the upper respiratory tract, that is, the nose, throat, bronchi, and sometimes, the lungs. The infection usually lasts one week and is characterized by fever, aches, nasal congestion, cough, sore throat, headache, or general tiredness. Flu passes easily from one person to another through particles or droplets that an infected individual usually coughs or sneezes, which are absorbed through the nose or throat of someone else. Symptoms usually begin three or four days later. A person is infectious from the day before he or she develops symptoms until seven days later. Because the virus survives well—even outside the body—in cold and dry weather, flu outbreaks tend to be seasonal. The World Health Organization (WHO) estimates that in a typical flu season, somewhere between 5 and 15 percent of the global population will be infected. Of these there will be about three to five million cases of severe illness and 250,000 to 500,000 deaths worldwide each year.[11]

For most people, flu is uncomfortable and potentially costly in time away from work or caregiving responsibilities. However, some individuals are at an increased risk for complications, including life-threatening pneumonia that can result from infection. These include people over sixty-five, young children, pregnant women, people with underlying health conditions, including asthma, emphysema, diabetes, and heart disease, and people who are immune-suppressed. It is also a vaccine parents feel is not as important as others.

Carrie thinks the influenza vaccine is important, but accepts that many families will reject it. She instead prioritizes evaluating risk and recommending flu vaccine for the children most susceptible to a serious illness, a strategy more persuasive to families.

> It certainly depends on how old the child is and what other underlying risk factors they have. So I spend most of my time focusing on convincing families of children with asthma to get their children vaccinated. And then also families that have very young children who are under the age of six months who can't become vaccinated. I say, one of my arguments is, "Well, you know, you're providing this young child with vaccinations for all other illnesses; this is an illness that can be equally devastating and can kill your child at this age. And so it's really something that you and your whole family need to protect that child."

This two-pronged approach requires speaking of each child as an individual and also addressing parental resistance to receiving a vaccine that may not seem pressing.

Parental doubts about the necessity of the influenza vaccine reflect the reality that calculations of flu death remain somewhat controversial. The Centers for Disease Control and Prevention (CDC), the national agency charged with monitoring incidences of illness, explain that there are several reasons it is difficult to know precisely the number of flu-related deaths each year. First, states are not required to report individual cases of seasonal flu or deaths of people over the age of eighteen years. Second, many deaths of people with flu occur one to two weeks after infection because the person develops a secondary infection (like pneumonia) or because flu complicates a chronic condition they already had, like congestive heart failure or other pulmonary disease. Third, given the subsequent complications, seasonal flu is seldom listed as the cause of death on death certificates, making monitoring difficult.[12]

The severity of flu varies by year, strain, and other factors. Reporting also varies, making it hard to calculate the community effects of influenza. One CDC report found that from 1976 to 2007, "estimates of annual influenza-associated deaths from respiratory and circulatory causes (including pneumonia and influenza causes) ranged from 3,349 in 1986–1987 to 48,614 in 2003." This translates to an annual rate of influenza-associated death in the United States that ranged from 1.4 to 16.7 deaths per 100,000 persons.[13] Mortality aside, annual costs from influenza are considerable, amounting to an average of 610,660 life-years lost, 3.1 million hospitalized days, and 31.4 million outpatient visits. Estimates of the total economic burden of annual influenza epidemics (using projected statistical life values) are close to $87.1 billion.[14] Children under the age of five years are among the most detrimentally affected by flu, generating about ninety-five clinic visits and twenty-seven emergency department visits per thousand children during the 2003–2004 season.[15] The mean direct cost per hospitalized child was $5,402, with annual expenses estimated from $44 to $163 million. Children with underlying health conditions were more likely to be admitted to intensive care units, which added significant expense.[16]

These costs matter to public healthcare systems, to public and private insurance where costs are shared, and to the families who must shoulder much of these expenses. For adults, flu vaccines may lower lost wages and work time (even as there is disagreement about the size of these cost savings).[17] As Carrie sees in her practice, where many parents work in inflexible jobs without sick time, lost work time matters to workers as much as employers.

Critics of CDC calculations argue that the conflation of flu-related deaths and pneumonia or other secondary infections resulting from flu might be misleading, or designed to cause panic so individuals seek out more vaccines.[18] Yet there is little disagreement that 90 percent of flu-related deaths in most years are to those over sixty-five (although notably, the H1N1 in 2009 looked different as it disproportionately affected young people). Although older Americans absorb most of the illness burden, children are also affected. Flu can kill even previously healthy children, as the story at the beginning of this chapter illustrates. As flu death in children remains rare, pediatricians must decide how to advise their patients. Most draw on their own experiences as clinicians.

One pediatrician's story illustrates how doctors come to feel passionately about flu vaccine. This pediatrician, who cares for hospitalized children, told me about a five-year-old child with flu in his care:

> Now the mother was really good about vaccination. I mean she vaccinated every year, including the flu. She vaccinated, . . . but this year she just didn't get around to it. [Her] child gets flu and pneumonia. Child comes in with face mask oxygen and then was on a ventilator, an oscillator, and a heart-lung machine. And I would say the odds are that child doesn't live. Now she just didn't get around to it this year. It's like the casual kill. And if you watch that mother for those few days, you would cry. Because it's exactly what you would have done. She couldn't leave the bed. She was just pacing back and forth. It was like she had just been hit in the face with this big, cold air. You sort of gasp. She was constantly gasping because she just couldn't catch up to the fact that her child was this sick. And she just hadn't given the vaccine because she hadn't gotten around to it, because she thought it would never happen to her. Because the odds are it doesn't happen to you. Until it happens to you.

Deaths from flu in children are rare. In 2012–2013, there were just over a hundred child deaths from flu. Stories like the ones above are horrifying and uncommon.[19] Of pediatric deaths, 90 percent are in children who did not have a flu vaccine, and 40 percent are in those who had no identifiable increased risk of complication. (Some evidence suggests that children who are healthy who die of flu do so faster than those who have preexisting identifiable risks.[20])

From a public health standpoint, vaccination against flu holds the promise of significantly reducing rates of worker absenteeism, emergency room visits, hospitalization, healthcare costs, and most importantly, lost lives. Even with disagreements about rates of deaths, costs, or lost worker productivity, flu vaccine provides protection from illness and more serious potential consequences, which makes arguments for vaccination seem logical. Yet there is significant resistance to flu vaccination on an individual level, even among those who seek out other vaccines.[21] Because of the commonness of flu and the rarity of serious consequences, parents feel dubious about claims of necessity. In short, flu just doesn't sound that scary, especially since most parents have had it. That perception is stacked against claims that the flu vaccine might be harmful long-term. For example, the website of the National Vaccine Information Center (NVIC), the largest U.S. advocacy organization opposed to vaccine mandates, explains,

> One consideration with the mass use of flu vaccine in healthy children is the removal of natural antibodies to flu which are obtained from natural infection. The question of whether it is better for healthy children, who rarely suffer complications from flu, to get the flu and develop permanent immunity to that flu strain or it is better for children to get vaccinated every year to try to suppress all flu infection in early childhood is a question that has yet to be adequately answered by medical science.

To parents who already question the necessity of vaccines and believe there are too many, flu vaccination represents the excesses of immunization policy and practice. Katie, a mother of two, explains, "I feel like [vaccines] are useful but I think they can be overdone." Reflecting on how her perspective has changed over time, between her first child and her second, she notes, "I think, I came from when I first had my first child [and thought] give me vaccines—vaccines for everything— vaccines for a cold! Anything you can to keep him safe, to thinking, well, maybe the same very things we think that keep us safe [don't]. It's like the whole part of it is reevaluating the way the immune system works."

There are no vaccines for common colds, despite extensive efforts to find one.[22] However, for parents like Katie, flu seems to be a routine illness, like the common cold, and one that can be combatted easily by children's bodies, making vaccination unnecessary and suggesting pharmaceutical overkill on vaccines.

John Landress, a pediatrician who encourages parents to follow the recommended vaccine schedule in his practice with a high portion of publicly insured patients, works to challenge conventional wisdom that flu is no big deal. He perceives parents as cavalier about flu: "I think a lot of it is, 'Well, you know, flu has been around forever and we all have gotten better from it and it will make my child stronger if they have a bad case; if they have to fight [it] off, it'll make them, sort of the old Methodist perspective of strength through infections.'"

He combats this by focusing on how infection moves through the body and becomes potentially lethal.

> I tell them a lot of the epidemiology of Colorado. And you know, last year, the winter before this, there were seven kids that died in Colorado as a result of influenza. And most of them died because of encephalitis [swelling of the brain] or mild carditis [inflammation around the heart], not because of a pulmonary death. But a lot of them died from mild carditis, and I think a lot of people don't realize that flu can affect your heart muscle. And when they start to realize maybe a vaccine protecting the heart muscle or the brain is really a pretty good idea, a lot of them sort of come around.

In these ways, pediatricians like John choose between emphasizing risk of catastrophic, albeit rare, complications and accepting parents' more pedestrian sense of the disease.

Culturally, there is a lack of precision in discussions of flu, which challenges physicians to address it differently in their practices. Frequently, sick people describe themselves as having flu, when it is more likely they have a severe cold. Stomach flu is not actually related to flu, and over-the-counter medications promise to manage the symptoms of cold and flu equally and interchangeably. The pediatrician Carrie Mathers, who strongly recommends the flu vaccine, suspects that part of the resistance to flu vaccine stems from a misunderstanding of the difference between influenza and the common cold. Although this confusion is common among many of her patients, she highlights how challenging it can be for Spanish-speaking families:

> Flu in Spanish translates to *gripa*, and I think that they think of that as a really bad cold and so they don't understand why flu is influenza and why influenza is important and what the risks are with influenza. And no matter how you explain it, even if you are really great in Spanish, it doesn't always translate to "This is a serious, vaccine-preventable illness."

With this in mind, Carrie considers how to communicate with parents who don't think flu vaccines are important. "So a lot of times parents are like, 'I'm tough, I don't need the vaccine for myself.' And I say, 'Well, I don't care.' I'm like, 'I honestly don't care if you get the flu or not for your sake. I care about your child who might die if you get the flu.'"

In her discussions with parents, Carrie also focuses on the challenges of caring for a child when adults become ill. "I say, 'Imagine that you have an illness that gives you high fevers, chills, rigors and puts you in bed immobilized for two weeks. How will you care for your two-week-old? Who else will do it for you while you're vomiting and coughing?'" As Carrie advises parents about vaccination, she draws on the risks of disease for the whole family and aims to persuade parents.

In contrast to Carrie's approach, Ben approaches the flu vaccines as only sometimes necessary, depending on individual circumstances. Rather than asking families about their work and caregiving responsibilities that would fall apart with infection, as Carrie does, Ben instead considers who might be most vulnerable around them and who they know who would be at risk of infection should their children become sick.

> I mean it comes up with things like the flu shot specifically if you have multiple kids in the family and there's a really young child. Or if you're, for example, I have several parents who are, like, daycare providers, so things like that. . . . Especially if you live with someone or have someone who is immune-deficient, you know, those could be real issues.

In Ben's approach, he returns to a view of risk as knowable and care for the people in a patient's network as a priority, but not necessarily the broader community or the other factors that matter with infection. This may in part reflect the kinds of employment and resources that families in Ben's cash-only practice have in comparison to those in Carrie's practice, who rely on wage work and have fewer resources with which to outsource carework. Yet as all doctors work to identify family priorities and vulnerabilities, and counsel them accordingly, they note the importance of an individualistic vocabulary to parents, even as they remain committed to public health. As Kevin explains of his role, "I think that in some ways that is ideal, where you get to know people and you can really individualize things. But I also feel like we have to weigh both." In striking this balance, physicians walk a thin line between consultant, advisor, and public health advocate. Balancing on this tightrope is not easy.

Conflicting Expertise in Pediatric Care

Pediatric primary care is not monolithic. Parents are also not a singular group. All pediatricians with whom I spoke expressed a desire to work with parents to find common ground in support of children's health. As Ben describes his goals,

> My whole philosophy about it is that I'm really not—I'm not dogmatic, I'm not here to push any view on anybody, and I'm here to just try to support them. So a huge part of that is communicating with them and trying to get to a place where, you know, I can speak to them and they can understand me and I can understand them.

Even with the time and resources Ben's practice offers, this is not always simple; Ben acknowledges that there are "definitely people that are tough to penetrate." Physicians see themselves as professionally trained experts in healthcare who can share that knowledge. They respect parents and want to maintain trust with them, but they do not perceive them as equally knowledgeable about vaccines and the illnesses they can prevent. This sense of expertise is also difficult to combine at times with the goal of maintaining a partnership in support of individual children.

Much of the disconnect between parents and providers tracks on to competing definitions of whose expertise matters—who ultimately calls the shots. Parents know their own children as individuals, while providers read journals, look at population-level data or empirical research about illness and immunity, and draw on clinical experience caring for other people's children. These are at core different forms of information and different ways of knowing, but are not equally valued by each side. As young physicians express increased awareness of the importance of patient autonomy, they accept different kinds of compromises, some of which they believe represent inferior care (as the next chapters explore). This increasing willingness of pediatricians, many of whom compete for private paying patients, to defer to parents as experts illustrates a transformation in medical care. As Barbara Loe Fisher, founder of the NVIC, the largest U.S. organization in opposition to vaccine mandates, writes optimistically to parents who reject vaccines:

> There is hope. At least 15 percent of young doctors recently polled admit that they're starting to adopt a more individualized approach to vaccinations in direct response to the vaccine safety concerns of parents. It is good news that there is a growing number of smart young doctors, who prefer to work as partners with parents in making personalized vaccine decisions for children, including delaying vaccinations or giving children fewer vaccines on the same day or continuing to provide medical care for those families, who decline use of one or more vaccines.[23]

Whether these changes represent shifts in how younger doctors view parents or pragmatic compromises in order to get children covered against some of the most devastating illnesses—or maintain a large roster of patients—is a complicated question to unpack. Overwhelmingly, physicians describe their efforts to educate and empower parents as central to their practices, while also providing the best care to children. Although most physicians aim to get children as close to fully vaccinated as is feasible, they have created more room for parents to participate in these decisions.

6

The Slow Vax Movement

When we at Age of Autism talk about ending the epidemic, the "to do" list seems almost overwhelming—funding a vax-unvaxed study, getting mercury out of flu shots, proving the HepB shot is nuts, wresting control of the agenda from pharma, fixing Vaccine Court (this time in the good sense of "fix"), establishing that biomedical treatments help kids recover, and on and on. But there's a shortcut to all this, and it goes straight through pediatricians' offices. The evidence is growing that where a sane alternative to the CDC's bloated vaccine schedule is offered, and other reasonable changes adopted, autism is either non-existent or so infrequent that it doesn't constitute an epidemic at all.
—Dan Olmsted, editor, AgeofAutism.com[1]

In routine pediatric encounters, parents are asked to weigh two perceived abstract risks—of adverse reaction or infection—and to consent to one, albeit with imperfect knowledge of how their child will react. An increasing number of parents—even those who eventually want all vaccines—are requesting self-designed or alternative vaccine schedules, rather than the ACIP one. In fact, between 20 and 25 percent of American parents opt for alternative or slow vaccine schedules.[2] As such, examining the goals, perceptions, strategies, and challenges of this group of parents is important for understanding broader issues of trust, expertise, vaccination, and public health.

Vaccine schedules are devised by the Advisory Committee on Immunization Practices (ACIP). This national committee comprises fifteen experts in fields related to immunization who are selected by the secretary of health and human services, eight ex-officio members from federal agencies responsible for vaccines, and twenty-six nonvoting representatives from other organizations. The committee is charged with providing the Centers for Disease Control and Prevention and other agencies with "advice that will lead to a reduction in the incidence of vaccine-preventable diseases in the United States, and an increase in the safe use of vaccines and related biological products." The ACIP is the only entity in the United States that develops written recommendations for routine administration of vaccines to both children and adults, which includes recommendations about "the age for vaccine administration, number of doses and dosing interval, and precautions and contraindications."[3]

When the ACIP develops vaccine schedules, members review all research and literature, including information on adverse reactions that have been reported, risk and severity of disease, and timing of vaccines in relation to each other. As one ACIP member explained to me,

> When it's a new vaccine on the market, you have to show that the safety in the immunogenicity profile of the existing vaccines don't interfere with your vaccine and vice versa. There are hundreds of millions of dollars' worth of studies, probably eight hundred studies out there on this. And because you have to show that, you can't just flop it into the schedule and hope for the best. I mean, you have to show that it works and it's still safe and there's no interaction. And you should see the level. Because remember, the pertussis vaccine can have five components. You have to show that you won't interfere with any of those five components, and those five components don't interfere with the immunogenicity of your vaccine. It's a massive amount of work.

The ACIP's schedule also aims to provide the best coverage with a limited number of well-care visits, which can be costly in time and co-pays for parents.[4] The schedule, which targets all children in the country with dramatically varying incomes, linguistic backgrounds, access to health systems, and resources, does consider this. Low-income children often lack consistent access to healthcare and may have parents with limited capability to bring them to frequent appointments, including work schedules, limits in transportation, or inability to pay. As a result, groups like the Immunization Action Coalition, a nonprofit that provides information to consumers and providers about immunization, advises practitioners who face parents' concerns that there are too many vaccines in the schedule:

> We strongly recommend that you do not defer any recommended vaccines. This would be a missed opportunity. No upper limit has been established regarding the number of vaccines that can be administered in one visit. CDC's Advisory Committee on Immunization Practices (ACIP) and the American Academy of Pediatrics (AAP) consistently recommend administering all vaccines indicated for the patient's age.[5]

Many studies show that children encounter more antigens each day than are in a vaccine—even ones containing multiple inoculations in one shot.[6] For example, the ball pit in many indoor and fast-food restaurant play areas contains much higher rates of bacteria and viruses than are in vaccines, but parents do not often question the cleanliness of those play areas.[7] Physicians who promote vaccination also spend considerable time trying to communicate these differences in risk to parents. For example, Rachel Herlihy, a physician who directs the Division of Disease Control and Environmental Epidemiology at the Colorado Department of Public Health and Environment, explains how parents' concerns about vaccinations often come from a sense that babies' bodies can't handle the vaccines. "That is simply not true," she argues.

> There is no such thing as overwhelming the immune system with shots. Even infant immune systems have an almost limitless ability to respond to new germs. And the number of antigens or germs in childhood vaccines is a drop in the bucket compared to what young children's immune systems are naturally exposed to every day.

Similarly, the pediatrician James Todd, medical director for epidemiology at Children's Hospital Colorado, argues, "The 'too many too soon' myth puts the health of our youngest children and their playmates at risk."[8] From the perspectives of those who aim to prevent infectious disease, these concerns represent a fundamental misunderstanding of how the immune system works and ignores bodies of systematic research that support the effectiveness and safety of vaccines, even in increasing dosages.

Medical providers and public health officials largely view the practice of giving vaccines as more nuanced than parents recognize, and believe that their methods are empirically sound. They also suggest that parents misunderstand the mechanism by which vaccines work. Parents often argue that giving the same "dose" of vaccine to a football player and a baby makes no sense and illustrates the lack of specificity in vaccine schedules and failure to adjust the dose, as is done with most every other medication. I asked the pediatrician and vaccine researcher Paul Offit why this was not a reasonable critique.

> They think about [vaccines] as a drug. It's not a drug. It doesn't have the volume of distribution. . . . You give it locally. It's taken up locally by antigen-presenting cells like dendritic cells, B cells. And then it's processed locally. Then you develop those effector cells, which travel. Therefore, it's not the whole body you're really talking about.

To consider this in another way, when someone is exposed to a virus in a droplet in the cough of an infected person, that is not metered, but both infants' and football players' immune systems respond to that antigen and develop a response. This fundamentally different understanding of how vaccines work in the body underscores parental distrust of vaccines.

Even arguing that vaccines are not medications, Offit insists that vaccines are actually calibrated to need and size in ways parents don't recognize:

> The influenza vaccine, its dose is different for a young child than it is for an older person, same thing with hepatitis B. The doses are not the same and it's not one-size-fits-all, because there's this tremendous list of contra-indications and precautions based on the individual child. That's why you go to the doctor to get it, for the most part, so they can know that. That's where all these footnotes come from. [*He flips through a manual.*] Right? I wouldn't call that a one-size-fits-all schedule.

This discussion illustrates how physicians may consider far more factors than parents realize and do, in fact, see each child as an individual, even as their bodies work in similar and patterned ways. Pediatricians are also encouraged to recognize the careful work and the total research that goes into evaluating population-level studies of vaccines, to trust the rigor of the scientific method, and to then support ACIP recommendations. As Herlihy explains to a room of pediatricians and pediatric trainees, "Hundreds of people contribute to the ACIP and ACIP workgroups to come up with the ideal timing of vaccination, so an incredible amount of brain power goes into the recommended schedule."

For providers who trust in expert knowledge generated by the ACIP, parental distrust is irrational, representing not just a misunderstanding of vaccine safety, but also a miscalculation of the severity of vaccine-preventable disease. As one pediatrician explains,

> I feel like because we've been successful in the past, not eradicating, but really decreasing the prevalence of these vaccine-preventable illnesses, people get so relaxed and so complacent. And it's frustrating when you're trained in understanding the complications and know that not only for this one child you're increasing the risk, but for the rest of society you're increasing the risk. So it's so frustrating to hear people say, "I don't want to do it just because. Just because I'm worried about some remote possibility of some complication," when the real complications of not vaccinating are so much more evident to me.

Pediatricians assert that their training to recognize complications and disease risk is more legitimate than parental fear of a rare risk of an adverse reaction to a vaccine, particularly in contrast to the risk of disease presented to that child and others. Pediatricians and public health policy makers see vaccines as an obvious choice, while parents prefer to make decisions that feel more intuitive and more relevant to their family.

From this perspective, parents see themselves as experts most committed to their own children's health and most able to assess what their children need. Few parents know what goes into creating schedules of recommended vaccines, but as the outcomes appear to provide a "one-size-fits-all" schedule, they see them as irrelevant and unable to honor their children's individual bodies and needs. They do not necessarily trust the expertise and population-level research that the ACIP uses to create the schedule, which does not necessarily seem relevant to their own children, particularly as parents insist that their children are unique.

The Unique Immune System and Rejection of Multi-Shot Series

Many of parents' anxieties about vaccines are driven by the schedule that recommends multiple or combination shots at one time, followed by boosters later, known as a multi-shot series against an infectious disease. Multi-shot series are given to increase the probability of seroconversion, that is, the production of immunity against a specific bacteria or virus, and to create long-term immunity. With each booster, the overall odds of becoming immune against the vaccine-preventable microbe go up. For example, 85 percent of children receiving one varicella vaccine against chickenpox will develop immunity with that one vaccine, but nearly 100 percent develop immunity after a second vaccine. For measles, 95 percent of children who receive the vaccine at twelve months (and 98 percent who are given it at fifteen months) will become immune, but practically 100 percent develop serological evidence of immunity after a second dose. Of course, a small portion of children will lose immunity over several years, requiring additional boosters, and some might never gain it, but multi-shot series increase the odds of immunity.[9] In short, some children will develop immunity with the second or third shot, rather than with the first or second, but it is not self-evident which children will need additional boosters.

Parents who aim to limit their children's exposures to medications, drugs, or other interventions—embracing therapeutic nihilism—object to giving their children boosters that might not be necessary if their child gained immunity early. Anna explains both the importance of personalizing vaccine decisions and the risks associated with too many vaccines: "Everyone has a different immune system. For some people, it may take three shots. For some people that might be why they react is because they got immunity that first time [and when] their immune system is getting hit with it a third time, their system freaks out, you know?"

Many parents want their children to have immunity against serious illness, but also as few vaccines as possible. To accomplish this, they reject the recommended timeline for vaccines and boosters and devise something more personal. In many cases, parents will consent to one inoculation and then, wanting to understand their own child's immune response, have their children's immunity levels tested by having a titer (blood test) performed that looks for signs of immune response. Bob Sears, a pediatrician and proponent of alternative vaccine schedules, addresses this strategy directly on his website. He writes, "Some kids don't need some of the booster shots at age five years because their original infant series may still be working just fine."[10]

Checking titers requires drawing blood from a child, sending it to a laboratory equipped to test for antibodies, waiting for results, and then either giving the child the vaccine if the test is negative for a certain level of antibodies, or deciding the vaccine is unnecessary if the antibody levels are sufficiently high to suggest adequate immunogenicity. Sears adds, "While this is a costly and time-consuming approach, some parents prefer it instead of automatically getting all the boosters." Despite time, cost, and pain of a blood draw, many parents see titers as an opportunity to make more precise decisions about vaccines for their children.

Titers promise personalization in medicine and are promoted by many popular websites. One is run by the osteopathic doctor Sherri Tenpenny, an outspoken opponent of the widespread use of vaccines. Her site allows individuals to purchase home testing kits to send to a lab with which she contracts. On her site, she cautions parents that "doctors may resist vaccine titer testing." Blaming the uniformity of medical approaches, she cautions parents: "Doctors are hesitant to adjust any clinical regimen they have adopted or is accepted as 'usual and customary.' All children are vaccinated with all doses of vaccine, regardless if the additional doses are needed to create an antibody response. Vaccination protocols should not be a one-size-fits-all healthcare."[11]

Tenpenny and others who promote titer testing (often through their own commercial services) offer parents a way of feeling like they are individualizing their child's health, even as they subject their children to additional needle sticks from blood draws and other expenses that are seldom covered by insurance. It is also unclear whether titer levels predict immune levels, what the baseline for each vaccine should be, or how well some antibody presence on titers implies a likelihood of successful immune response.[12] Titers also rarely meet legal requirements for school attendance, a common question on listservs of those who want to opt out of the entirety of vaccine schedules. These costly tests promise a tool with which parents can challenge mainstream pediatrics, and seemingly return power to those who can afford them.

From a medical standpoint, parents' belief in the uniqueness of each immune system is overstated, because in most ways, immune systems respond similarly. Yet different children do develop different levels of immunity based on vaccination, underscoring the logic of boosters. The recommendation to provide boosters is in part historical and in part pragmatic. It is clear that some historic vaccine failures—that is, waning immunity or failure to elicit an immune response from a vaccine—were due to problems of vaccine storage or heat exposure. Since 1979, the chemical stabilizer used in vaccines has been better and makes vaccines less likely to fail (but also heighten parents' concerns about risks of vaccines).[13] Pragmatically, the small rates of vaccine failure when aggregated hold the possibility of compromising collective immunity and presenting an unknown risk to children whose parents may erroneously believe they are protected. From a public health standpoint, titer testing is inefficient in terms of time and expense, and arguably leaves children unprotected for longer.

These are not parents' primary concern. As parents seek out testing strategies to avoid medical interventions or deviate from the ACIP schedule, they rarely consider the health of others. Because of this myopic view focused on one's own child and the ways that child is unique, mainstream providers—particularly those who aim to see a wide array of patients with varying means, incomes, resources, or family backgrounds—view these parents with some frustration. With the competing goals of individualized care and public health, providers differently support or reject parent-dictated vaccine strategies.

Individualized Schedules and the Parent-Driven Slow Vax Movement

Parent-driven vaccine schedules are increasingly common; they also provide a point from which we can most clearly see the disconnect between parents' views and vaccine policy. From the perspective of those who develop the official schedule, these self-designed vaccine schedules do not and cannot account for the many interactional effects the ACIP considers; they do not evaluate possible interactions between vaccines or how some combinations might increase or decrease vaccine efficacy. Ironically, some delay of certain vaccines might increase the likelihood of adverse reactions or complications from the vaccine.[14] More basically, vaccine proponents see these alternative schedules as increasing the window of time during which young children are most at risk of infection, without improving health outcomes.[15] Since their goal as federal advisory members is to protect the entire population, they see these alternative schedules as ill-informed and potentially dangerous.

In contrast, parents who see themselves as experts on their own children trust their intuition more than they trust science and the outcomes of the established scientific method. In strategizing their own children's vaccines, parents draw upon a wide array of books, articles, blogs, conversations with friends, and discussions with an array of providers. Heather's explanation of her process illustrates the laborious efforts of parents to become self-taught experts—even as the resources on which they draw are not necessarily seen as equally credible. Piecing her strategy together from a variety of sources, Heather explains that she consented to the vaccines against "the diseases that I felt were the most serious and also the ones that had been the best track record of reaction, may be safer, and things that I didn't feel he had a high likelihood of catching, I put off." Heather identified the vaccines she believed were the most likely to cause an adverse reaction and then, she explains, "I tried to space them out so that I didn't do two really reactive ones all at once . . . like the DTaP I did by itself, because I just wanted to make sure that was all that he had to deal with at the time."

Physicians would see these efforts as well-intentioned but misguided. For Heather, though, they represent an effort to be informed, diligent, and cautious. Although many parents share their own strategies with each other (particularly in online discussions), some alternative vaccine schedules are promoted and sold, and are more prescriptive. Taking the case of the best-selling one, we can see the goals, limitations, and professional responses to these efforts.

Dr. Bob and the Vaccine Book

Of the many sources to which parents look to craft their own schedules, the best-known and best-selling is *The Vaccine Book: Making the Right Decision for Your Child*, by Robert "Dr. Bob" Sears. A pediatrician who sees himself as crafting a space between ACIP recommendations and parents' goals, Sears has been vilified by mainstream pediatrics, but also not embraced by those who most passionately distrust vaccines. As such, Sears and his role in this issue deserve more focused examination.

Dr. Bob, as he calls himself, comes from a family of pediatricians. His parents, Bill and Martha Sears, a pediatrician and nurse, have written dozens of parenting advice and children's picture books. The senior Dr. Sears also serves as an advice columnist for several parenting magazines. Bob practices with his father and older brother, who is also a pediatrician as well as a television talk show host on the syndicated program *The Doctors*. In practice, Dr. Bob does not accept insurance and instead touts a cash payment schedule that he explains allows him greater flexibility to spend time with his patients and their families, without intervention from insurance companies.

The Vaccine Book is Bob Sears's most successful book. The book uses accessible language to provide a framework to those who want to opt out of vaccines or rework vaccine schedules. As Dr. Bob writes, "As I see it, vaccination isn't an all-or-nothing decision. There are many choices that can be made. Some parents choose to get all the shots, others only choose some vaccines, and a few parents will choose no vaccines." Sears continues in his book to explain that while vaccines are important, "You as a parent are still entitled to know what you are giving your child." Advocating parents' responsibility to make informed health decisions, he suggests that vaccines are no longer an automatic part of childhood as they once were. Rather, "today's parents are taking a more active role in making choices for their child's healthcare."[16]

Sears's book explains that there are twelve vaccines in the vaccine schedule and that parents have twelve separate decisions to make. He writes,

> If you choose to vaccinate, this book will answer your questions about how to proceed in the safest manner possible. Should you get all the shots together as they are recommended, or should you space them out a little bit? Are there one or two shots you might delay for now or skip altogether?[17]

Sears believes that not all vaccines are equally important, but in general supports their use. He explains, "Vaccines are beneficial in ridding our population of both serious and non-serious diseases. But families do have the right in our country to take their chances without vaccines." In these ways, he supports vaccination but also sees himself as an advocate for parents' rights, families' individualism, and the uniqueness parents might see in their children.[18] Dr. Bob insists that parents are indeed the expert on their own children.

Sears claims that he developed these recommendations after reviewing research, examining package inserts that come with vaccines, reading the AAP's Red Book (a manual of recommendations for diagnoses, prevention, and treatment of infectious disease published for pediatricians to use in their practice), and drawing on his personal clinical judgment. His interest in vaccine safety came, he recalls, while he was in medical school in the early 1990s. Learning about vaccines, he felt that there were questions about the research on long-term safety. As Sears explains to me when we spoke, "There's just no long-term safety research. But then again, I'm one of the very few doctors that sees a problem with that. Almost every doctor feels that the current system of just reporting reactions when they happen, counting those reactions up, is perfectly adequate."

Sears positions himself as an advocate for parents and as the rare physician who questions other providers and the systems of regulation. His explanation to me of vaccine research illustrates this view.

> Vaccines seemed to have some very strange exemptions from mainstream science. . . . Like for example, when a pharmaceutical company makes a medication, you first have to study it in animals to prove that it's safe, animals that they can actually kill and do autopsies on. But vaccines are not subject to the same criteria, they don't have to study vaccines in animals; . . . there's no requirement for the companies to do those studies. So we've never been able to monitor any sort of internal toxic effect that we might be able to find on autopsies.

Sears points to the profit motives of pharmaceutical companies, which he suggests interfere with good science. More generally, he views other pediatricians as unsupportive of parents who are uncomfortable with vaccines, and sees his role as giving parents power to make their own choices. In thinking about this role he has carved for himself, he reflects on how he sees himself as different from other providers: "It's nice to be able to be guiding and influencing so many people, especially when they have nobody else to guide them, you know, because other doctors won't openly discuss these issues."

In these ways, Sears positions himself as a voice of common sense and accepting of parents' claims of expertise. As he explains to me, "In regard to vaccines, I'm exactly where I wanted to be and where I thought I would be—just being a voice for alternative ways to do it." Sears's recommendations in his book differ from those put forth by the ACIP and encouraged by the American Academy of Pediatrics. As a result, Sears has not received much support from vaccine policy makers or practitioners.

Questions for Sears

Criticisms of Sears's schedule are multifaceted. Although all reference his lack of skill in interpreting research on vaccine safety and efficacy as well as his lack of qualification to challenge ACIP experts and large bodies of research, these critiques also often weave in details about his persona and practice style. For example, I have heard several lectures and discussions by medical experts that, in the course of critiquing Sears's self-designed schedule, also reference the biography he provides on his website, which reads, "In his spare time Dr. Bob enjoys surfing the California waves, mountain biking, playing bass guitar with his teenage son guitarist, and trying to keep up with his three children."

These details are not inserted by chance. Rachel Herlihy, who in her capacity as a preventive medicine physician for a state department in charge of public health, speaks publicly about vaccine utilization and the problems of alternative schedules, and educates other physicians. In one pediatric hospital-sponsored lecture, she takes on Sears specifically: "Okay, so who is Dr. Bob? We are going to spend some extra time talking about Dr. Bob because I think he is a bit different than the rest of those alternative vaccinator/anti-vaccine folks in that Dr. Bob is a pretty mainstream guy." Unlike many other opponents of vaccine schedules, Sears is a board-certified pediatrician still in practice. Herlihy highlights why his biographical information is important:

So the reason I put this extra information on here is because Dr. Bob is an appealing natural guy. I would probably like being neighbors with him. We'd go biking. He sounds like a cool guy. I would probably run into him at Whole Foods and we would talk about organic apples.

Sears's biography does present a version of himself as likeable, not unlike those provided by many pediatricians on their websites. However, as Herlihy and others detail Sears's hobbies, interests, and likeability, they do so in ways that emphasize the frivolity of his lifestyle and the concurrent lack of training on vaccines and science.

Some critics of Sears present him as a well-intentioned pediatrician who is simply misinformed, and thus dangerously undermining decades of research and federal policy. Paul Offit, a vaccine researcher and director of the Vaccine Education Center at the Children's Hospital of Philadelphia, explains to me of Sears, "I think he's a nice guy who's trying to find a middle ground. My sense of him. He's wrong, I don't think he understands the science at all, and he waves the big pharma flag whenever he gets the opportunity to." He continues with respect to the Sears schedule, "Well, it's certainly not science-based." Sears's schedule, Offit suggests, has been successful because it "appeals to that fear, and the fear is easy."

Others also object to how Sears legitimates parental fear and allows it to trump research and science. For example, Herlihy explains,

> I think the most harmful thing that I see in his book . . . is these pro-con lists that he has. . . . Pro: these are the reasons for giving this vaccine: *your child won't get measles or give another child measles.* Cons: which are things like, *some parents feel, some parents' instinct is, some parents believe,* or *some parents have hunches.*

She acknowledges the utility of pro and con lists when making decisions, but criticizes the bases of Sears's lists. The pro lists, she suggests, are based on information from science, whereas the con lists represent "hunches, beliefs, and feelings." She notes, "Unfortunately, the con lists are much longer than the pro lists. And I think that is what parents are seeing and basing their decisions on: these lists, the length of these lists."

Like Offit, Herlihy suggests that Sears is also well-intentioned, wrong, and dangerous. These critics accept that Sears may not be malicious, but argue that the results have nonetheless been harmful to consensus on the importance of vaccines. Herlihy continues,

> He states that his intention is to give options to concerned parents, to convert non-vaccinators to at least partial vaccinators. Unfortunately, because of these anti-vaccine messages that appear and the lack of acknowledgment of some good science that exists, he misinforms his audience on a number of issues. And so in reality, what happens here is that he converts probable vaccinators to partial vaccinators and non-vaccinators.

These characterizations of Sears cast him as validating an unscientific position and in doing so, stoking anxiety about vaccine safety rather than reducing it.

Financial Incentives and the Slow Vax Schedule

Other providers are even less generous and presume that Sears has other motives, not least of which are financial. Certain incentives are inevitably built into the slow vax schedule and are often cited by policy makers and practitioners as a serious concern. ACIP members must create schedules they believe are safe and necessary for all children, irrespective of their insurance status or access to care. They aim to recommend vaccines at a population level, with full knowledge that agencies will have to fund recommended vaccines, parents will have to potentially miss work to bring children to appointments, and clinics will have to maintain stocks of vaccines, which can be prohibitively expensive. They also hold off on making universal recommendations if those vaccines cannot be reasonably delivered to all children.[19] Thus, the schedules represent a desire to provide maximum vaccine coverage to as many children as possible, affordably as possible, on a schedule that is workable for low-income families who may not have adequate access to primary care.

The slow vax schedule generally and the Sears schedule specifically require additional appointments, co-pays, and visit fees. Parents also must take time to bring children to these additional appointments, which carry the risks of exposure to whatever illnesses linger in the waiting rooms of pediatric offices. In contrast to the ACIP schedule's efforts to limit expense and maximize uptake, slow vax schedules do not do this, nor do they try.

Seeing the added expenses built into slow vax schedules, critics highlight how Sears has financial incentives to promote them, particularly as he accepts only cash payment for his services rather than insurance reimbursement. Because parents commonly reference "the Sears schedule," every pediatrician I interviewed had opinions about Sears and his book. For example, one primary care pediatrician who faces inquiries from concerned parents in her practice explains,

> Yeah, he's a financial genius who is preying on people's fears, and when people ask me about that all the time I'm like, "Well, I think he's a really smart man, who is making millions of dollars, but he's a general pediatrician. . . . He's done no studies. He's done no fellowship. He has done no extra training. He made it up. A singular guy in Beverly Hills, or wherever he lives—Fancyville, California—made it up, and is making millions of dollars trying to scare you. That's what I think."

Another pediatrician sarcastically explains that Sears is thoughtful, adding cynically, "He's thoughtful of selling his book, making money." Yet, another pediatrician describes her exasperation with parents who ask about the Sears schedule, but also believe erroneous claims that pediatricians are financially incentivized to give vaccines. "This guy that invented it has his own practice where he only takes—he doesn't take insurance— you have to pay out-of-pocket per each visit. So, 'Hey, you get to come back every month for a new vaccine. I'm getting tons of money from all your visits' and those are the people who are profiting from these weird vaccine things. And so that to me is illogical." Unsurprisingly, Sears receives no support from mainstream pediatric organizations.

At core, Sears supports vaccination, but would love to see parents have greater flexibility and choice. He explains to me, "I don't mind if they keep the mandates, as long as they would give personal exemptions for all fifty states." Sears's schedule is informed by a consumer-based logic that he views as unproblematic. "I just decided to come up with a different way that parents could vaccinate, that I felt bypassed a lot of the possible worries with the current schedule."

This willingness to tout vaccines as still the right choice, even as they are administered in a different order or time period, limits his ability to be seen as an ally by those who most resent vaccines and opt out altogether. At a conference hosted by the NVIC, which opposes vaccine mandates and encourages parents to buck professional advice, Sears was invited to debate Lawrence Palevsky, a self-described holistic pediatrician who rejects vaccines and according to his website, instead "utilizes a holistic approach to children's wellness and illness."[20] In this environment—heavily stacked against all vaccines—Sears was the pro-vaccine representative on the panel, a role that AAP and ACIP supporters would be surprised to see.

Alternative Vaccine Schedules and the Repositioning of Medical Knowledge

The slow vax movement generally and Sears's book specifically aim to address the concerns parents express: that children are given too many vaccines at once, which might overrun their immune systems, vaccines may not be safe, and the schedule doesn't consider children's individuality. We see support for "slow" movements elsewhere, in the slow food movement, which challenges fast food's inferior nutrition and rushed family interaction around meals, arts and crafts movements or do-it-yourself (DIY) efforts that challenge production line consumption, or anti-technology movements that aim to slow down the pace of life to more natural rhythms. In each, there is a tacit belief that slower is more cautious, and thus superior.

Slowing down the vaccines and spreading them out comes then to be seen as a prudent measure. Katie became interested in an alternative schedule as a way to have her son protected while also limiting the risk of an adverse reaction. She had read a book in which, she recalls, the author recommended "staggering them a little bit and not getting all of them in one day." Katie's goals for unbundling vaccines are diffuse:

> Well, there're two things. One is, if your child has a reaction to one of them, you know what it is. And that's one of the reasons not to do, like, five vaccines in one day. And then the other thing too is it is probably

overwhelming, you know, in my view it would be overwhelming for your immune system to get, like, six doses of vaccine in a day.

Katie does not provide evidence that five or six vaccines in a day *do* overwhelm a child's immune system. Instead, she explains that in her view, it *seems* like it would. Like Katie, parents craft their own strategies to find ways of consenting to some vaccines that *feel* individualized and safe, while rejecting others on the same basis.

Negotiating Vaccine Schedules in Clinical Encounters

Parents, particularly those with higher levels of education and resources, often enter pediatric visits with their own agendas.[21] Many develop their own vaccine schedules and present them to their children's doctors. Not surprisingly, physicians have different levels of receptiveness to these plans. Some parents describe their doctors as respectful of their efforts, while others relay that they are not. Leanne Boggess, for example, believes that her pediatrician is supportive of her efforts to conduct her own research and develop her own plan. She also accepts that her doctor shares the goal of protecting her children, explaining, "I think we both feel the immunizations can be very helpful if the body has time to handle them properly." Leanne feels respected by her physician, making her more willing to trust her doctor's professional judgment, which, she notes, includes "explanations of what things are, what our children are more at risk to here." That, she indicates, led her "to make those decisions to follow her advice or her recommendations." Most parents with whom I spoke also, like Leanne, describe their efforts to educate themselves as "research," while characterizing doctors as voicing an "opinion" or "recommendation." In so doing, parents notably relativize the terms and upend the hierarchy by placing their own sense of expertise above that of professionally trained doctors.

Parents' varying experiences with pediatricians underscore one clear fact: pediatricians expect to engage in lengthy discussions about vaccines with parents, with one study suggesting that more than 75 percent of physicians encounter requests for alternative vaccine schedules.[22]

Several providers note that even though the schedule presented in *The Vaccine Book* is light on research and comes with additional costs to implement, they often see parents who request "the Dr. Sears schedule" or "the extended schedule." One pediatrician remarks, "Oh, you bring it up [with other pediatricians] and their eyes go in the back of their heads and they're like, 'Ugh! This Dr. Sears extended vaccination schedule just really bums me out.'" The resonance of the Sears book is difficult to separate from his prominent family, or the "Sears family dynasty," as one provider characterizes it. Herlihy specifically considers how Sears's family name has added more legitimacy to his schedule than to the many others also available:

> I think [the reason] Dr. Bob has been more harmful than some of those other providers is the fact that he comes from this very well-respected family that is out there in the media. There's a TV show. They have this website. If you go on Babies R Us, every single product in the store is endorsed by the Sears family. So it is mainstream.

The centrality of the Sears family to the world of parenting advice, Herlihy argues, has contributed to a more fundamental cultural change. "What I think has happened here is that [Sears] has created a new social norm around alternative vaccinations. So because he is so mainstream it's created this sort of comfort for parents that this is the right thing to do, this is a normal thing to do."

As parents weigh expert advice and hear stories of disease risk, the approach of Sears and other supporters of alternative schedules might feel more validating because it addresses parental fear directly and treats it as valid and important, even if their recommendations are not necessarily grounded in science. Offit suggests that although it is an appealing vocabulary, it is not safer or better:

> I give them credit for using the word "alternative." It's a good word, sounds like "reasonable alternative," "alternative music," "alternative energy." But it's called what it is: it's a delayed vaccine schedule with no benefit. None. And it shows you how little [Sears] understands what goes into making the schedule, that he believes he can sit in his office and come up with his own schedule. And this is almost laughable.

Many pediatricians observe a widespread new cultural expectation that good parents question vaccines and challenge providers. They face these interactions daily, and prepare for them in different ways. The pediatrician Kira Watson expects patients to raise questions about vaccines. Her impression is that parents are told before pediatric encounters to be suspicious of doctors' agenda around vaccines and her goal is not to provide evidence to support those suspicions. She sees the parents who bring their children to her office as feeling compelled to challenge her expertise. She imagines they think, "What I've been told by the Internet, my girlfriends, whoever, is that I need to question." Yet even as she anticipates these questions, she describes herself as willing to spend as much time as parents want discussing vaccines and their concerns. Her role, she explains, is to help them understand why vaccines are important and that the risks are minimal compared to other risks, including vaccine-preventable disease:

> I think part of that education, part of maybe why I'm more successful convincing folks to get vaccines is that I take the time to reorder what is disordered in their thinking and that somehow this is a threat, and it's not. These other things are threats. You know, children used to die a lot. You know, getting through childhood used to be, like, a big deal, and now it's not.

The pediatrician Carrie Mathers also describes her frustration with having to discuss alternative schedules. Yet she admits that she and her colleagues recognize that getting children some vaccines is better than none; they will, as a result, be flexible, even though they see parents as ill-informed:

> If it's going to get them some versus none, I'll do it. I try to explain it: "It doesn't really help your child, you're kind of putting them at increased risk by not getting those vaccines on as soon as possible, it's more expensive, . . . it's more dangerous, it's more pokes for your kid at different times, and it just doesn't do anything positive."

Although questions arise less often in her clinic with publicly insured patients, Carrie knows that her colleagues who see privately insured families share her approach. "They do it, partly because it's good customer service, because that's what the families want, and you want to develop that relationship with the families."

Pediatricians with whom I spoke, all of whom are parents themselves, acknowledge that watching children get vaccines can be stressful. However, they insist that delaying vaccines is a poor strategy for dealing with those emotions. One pediatrician acknowledges parents' fears, but communicates how delaying vaccines carries its own risk. "It's hard to watch your child get so many shots at once. It's hard to watch them get so many shots in the first years of life. And so this sounds much better. But the fact of the matter is all you're doing is increasing the period of time during which you're putting those kids at risk."

The pediatrician Julia McMichaels also sympathizes with parents' emotion, but focuses on the risks of not vaccinating. She describes her strategy as "just telling [parents] that the more time your child is unimmunized, the more chance they have of getting sick, and there's no harm in doing this [vaccination], and then negotiating a little bit," so they will consent to at least some vaccines, or the ones Julia suggests are most pressing.

These negotiations are increasingly part of pediatric practice. The pediatrician Kevin Sato describes his approach:

> I'll say, "Here are the vaccines that are typically given at two months. Which ones are you comfortable doing today? What are you ready to do? These are the ones we recommend." If they have questions about them, then I'll talk about, "Here's this vaccine. This is why we do this one. This is why we do this one. If you want me to prioritize them, I'll tell you that there's not zero risk from skipping the hepatitis B, but here's the three that I think are the most important," and have a careful conversation about that.

Kevin believes that parents need help understanding necessity and risk, and tries to indicate which diseases are most serious at which ages.

> I think people want to know, is this a life-threatening illness? Is this potentially going to kill my child? And if they ask that question, we have to answer honestly. Some of them, no. Whooping cough? Maybe not, but it could. And it might neurologically devastate your infant. We have to talk about that.

Kevin is willing to rank the vaccines he sees as most important, assuming parents have already considered vaccines and are ready to discuss them. However, he notes, this is not always the case. "A lot of times those families just aren't ready; if they haven't thought about it at that point, I don't want to pressure them into making a decision in a twenty-minute visit."

Kevin is willing to defer to parents as experts on their children, even if they know very little about vaccines. Kira also strategizes her advice to patients, stressing the importance of vaccines, while also respecting parental experience. She believes strongly in the reliability of the ACIP vaccine schedule and likes to follow it. However, she also recognizes that in her practice, which is 80 percent privately insured and has a high percentage of parents who are college-educated, those most likely to question their children's healthcare, she must communicate to parents how she sees their children as unique and how she considers their individual needs in her recommendations.

> It comes down to, I need them to trust that what I am telling them is in the best interest of their child. So I won't try anything that will potentially jeopardize their perception of trust. Because I truly am, like, I truly don't want to go visit them in the ICU, I truly don't. I truly want them to be healthy and wildly successful. And they don't know what I know. So that's what my job is, just to tell them what I know about what the real risks are. . . . I have no other agenda, other than the health of the child.

Kira describes herself as respectful of the parents in her practice and invested in maintaining a strong relationship with them. She is proud that only a small number of patients in her practice are not fully vaccinated. She unapologetically aims to convince parents to vaccinate, and says she is direct about the harms of not vaccinating. She tells parents that she has been to funerals for children affected by pertussis and pneumococcus, and that while she has not seen Hib, there was an outbreak recently that killed four children. She tells parents it is their choice, but also acknowledges that she puts it in terms that are "very grim, [because] children died." She does so, she explains, "Because I think nobody says that on the Internet." These stories, she recognizes, are often more compelling to parents than are statistics or national studies that are often presented in support of vaccines. In doing so, she sees the power of stories of individual children devastated by infectious disease as able to combat the stories parents hear of children who were reportedly harmed by vaccination.

Communicating her respect for parents' authority, the importance of her relationship with them, and the importance of immunization is a delicate balance. Kira uses one example to show how she works toward this:

> It's interesting. I saw a mom of eighteen-month-old twins, and it has been a road to get these kids vaccinated. And at the end of every visit I'm like, "All right, look me in the eye and tell me you don't feel bullied, because that is not my intention here. My intention is to protect your children. Do you feel that way for me? Because if you don't, then we have a problem." And so I will ask, after every visit, I will say, "Before we vaccinate, do you still feel comfortable that I am trying to do right by your children? Because if you don't, I shouldn't do the vaccines today because that won't feel good when you go home."

Pediatricians often reference the balance between communicating their strong recommendation, informed by professional training and experience, and supporting the clinical relationship between them and their patients' families, which might require deferring to parents' plans. The question of how to build and maintain trust with patients' families was of central concern to every provider in this study. Yet they each had to develop their own strategies to maintain trust and recognize the individuality of their patients, which helped them position themselves between individual care and public health goals of disease prevention, albeit to sometimes different ends and levels of success.

Sarah Cazan became a pediatrician because she wanted "to partner with people" and support their goals for their families' health. Yet providing this individual level of care became more complicated as her practice grew to include hundreds or thousands of children. In one poignant example, Sarah recalls a baby in her office who contracted pertussis in her waiting room from a family that rejected vaccination. She recalls, "She got sick at two months and I was worried about her neurologic prognosis. . . . Nobody could do anything for her. I mean, all you could do was stand there and watch her, gasping, not gasping, turning blue." As a pediatrician committed to supporting each family's plans,

Sarah struggles to best balance each family's rights to shape their own healthcare, with the risk their choices might present to others in her office. "I don't know what you do about that, . . . but it's tricky."

Physicians work to find ways to connect emotionally with parents, build a relationship of trust, provide advice that is scientifically valid, and support parents' sense of their own expertise. As they do so, they find themselves working to find compromises to best protect the children in their care and to acknowledge parents' fear, even when it means accepting alternative schedules and sometimes the infection of other children in their waiting rooms. These efforts may require compromise from all parties.

The Limits of Individual Vaccine Plans

Parents frequently want the ability to implement the vaccine schedule they feel makes the most sense. They often expend considerable energy designing these schedules. Despite their hard work and deliberation, many of their vaccine goals are inaccessible for organizational reasons, including finding a provider who supports their plan, accessing unbundled vaccines, and costs. These constraints are worth considering, as they show how not everything is personally negotiable, even as parents claim their expertise.

First, many parents describe feeling dissuaded by providers from following their own plan. Although physicians I spoke with describe their efforts to work with parents, many parents did not perceive providers to be flexible. For example, Heather, a parent, recalls,

> I had this doctor, . . . she said she would go along with my plan, but every time I went in, she'd, like, give me a lot of pressure and, like—she tried to talk me out of [waiting]. . . . So this time I caved and she kept saying, "Well, we can do it in a combination shot and then he won't have to get it twice." And at that point, I was going in extra just for the vaccine and paying co-pays and all this, and so I'm like, "Okay. Let's just do it." And, of course, later on, I'm kicking myself.

Parents like Heather sometimes experience medicine as highly prescriptive and inflexible: patients should stay "on track" for predetermined well-care schedules that may not represent what parents feel they and their children want or need. Even when their children tolerate the vaccines without incident, the experience of being dissuaded from following their carefully constructed plan can feel disempowering.

Second, even when providers are flexible and cooperative, there are organizational barriers, including production and distribution limitations, to their self-designed schedules. For example, parents who want a single vaccine often discover it is difficult to obtain one without the other vaccines with which it might be combined into a single injection. Pediatric practices have varying abilities to keep vaccine in stock. There are several routes to buying vaccines, but each requires a significant financial investment. The AAP encourages practices to also buy insurance on vaccines, in case refrigerator malfunctions or power outages jeopardize supply.[23] Unless practices have a very high volume or are committed to maximizing patient choice, they are unlikely to keep different combinations of vaccines on hand, and may be able to buy only certain kinds, depending on whether they participate in a buying group to limit costs.[24] Practices also aim to manage supply to limit waste, a more significant issue as vaccines have become a larger investment with uncertain reimbursement. As the physician Sean O'Leary and his colleagues detail, "The cost of the vaccines needed to fully vaccinate a child through age 18 in the private sector in the mid-1980s was ~$50; in 2000, it was ~$600. In 2012, that cost was between $2250 and $2500, depending on the products used." As a result, the authors explain, "The cost of vaccines has gone from a minor consideration in the overhead of a private pediatric practice in the 1980s to one of the top overhead expenses, largely because of new vaccines, thus magnifying the risk to private practices of uncompensated costs related to vaccines."[25] Given the sizeable investment in vaccines for practices, it is unlikely that physicians will carry multiple formulations of the same antigen unless they have a particular reason to do so. So a parent who wants only, for example, a tetanus vaccine, without the diphtheria or pertussis with which it is commonly distributed, may have a hard time finding it. Overall, practitioners have neither a scientific nor logistical reason for providing multiple options, frustrating parents' plans.

Parents often describe their frustration with this. One mother recalls of her stunted plans, "I wanted to get the MMR separate and I spent a lot of time—I spent a lot of time trying to find it. I called a bunch of different organizations, you know, health departments and stuff like that. I could not get a hold of it." Unsuccessful, she consented to her son receiving the combined measles-mumps-rubella (MMR) vaccine, which her son tolerated well. Despite efforts to craft the perfect individualized schedule, the ways private practices stock vaccines limit parents' abilities to implement their own plans.

Third, patients who change providers may face challenges in finishing a sequence, as vaccines might vary from one practice to another. Lauren, for example, wanted her daughter to complete the series of tetanus vaccines she had begun with one pediatric practice at the age of three years.

> She's had two and she needs one more. And I made an appointment for her four-year checkup with another doctor and I specifically called and asked them "Do you have this tetanus booster? It's not the DPT, it's just the DT." And they're like, "Oh yeah. We have that." And of course I go through this long, horrendous long wait and this doctor appointment, . . . and then at the end she's like, "Oh no, we don't carry that vaccine." So I don't know how to get it for her.

Faced with these limitations, parents have to make a decision to accept the combined vaccines or reject them altogether. These can be challenging choices for parents who have invested time and energy into designing what they believe is the best schedule for their child.

Some providers recognize how emotionally laden vaccines have become for some parents and work with parents accordingly. Kira explains her view of parents in her practice and her approach:

> Some parents who are interested in alternative schedules just want to feel like they're in control, that they had some power in the decision. And I'm fine with that because I can catch up the things that are—like, if you're not internationally traveling, polio is not an immediate threat to your child in the first year of life. So I'll let them control that. They feel good. I feel, I get the kid protected [against other diseases], and then we'll approach it down the road.

Yet even Kira's ability to grant parents control is contingent on the availability of the vaccines in the forms and timing parents most want.

Slow Vaccines and Parental Control

Slow vaccine movements—Sears's and others—can be understood in many different and opposing ways. For parents they can be a way to assert parental expertise, ensure individualized care for their children, and reject mainstream recommendations that seem impersonal. For providers, these movements represent an effort for parents to claim more control over their children's healthcare. They present new challenges to professional authority and require providers to offer new tools with which to manage parental fear of vaccine safety or claims of expertise. For others, these schedules, with the extra time, appointments, and costs, represent the worst of medicine: potential profit motives for providers and wasted healthcare expenditures that provide no improved care—and arguably worse care. These new interactions present new challenges to the relationship between parents and providers in healthcare settings.

The option to alter vaccine schedules—and physicians' widespread acceptance that they will need to have these discussions in their practices—marks a fundamental transformation of preventative care from a more uniform public health system into menus of individual choices. The parents in this study represent those most committed to resisting vaccines and communicating their views. Yet we should not lose sight of the reality that about 20 percent of American parents deliberately delay vaccination, even if they are less purposeful in declaring a self-designed schedule.[26] It may be that the view that good parents should question experts about vaccines has become a new cultural norm. This trend may represent a broader attachment to processes that are "slow" and "alternative" as superior. These slow vaccine schedules reflect some acceptance that vaccines are important and successful in protecting children, alongside a seemingly contradictory general distrust of medicine and scientific expertise. The outcome is that parents are increasingly choosing self-designed schedules over the ones put forth by national experts and that this represents failure of government agencies and professional organizations to communicate the hard work that goes into vaccine schedule research and development. As a result, parents rely on their intuitive sense of safety and self-guided education to make choices they feel are the best for their children, and are increasingly calling the shots.

7

Finding Natural Solutions

Our bodies are Organic!! Everything we need to cure them,
ARE ORGANIC TOO!!!!
—Parent blog post

A friend recently traveled with her teen daughter's soccer team to an out-of-state tournament. Upon returning from several days of the girls sleeping, eating, and playing in close proximity, one girl was hospitalized for meningitis. Although my friend initially panicked, she remembered that her daughter had received the meningococcal vaccine as she entered middle school and was protected. Although no vaccine is 100 percent effective, most are highly effective at preventing infection and provide assurance to parents. For this friend and others like her who consent to vaccines, the decision to trust government agencies, regulatory bodies, and professional clinicians provides a sense of reassurance; by following expert advice, they ensure that their children are safer.

For other parents who question vaccines, immunization represents a process of choosing either the risk of disease or the risks associated with complications from vaccines. Seeing no perfect option, parents who distrust vaccines focus on other ways to control risk and uncertainty in their children's lives. So while parents reject vaccines, they embrace other parenting practices they view as promoting health, which they believe also render vaccines less important. This chapter explores these strategies, which include natural living, breastfeeding, commitment to organic or natural foods, and control of social interactions. It is worth acknowledging that these practices—as deliberately crafted as they may be—are not likely to provide total protection against infection. Instead, they provide a sense of control over mechanisms of possible infection that are otherwise uncontrollable.

Illness Prevention through Natural Living

Parents in this study, overwhelmingly mothers, largely see their children as healthy, even as they sometimes also view them as fragile. They communicate confidence in their decisions to opt out of vaccines because they trust their ability to keep their children well through practices that are resource- and time-intensive, but which they see as a personal choice for the good of their children. Because these parents see health as a state of being naturally immune to infection (and illness as being vulnerable), they perceive vaccines as unnecessary. Parents challenge more traditional forms of authority held by pediatricians by asserting their sense of control over their children's well-being, particularly around feeding practices. "Feeding the family" is gendered work that is both a material and interpersonal form of carework.[1] In the stories mothers communicated to me, feeding—that is, the production, preparation, and delivery of sustenance—was key to both their mothering and attention to healthy living. Those who rejected vaccines for newborns expressed confidence in the power of breastfeeding to confer immunity. They also cited their efforts to manage food and nutrition as the foundation of their children's health. By defining feeding practices as the center of health promotion, mothers communicated their commitment to their children in stereotypically feminine ways. At the same time, they fail to acknowledge how these choices are resource-intensive and not equally available to all mothers and children.

One online discussion of mumps was particularly informative. A mother who chooses to reject all vaccines posted this question: "My son is entering his teen years. Though not vaccinated so far I have to confess a concern over the effects of mumps. I would hate for him to become sterile should he get mumps. What does everyone do about this? Any advise/suggestions [sic] will be gratefully received". Another mother replied with advice. First, she addressed the rarity of mumps exposure:

> My understanding of sterility by mumps is that even *if* our sons were to catch it, the likelihood of it going to the testicles is HIGHLY unlikely and then the risk of going sterile is usually—on the VERY rare occasion that it happens—in *one* testicle, leaving the other one unharmed. We are talking minuscule numbers.

Yet as she continued to consider risk, this mother broadened her advice to identify other risks that she sees as more salient and that result from parenting practices, foods, or use of technologies that are incompatible with "natural" living, adding, "Personally, I am not worried about this at all. I think the risk of sterility from GMOs, laptops on laps, cell phones in pockets and other sources is much more likely."

Lifestyle matters, but parents often return to the importance of nutrition in managing risk. One mother writes to the mother concerned about her teen son's risk of sterility, suggesting she can mitigate risk through feeding—and that real risk belongs to those with poor access to nutrition.

> Another thing to keep in mind is that when healthy people get sick, they can fight things off better than already-sick-from-bad-diet people. Eating properly is the key to overcoming illness. Vitamin A is a huge help in fighting viruses and finding ways of adding organ meats is a great way to get vitamin A into the diet. I realize it can be difficult to control the diets of teenagers, but at least you have a say about what he eats at home. Give him a good, balanced diet at home and hopefully he'll remain strong enough to fight off anything that might come his way.

In these responses, mothers communicate various strategies to define and manage risk. First, they use the language of medical authority to speak to the probability of infection, which is rare. Second, they identify risk as existing in more banal activities in daily life—including laptops, cell phones, or junk food teenagers might consume away from home—which in turn characterizes vaccine refusal as the least risky of daily choices among myriad others. Finally, they suggest that parents can reiterate their authority over health decisions and their power through time, money, and supervision.

Breastfeeding and Nutrition as Good Mothering

Breast milk is widely touted for its superiority over formula because it contains antibodies to illnesses the infant's mother may encounter. In promoting breastfeeding, government agencies frequently describe the immunological properties of breast milk as a rationale for why "breast is best." As the American Academy of Pediatrics explains,

> Human milk . . . contains many substances that benefit your baby's immune system, including antibodies, immune factors, enzymes, and white blood cells. These substances protect your baby against a wide variety of diseases and infections not only while he is breastfeeding but in some cases long after he has weaned. Formula cannot offer this protection.[2]

Parents are aware of these kinds of claims of the superiority of breast-feeding to formula and have in virtually all cases prioritized practices they see as more natural, of which breastfeeding is one. Using this logic, vaccines are crafted as unnatural. Parents are routinely asked to consent to vaccines within hours or days of the birth of their babies, as is the case, for instance, with the vitamin K injection to protect against a rare but serious blood clotting disorder. For many, these interventions seem unnecessary or redundant to the protection breastfeeding provides, and notably, all of the mothers in this study had breastfed babies, with more than half nursing for between one and five years, longer than experts recommend. Astrid Villa explains, "You have this tiny little infant that's just been born, I'm breastfeeding already, which is providing the immunization from my breast milk, . . . and she wasn't gonna be in any environments when she would potentially be exposed to any of these things, so why would we do that?"

Gabriela was also uncomfortable consenting to newborn vaccines. Highlighting her sense of authority through intuition as a source of decision making, she explains,

> I just—I could not fathom injecting a foreign substance of any kind into the bloodstream of my infant. It just didn't resonate or feel right on any level, and so I did research because I needed to make sure that my instincts were going to be safe enough, because I definitely was torn. I'm not totally anti-vaccinations or vaccines at all. . . . I wanted to wait until he was two so his body just had a chance to really have the strength and have the immune system to have everything on its own.

As she made the decision to delay vaccines for several years, she derived confidence from her intuition and her mothering to keep him well, explaining, "I just—I needed to trust breast milk and our lifestyle and everything else, and just felt like it was really important to keep him safe from those things."

Mothers' certainty that breast milk will protect their children, alongside their desire to control disease risk through nursing, however, does not mean that it works. The AAP specifically outlines the kinds of infection breast milk protects against, none of which are vaccine-preventable diseases. For example, the AAP statement on breastfeeding notes,

> This defense against illnesses significantly decreases the chances that your breastfeeding baby will suffer from ear infections, vomiting, diarrhea, pneumonia, urinary tract infections, or certain types of spinal meningitis. Infants under the age of one who breastfed exclusively for at least four months, for instance, were less likely to be hospitalized for a lower respiratory tract infection, such as croup, bronchiolitis, or pneumonia, than were their formula-fed counterparts.

Breastfeeding indeed reduces the incidence and severity of some illnesses, particularly respiratory and gastrointestinal viruses, because mothers who encounter those same strains at the same time their babies do build immunity, and those antibodies enter breast milk and are available to the nursing babies. Yet hearing the many immune-supporting benefits of breastfeeding, most parents believe that the benefits are much more expansive. And while breastfed babies are *less likely* to experience a range of sicknesses or hospitalizations, mothers often assume that breastfeeding protects completely against illnesses, providing what several parents (like Astrid) referred to as "immunization from breast milk." Steph's description of her surprise when her infant son developed an ear infection illustrates this: "He got an ear infection. I didn't even know what it was because [my other son] never really had one and, you know, if you breastfeed your babies, they're not supposed to get ear infections, supposedly." Here Steph provides an example of how parents conflate reduced risk of certain infections—promised by organizations like the AAP—with assurance of no risk.

Although claims of the superiority of breastfeeding have come under scrutiny,[3] mothers who reject vaccine recommendations perceive breastfeeding as protective. As some mothers were inclined to see breastfeeding as protecting completely against all illness, many also assume erroneously that their own immunity from past illness or inoculation could be transmitted to their children through breast milk. For example, several mothers falsely believed that their own childhood polio vaccine could protect their children through breast milk. Breastfeeding is a privileged maternal practice, disproportionately available to women who do not work for wages or have autonomy and flexibility in employment.[4] Yet for mothers who distrust vaccines, breastfeeding also marks their maternal commitment to their children's health, their perceived control over risk of disease, and their efforts to ensure health without having to defer to the generic medical recommendation that vaccines represent.

Breastfeeding also marks caregiving in highly gendered ways, as food is literally produced in the maternal body. Consistent with research that suggests that intensive mothering practice begins in pregnancy, as women's prenatal health is causally related to children's health, mothers rely on their sense of their own prenatal health in justifying vaccine refusal.[5] Illustrating this, Paula explains why she did not feel compelled to consent to infant vaccinations: "I had an extremely healthy pregnancy with her. Loaded up on all the vitamins and protein powders. . . . I was healthy and she was really healthy." Thus, women perceive management of their maternal bodies—and deliberate efforts and ability to access sources of nutrition—as superior to medical interventions that physicians, government agencies, or pharmaceutical companies might recommend. As they see it, if a mother is healthy, her child will certainly be.

Healthy Bodies through Healthy Food

Many mothers also express confidence in their ability to mitigate risk of disease by managing their children's nutrition more generally. In claiming the superiority of homemade baby foods or organic products, they communicate their confidence in their ability to protect against illness through individual feeding strategies, as well as their acceptance of the moral and maternal responsibilities inscribed in healthism.

Lauren, a mother of four, explains the role of food in her decision not to vaccinate: "We also are very conscious about how she eats and how, you know, that she eats mostly organic food. . . . I made all of her food at home the first—when she started solids, and so we try to keep her immune system strong in that sense as well." Although there is no evidence that organic foods increase immunity to disease, mothers like Lauren describe their superior care by referencing their commitment to consuming high-quality, expensive foods and time-intensive ways of preparing them. Seeing feeding as inextricably linked to immunity, mothers consistently articulate a strategic intentionality in their choices as evidence that they are responsibly managing their children's health without vaccines.

Tara, the mother of an unvaccinated child, insists that she avoids toxins by managing "everything we can control" through organic and unprocessed foods. As we sit in a local vegan restaurant, she confidently explains,

> We finally just moved into a house where we're growing our own organic garden, which is nice. But we buy local as much as possible and organic. We don't do premade. We make our own rice milk. We make a lot of our own stuff. We don't do additives, food colorings. When we make Halloween cookies, we make food coloring out of beets and semolina and carrots.

Lauren and Tara, like most mothers I interviewed, articulate the importance of feeding the family as core caregiving responsibilities and key aspects of successful mothering. In claiming the superiority of homemade baby foods, breast milk, or organic products, mothers communicate their confidence in their ability to protect against illness, reiterate their sense of expertise and control, and highlight their advocacy for their children. They see these demanding and time-consuming practices as replacing the need for vaccines and protecting children from disease without expert intervention. They also locate control for children's health with women, emanating from mothering practices that require the time, skill, and resources that come from privilege. Responsible only for their own children, they do not reference the privileges of their access to time or food compared to children in other families.

Healing through Nutrition

Some mothers express how food management did more than provide preventative care, but also could provide medicinal care. For example, Heather believes that her son's health declined after receiving infant vaccinations. At age two years, he developed asthma and allergies. To address this, she began changing his diet. She describes the improvements to her son's health, and how managing his food and nutrition and seeking out healthcare from an alternative provider who believes in the importance of nutrition have made the difference:

> That could partly be his age and it could partly be changes that we've made in our family lifestyle as well. We've done a lot of changes with our diet. I have him kind of on an anti-inflammatory diet for his asthma and [have] gotten a lot of supplements going, like fish oil and Juice Plus. . . . And [we've] been to see a doctor who specializes in those things as really kind of a natural approach to things, and he got us on some supplements.

Similarly, Katie treats her five-year-old son's eczema and lack of concentration in school through diet modification. She explains,

> His behavior is markedly different. When he has a lot of milk, he's totally zoned out. Like, la la land. It's almost like he's drunk when he has milk, . . . which, I think, it's a leaky gut thing. It's almost like [it's] released in his body like an opiate. So I've seen—and even my sister said—she's like, "I kinda thought you were crazy," but then she saw the difference in him after he had a bunch of milk.

Katie continues to explain her belief in her nutritional strategy, which also includes eliminating gluten, even as she does not get support from her family. "Yeah, people in my family think I'm kind of crazy. But you know, I've always sort of marched to my drummer, so it makes it easier to, you know: 'Oh, look at Katie! Crazy Katie has her children on a gluten-free diet; that's so crazy.'"

Katie's husband disagrees with her efforts to consult occupational therapists, nutritionists, or other providers outside mainstream medicine, as well as her choice to opt out of vaccines. He resents the additional costs and doesn't see evidence that any of these modalities work. To support these consultations, Katie works sporadically as a freelance writer and uses her earnings for her son's care. She also reports that her mother often undermines her efforts when she goes over to visit: "She's giving them milk and chocolate and everything else they're not supposed to have." She elaborates, "Well, my mom thinks I'm weird. You know she's—she's very freaked out, like I—my son doesn't—is off dairy and she will purposely give him milk in front of me, because she's like, 'I've never heard of a child who can't drink milk. That's just your crazy thinking. Like, I don't know where you get these ideas.'"

Katie articulates her advocacy for her son by managing his diet, even as she is undermined and criticized for doing so. Her willingness to work for wages solely to fund her son's care suggests that finding support for diet management is significant to her. She describes her son's health challenges in terms of "leaky gut," a pseudoscientific explanation based on the discredited research of the British physician Andrew Wakefield, who most famously erroneously claimed a causal relationship between the MMR vaccine and autism through the gut. In choosing to breastfeed, manage nutrition, and seek out dietary solutions for allergies, mothers like Katie articulate a view of themselves as committed to their children's health and willing to advocate for it, even as they are challenged or undermined.

Managing Risk from Imagined Gated Communities

Many parents share the view that supervision is a way to guard against infection. Through intensive mothering practices, they evaluate risk and their individual ability to mitigate it through vigilance, as viruses or other sources of vaccine-preventable illnesses (and those who might carry them) can be spotted and avoided. Heather explains that her children do not need all recommended vaccines because her caregiving limits potential exposure: "I was at home with them; they didn't have to be in daycare. We were kinda attachment parenting-style, where I really didn't separate from them at all. . . . Because of our lifestyle environment, [they're] low-risk for some of these things." Most mothers like Heather identify childcare staff and children who attend childcare as potential vectors of infection. They communicate their pride in practicing attachment parenting (where mothers closely bond with their babies and prioritize physical contact and responsiveness day and night) and they value their abilities to avoid childcare settings, large or crowded spaces, and places where strangers may congregate.[6] From their self-described commitment to care for their children's bodies themselves, mothers emerge as accomplished risk managers, even as they rely on privilege to protect their children from these settings.

Although parents feel that they can control disease exposure, some anticipate that this will become harder as children age or travel, when they will have less ability to monitor their social worlds; they know that children will encounter increased risk of exposure as they will potentially interact with more people. Lauren, for example, explains that her seven-year-old son wants to be a missionary and that illness, therefore, "is going to keep cropping up" in his life. Travel presents particular new challenges to parents' abilities to manage social contact. Molly, for example, admits she would reconsider her decision to opt out of all vaccines, depending on what countries she and her family visit. Although she feels she has thoroughly researched disease and vaccine risk in the United States, she acknowledges that this information doesn't apply equally in all contexts. "Well, because I'd probably have to do all new research. . . . Where are we going? . . . Where are the outbreaks in that country and what are they of, and are they people that we'd be exposing ourselves to on a regular basis?" Similarly, Tara considers how travel would change her plans. She insists,

> The only way I would consider a vaccine for him would be if we were going to travel to Africa or somewhere where there was a real—and it would have to be a real—imminent threat. And we probably would choose to just not go there until he's a certain age, until his body has developed to a certain point.

In more general terms, Gabriela doubts that her preschool-aged son needs vaccines. She explains, "I feel that at this age and his exposure to the world, it's not [necessary]," a view that would change, she notes, "if we travel more and as he gets older." Yet, as they began planning a trip to Europe, Gabriela approached her physician to discuss what they might consider in terms of disease risk when traveling abroad. She recalls, "We started talking to her about what we would need. We were flying through London. That's one of the, you know, biggest—everyone in the world stops through Heathrow, and so she said, 'Well, these are the things that he'll be exposed to there. You need to be aware of that, including polio.'"

Although Gabriela considered the advice, she opted against vaccination: "Again, I decided to trust the fact that he was still primarily nursing" and not vaccinate. Yet Gabriela did seek out one vaccine, against tetanus, despite her discomfort with vaccines. Notably, tetanus is a disease that is not contagious—providing no herd immunity—but is ubiquitous in soil and the environment. She explains her reasoning: "We did do one shot of the DTaP before that trip because he was starting to be so active outside and digging in the dirt constantly and, you know, walking and moving and that the DTaP was—I just wanted to be safe. That's— that's the only one I was able to do."

Gabriela is certain that polio is a terrible illness and believes that if her son were facing sustained risk of exposure, she would want him to be vaccinated against it. She explains, "If I was going to travel with him someplace where there's polio or some of these really devastating diseases, I would definitely weigh the vaccination as the safer option than the exposure." In thinking about this choice, Gabriela considers parents she knows who make different choices. "I have friends who have not chosen that. I have friends who live in India with their babies and no vaccinations, but they feel so powerfully about that that I feel like they're safer than I would be with any doubt in my mind." Noting her belief that intent and desire protect her child, she continues, "I have to really, truly believe what my choice is for him to be safe."

In these narratives, parents place their children at the center of their risk calculus, and consider their ability to manage disease risk, which becomes more complicated as they envision travel to foreign countries, where it seems less controllable, more common, and as potentially demanding new strategies. Even as disease avoidance becomes harder, most parents express confidence in their abilities to manage it. Elizabeth, a mother whose children received no childhood vaccinations, faced these issues directly. Her process of changing her views on vaccine risk and necessity is informative.

In describing her decision to reject vaccines, Elizabeth explains that she and her husband "have a pretty ideal situation," in that they both worked from home while also employing a nanny. She compares her own situation to some of her friends "who knew in six weeks their kid was going into a [large childcare center] kind of environment where maybe your risk factors are higher." In assessing risk in her home, she feels secure with her decisions. Yet, as she began planning a meditation journey and vacation to India with her now-school-aged children, she recalibrated her thinking. She explains of her children, "They've traveled quite a bit outside of this country, but never to a Third World country—you know, that is in your face even more. So now we definitely feel like, 'Oh, they need to be fully vaccinated. I'm not gonna take them to India and expose them.'" Elizabeth's shifting perceptions of vaccines, like those imagined by others who provide similar descriptions, illustrate the subjective meanings of disease risk and vaccine benefit. As Elizabeth reflects on her "ideal situation," she references the class privilege that allows her to secure an in-home (presumably vaccinated) nanny who could shield her children from infectious disease, as well as the choice to travel for her children's enrichment. These choices underscore how access to resources shapes her views of healthcare as a consumer product, with vaccines serving as a kind of technology to be used according to individualized assessment, and facilitated by privilege. Disease remains uncertain, but parents have confidence that their ability to identify risk, to choose when vaccines might be beneficial, and to use them on a schedule of their own design serves to manage these unknown variables.

As parents articulate their abilities to assess potential infection and protect their children from exposure, they draw on racialized narratives of disease. Perceptions of disease risk often represent anxieties about race and difference.[7] The historian Leslie Reagan writes, "Infectious diseases have never been confined to the body, for diseases are only understood through culture and history."[8] These parents trust not only their ability to maintain social distance from others who might carry disease, but also their ability to use their privilege to discern when exposure to others might happen and under what terms. This is not to deny that disease risk looks different in different places, or that, until recently, wild-virus polio was present in India, while no case has been recorded in more than thirty-five years in the United States. Rather, this view of disease ignores epidemiological data that the majority of outbreaks of vaccine-preventable diseases originate with unvaccinated children in the United States and those who have traveled in Northern Europe.[9] Parents view their own children as consumers of travel and resources, but also as vulnerable to infection presented by others. Notably, none consider how their children might present risk to others—particularly to children with fewer resources or less access to care, including the undervaccinated, in the United States or abroad. These questions remain pressing to leaders in other countries, particularly those who host international events, like the Olympics or World Cup tournaments, but are outside the view of parents who cannot imagine their children presenting risk to others.[10] In so doing, they both claim privilege and then deny it exists by resituating risk management as individual processes that good parents take seriously.

The explanations parents offer for rejecting vaccines illustrate the importance parents assign to managing their children's worlds and the invisible privilege it takes to do so. They construct imagined gated communities, which, like their material counterparts, serve as symbolic and political ways of creating a safe haven from those deemed socially undesirable, while allowing parents to align themselves with those they imagine share their values, ideologies, and lifestyle.[11] Vaccines are, at core, a technology of containment and a guard against both biological and social contagion.[12] Parents who refuse vaccines aim to create a domestic sphere free from both state regulation and disease risk, neither contributing to public health nor acknowledging the broader communities in which they live. This parenting project, which focuses solely on one's own children, allows parents to ignore how their unvaccinated children benefit from other people's vaccinations and how their children might present risk to others.

One would assume that parents who see vaccines as risky would discourage their use more broadly. Some did, but most parents I spoke with were more willing to assume that all parents are experts on their own children and should thus make their own decisions. As Lauren explains, "I would never ever tell anybody what to do because [what] if their child dies from measles or my child, you know, gets brain damage or dies of anaphylactic shock from vaccinating . . . I don't push my opinion on anybody." As such, vaccines remain an individual choice informed parents should make.

At times parents characterize other parents as inferior as a way to distinguish themselves and valorize their own practices. They often see other parents as failing to actively manage their children's social worlds in order to optimize their health or manage risk and uncertainty. This is most observable as parents consider whether vaccines are appropriate for other children, even if not their own. For example, one mother of an unvaccinated toddler explains,

> I think there are some vaccines that maybe some kids, maybe it's okay for them to have, because maybe their parents don't at all—aren't at all educated and don't—and compromise their systems. If you have a kid they're going to be putting on antibiotics their whole life, their immune system, there's already compromise. So maybe they do need to rely more on outside sources, because that is being done to them.

In accounting for how some children might need vaccines, parents can see the use of vaccines as a sign of weaknesses in other parents, or a necessary crutch for those who fail to raise a disease-free child in a social world they have imagined as potentially free of risk. These seemingly uncommitted parents may lack financial, social, or educational resources to support the foods and lifestyle components parents who reject vaccines view as essential. They also may trust expert recommendations, which can be seen as a lack of independence. Yet as parents intensively manage their children's lives, they can criticize others for lacking the same individualistic commitment to their own children, which in turn serves to celebrate their own superior care and commitment.

Risk and Perceptions of Control

Throughout all these strategies—breastfeeding, managing nutrition, monitoring social contact, assessing potential vulnerability—parents overwhelmingly express a desire to manage their children's health, despite the reality that not everything is entirely controllable. In this context, vaccines represent one individual choice that is within a parent's control. Just as parents describe their choice to reject vaccines in an unmanageable world of potential toxins, they may also reject vaccines because they overestimate their abilities to safeguard their children.

Throughout parents' narratives of health promotion and disease avoidance, we see how vaccine choices represent their perceived ability to manage uncertainty though individual effort.

Physicians who recommend vaccines often express frustration that they cannot convince parents that much of their children's infection risk is well beyond their control. Kira, a pediatrician and mother of young children, suggests that parents' efforts to manage and limit vaccine uptake represents a broader effort to control children's lives. Identifying the reality that vaccine refusal is most often practiced by white, college-educated mothers, many of whom have waited longer to have children so they could finish their education, she observes,

> I think there is something very real about women delaying childrearing, and the women who delay childbearing are educated and professionally successful. And how they have gotten to their education and professional success is through study. So they feel like if I just "study parenting," study these medical decisions, study it as hard as I've done in my real life, I can know X, Y and Z. And it's not true about pediatrics, nor is it true about parenting. I mean it's trial by fire. Like, you don't know until you know. I tell folks, at four months you may or may not have a good sleeper and you didn't control that; that was your baby. You don't control the baby that you have. And that's a very difficult concept, I think, for successful women, that they can't control this.

Kevin, a parent and pediatrician, also describes his efforts to educate parents about the limits of their own abilities. Noting parents' belief that breastfeeding or social management can protect against illness, he explains, "My basic response, without being judgmental about it, is that breastfeeding, not being in daycare, decreases your risk, but it's not zero. You go out and you're amongst people and your risk is slightly lower, but it's not zero." As he counsels parents, he explains that social interaction is inevitable, as is disease risk. "You can't live in a bubble."

Sarah, a parent and pediatrician, sees much of the dilemma over vaccine choice to be a problem of contemporary parenting. She explains, "That's just a consequence of parenting that sort of goes along with all of this, that we want everything. We don't want to get sick, we don't want to suffer, but we don't want to suffer the consequences of treating every illness and preventing every illness either."

Parents often referenced the lack of certainty in their children's lives, yet saw vaccine risk as something they could control. Some acknowledge how information about risk is intrinsically imperfect, requiring them to make the best decisions possible with the information available. Molly, a mother of three unvaccinated children, describes her lack of faith in expert calculations of risk and the importance of choice—not just for vaccinations but for all parenting decisions. Molly sees many places where experts tell parents they are creating risk by not following expert advice. She describes these messages: "'You're choosing not to vaccinate, you're putting your child in danger. That's not okay.' And yet, it's my choice if I want to take the risk of having a home birth or if I want to take a risk of having a hospital birth. I feel like that has to be my choice as a parent to make."

Molly acknowledges some of the inevitable uncertainty that accompanies parenting choices. "I could make a wrong choice, and every day I'm faced with that, you know? 'Am I driving the right way to school?' It gets overwhelming. Corn syrup? . . . 'Wow, I just gave my kid two suckers. What?' You know, so it can become all-encompassing." Yet, even as Molly and others acknowledge the limits of perfect knowledge of risk—for them and experts—they return to the belief that they are the best qualified to make these determinations. If risk is unknowable and uncontrollable equally to them and those who recommend vaccines, parents claim expertise and focus on the ways they can individually maintain control and promote health: through diet, breastfeeding, social contacts, or evaluation of possible vulnerability. As parents, they are uniquely qualified to manage uncertainty for their children. As such, they insist it is their call to make.

8

Vaccine Liberty

We stand at the moment, I believe at a defining moment in the history of this country. I think future generations will remember that this was the beginning of the end of the first republic of the United States of America. When a government and its politicians sold out the constitution and the people of this country to the properties and the pharmaceutical industry, and the parasites and the carpet baggers that attach themselves to that industry in the interest of profit with the illusion of public health. While just behind the curtain is the sickest group of children in any developed country in the world. A group of children who apparently need to be sustained by the candy-coated offerings of the very industry that I believe put them there in the first place. We will not stop until this fight is won. . . .

You have had something taken away from you as a people. And I am not talking about your rights in SB277. I believe it is your innate instinct for the well-being of your children that has been usurped by pediatricians and doctors who think they know better when they do not. There is no one who knows a child better than her mother. . . . So my message to you, please people, is you must go back and you must trust your instincts. You must believe in yourselves as you have never done before. And do not let that be taken away from you. Because everything I have learned about vaccine safety and about autism in particular comes from you. It does not come from my profession. All they have taught me is what we don't know. What I have learned from you is what we do know and what we should know. And what we should continue to pursue.

. . . This is not a time to be frightened of anything at all. And I speak to my colleagues in particular. If in this battle, if you leave yourselves a lifeline, if you are concerned about your respectability, about what the mainstream media or

the bloggers say about you, about what your colleagues say about your status in this profession, then you are lost to this cause. You have to cut all of the lifelines. Because if you don't, you will take the way back. If you cut those lifelines, then there is only one way and that is forward. . . . So do not fear. This is not a time to be afraid. Trust your instincts. I have been in this for 20 years and I will fight this battle until I die. Because your children are worth fighting for.
—Andrew Wakefield, Health Freedom Rally, Santa Monica, CA, July 3, 2015, in response to California's SB277, which removed personal belief exemptions to vaccinations from state law.[1]

How do parents who reject recommended vaccine schedules deal with the negative feedback from other parents, friends, doctors, schools, or even their own family members? Such challenges informally communicate, sometimes aggressively, that parents have violated important social rules by rejecting vaccines. Social vitriol is a common topic on online discussion boards between parents who opt out of vaccination. For example, one mother writes of her challenges deciding when and to whom to disclose her decision to opt out of vaccination:

> I'm actually having a hard time too, especially with sharing our choice if anyone ever asks, most of my really close friends and family just respect it and leave it alone (maybe secretly think we are nuts, but i'll take that). . . . I'm tired of feeling nervous or anxious about this conversation coming up with play groups or new friends, parents who may be uncomfortable, or attack me because "their kid is in danger."

Another mother notes similarly, "Our son is 2.5 and we haven't vaccinated, nor do we plan to, but am I the only one who feels bullied about having made this decision? Or even scared?"

In online discussions, mothers frequently post about their experiences of receiving negative feedback for their vaccine choices. These exchanges often follow particularly high-profile news stories—for example, those covering recent outbreaks of vaccine-preventable illnesses and identifying pockets of children with very low vaccination rates. The public comments posted in response to these online news stories insist that vaccine refusal creates risk in particular communities, a hurtful proposition to parents who reject vaccines but don't see their individual choice as affecting others. Illustrating this, one mother described a sense of shock that one of her friends posted on Facebook a news article about record-high rates of measles.

> The friend who posted this does not have children, and the article posted is probably the only vaccine-related article they've read this year, and sometimes I feel that the entire pharma-medical industry keeps their pockets full by fear-mongering. We are definitely in the minority in our circle of friends and are okay with that, but wow, sometimes it is just exhausting.

Referencing the same article, another mother writes, "I had two FB friends post the article, and each had about three responses. It felt like a bit of a witch hunt with responses such as 'I am so nervous when my infant is around unvaccinated kids, my oldest is vaccinated so she is ok' and 'the Jenny McCarthy theory was debunked.'"

Social media often provide an outlet for social disapproval, where opinions can be freely posted and shared without actually seeing those they criticize. One woman explains,

> A FB friend (who also happens to be a former coworker of mine from when I worked for big pharma—and he still does) posted this [measles story] today too. Along with some angry comment about "stupid people who dont [sic] vaccinate." My children are not vaccinated and I won't be bullied into it.

As rates of vaccine-preventable disease increase, blame placed on those who don't vaccinate has grown in noticeable ways. The pediatrician Kira Watson also notices this trend and relates of her medical practice,

> I'm starting to get more [questions] with [increasing rates of] pertussis in the last six months being such a hot topic in Colorado. I'm starting

to get more of this question. I didn't used to get it: "What percentage of your practice is not vaccinated in the waiting room?" which I think is an awesome question. So that tells me people are really thinking about it differently than maybe even five years ago.

Although parents share experiences of facing anger from those who disapprove of their choices, there is disagreement among them about how to best manage it. On one hand, some advocate for parents to politely smile and ignore critics. One mother suggests in a forum,

> I think it's to the point where we need to keep quiet about our health choices if we are not within a like-minded community. I used to feel like I was a rebel and was educating people when the subject came up (not lecture-y or anything, just sharing in a simple way to show that "normal" people are thinking about these things), but now I just nod and smile if I am with a group that might not accept my views.

Another mother agrees, "Good input, especially about keeping our mouths shut and just smiling. Otherwise it's just a problem. I'm sure most of us deal with it within our own family circles too. I have a retired [physician] mother in law; imagine how she feels about our choices!"

Parents perceive a division between those who are sympathetic to the position that vaccine choice is personal and those who are not—who see vaccine refusal as a rejection of public health and a willingness to introduce risk to others. Parents' forum comments also represent the varying strategies they believe parents should use to manage information about their choices. In contrast to those who suggest smiling and keeping quiet, others insist that parents who reject vaccines need to speak out about their choices to educate others. One mother of children who received some vaccines before she began questioning vaccine safety explains, "How I wish that someone cared enough to enlighten me. If someone would have just shared, I would not have made all the mistakes I made. The only people that were opening their mouths and giving me their advice & telling me what to do were the wrong type of people."

In thinking through how to respond when others confront her about her vaccine choices, this mother describes her plan to dismiss them by accusing them of following recommendations blindly: "I've decided that if anyone should outright attack me, I am going to 'baaaa' them. I'm going to just not bother w/justifying myself and just tag them for what they are: 'Oh, sheeepy, sheepy, sheepole, so sad that you're a sheepy. Baaaaa, baaaaa.'" Sharing this view that those who follow expert recommendations are less enlightened than those who reject vaccines—and are proverbial sheep—another mother offers, "We are fierce, independent thinkers and intelligent. Tough skin comes with the territory, without that you cave. I think we have it as our duty to keep our mouths wide open. If people don't like what we say 'Forget them! You did your part.'" As she recalls another woman who had shared her own process of coming to reject vaccines, she relays a sense of gratitude:

> I never knew or met anyone who didn't vaccinate their child, until I met a chiropractor who kept those books around her office. She had monthly "Vaccine Talks" that were decidedly more on the "think again side". She asked us to put as much research into both sides as we would into buying a new car or house. . . . She put the seed into my head. What would I have done if she kept her mouth shut?

From this experience, she explains, emerges a sense of obligation to proverbially pay it forward. This obligation overshadows any personal discomfort or disapproval she may face.

Social media also become a resource for those who feel an obligation to speak out about their own decision to reject vaccinations. One mother suggests,

> FB is the easiest place to be completely frank about these things. I never hesitate to stir up trouble on web boards *when new moms ask* or seem to be searching. To not be completely obnoxious, and not cause too much trouble, I rarely say anything unless someone specifically asks a general question at mom's groups about vaccination and even then, often I don't say anything unless I'm asked directly.

This shared sense of obligation to speak out affirms parents' sense of themselves as not necessarily stigmatized, but rather, wise in a world of others who remain unenlightened.[2] In response, parents collectively advocate for what they see as the higher moral ground. Despite the discomfort that comes with disapproval—of feeling stigmatized—they re-cast their views and actions with a shared sense of self-righteousness and a duty to speak out. In doing so, they often find themselves feeling vindicated as others behave badly. For example, one mother writes,

> Yes, the vitriol is depressing—unnerving, didn't realize it was that bad out there. Most people I know say things behind my back & then I hear about it later. At this point, they are way too afraid to say snide/nasty things to my face. I've heard 2nd hand, the "you are irresponsible, selfish parents . . ." But, yeah, I hear it second hand, and I know exactly who in our family/friends have said what, and eventually, they realize I know what they have said. And, when they realize that I know, they are the ones that are squirming.

In each of these narratives, parents understand themselves as indepen-dent, thoughtful, and deliberate, in contrast to those who mindlessly ac-cept expert advice. None of these negative interactions inspired parents who reject vaccines to question their views. Rather, these critical interac-tions served as further evidence that they were on the right path in ques-tioning vaccine recommendations and the providers who offer them.

Navigating Disapproval in Medical Systems

Parents who reject vaccination often want pediatricians to help care for their children in other ways, beyond immunization. Parents enter these encounters understanding that they will have to manage information about their rejection of vaccines. For example, one mother refuses to go to public health clinics because of their insistence on vaccination. She explains, "I've heard that they'll send you card after card after card that you're late, you're, like, delinquent, and I have four kids and it would be, like, filling my mailbox." Instead, she has found doctors who are flexible about vaccination, but many do not accept insurance and demand cash payments. She explains, "I'm at a loss. . . . I went to this other doctor [but] he doesn't take insurance, so it's quite a pretty penny out of our pocket."

Parenting blogs and neighborhood listservs are filled with requests for advice on where to find "vaccine-flexible" pediatricians, with many listing replies about doctors they like or advise avoiding. One mother recommends more optimistically that parents should schedule a meeting with a pediatrician and then "ask your pedi if he/she vaccinated their own children. You may be surprised at the answer as many don't or they delay, separate etc." These replies identify the larger landscape in which networked parents, those more likely to have resources, approach physician selection as they would a service provider to be reviewed and vetted.

Outside the well-care context, when children are injured or sick, parents often find themselves in encounters with doctors with whom they do not have a relationship. In many of these interactions, parents experience doctors as inflexible and unwilling to adopt treatment protocols that are out of the ordinary. Although they identify this inflexibility in other arenas, it appears most clearly in the context of vaccine decisions.

In one example, Lauren, a mother of four unvaccinated young children, describes feeling surprised that her infant's croup was taken seriously and treated immediately at the emergency room:

> She didn't even make it through triage because she was, like—I don't know, she was turning blue or she was choking so bad the nurse was like, "Come with me" and he's, like, yelling for the doctor and the doctor comes running in and he's grabbing her out of my arms and laying her down and they're immediately getting steroids . . . and then getting out the nebulizer and nebulizing her. And they were so nice to me. It's the nicest treatment I've ever had, and I thought, "Wow. I'm always coming [here]. Wow. Like this is the best emergency room doctor ever. This is the first time they've been treating me like a human being."

When her son came down with the same illness a few days later, Lauren rushed to the same emergency room, thinking, "We're just going to go to the hospital; hopefully we'll get the same nice man to give the steroids." This time, with a toddler whose symptoms were less serious, they were stopped at triage and asked many more questions, including about vaccination. Lauren then asked for the same physician who had been kind a few nights prior. "Sure enough, he walks in and I'm so happy and he's—you know, because he was so friendly—and he doesn't even look at me." Lauren tries to get his attention. "And I'm like, 'Excuse me, excuse me, but do you remember me? I was just here three nights ago?'" As she recalls, he then looked up from her son's chart with a look of confusion. "I don't understand—why is it that you vaccinated your daughter but not your son?"

In that moment, Lauren understood the difference in the treatment she had received. "Wow. This just explains everything to me right there. And I said, 'We didn't vaccinate my daughter—why do you think we did?' And he said, 'That wasn't on the chart. I would have noted that.'" Lauren explained to him they had not gone through triage or patient intake. "Nobody ever asked me because they whisked me right in." She remembers his look of disapproval. "And he said, 'Nobody ever asked you that? . . . Well, that's a problem,' or something and he is just nasty."

Rather than reassuring her this was the manifestation of "a nasty virus going around," as he had with her daughter, he instead expressed concern about more serious issues, including diphtheria or epiglottitis, a symptom of haemophilus influenzae B or Hib, both vaccine-preventable. "We are going to admit him to the hospital. We are going to take all these X-rays. We are gonna do all this stuff."

Lauren argued that the response was ludicrous. "Oh, come on. Like, my daughter was just in here. She was far worse off. You told me, 'I'll see you in three days,' and here I am three days later." She insisted that her son's symptoms did not look like epiglottis, and that diphtheria was un-likely. The physician admitted that his symptoms did not look like Hib, but could nonetheless be the beginnings of it and had to be ruled out. He was unrelenting. "And so he is just nasty and he's like, 'We're admitting him to the hospital. This is what we're doing because you didn't immu-nize.' He was just flat-out, this is the way it's gonna be."

After experiences like these, many parents describe their efforts to steel themselves for future interactions with healthcare providers. Lau-ren, for example, describes her preparations before she takes her son to the emergency room, particularly after experiences like the one de-scribed above, in which an emergency room physician treated her better when he believed that she had vaccinated her kids.

> So I go through and I read all the symptoms for everything so that I'm, like, fully brushed up. . . . And it's been sad because there's been times where I would have, like, rushed my child to the hospital, but I seriously

feel like I need to get out a book and find out, can they possibly blame this on me and not immunizing, and how do I defend myself?

In preparing for providers' disapproval, parents like Lauren see themselves as adversaries to those they must also rely upon to help their children, particularly in times of crisis. They enter these encounters with a view of medicine as inflexible and identify ways to navigate around providers, while maintaining a sense of themselves as good parents. Lauren participates in a broad network of homeschooling families who do not vaccinate and whom she regularly asks for guidance. "I've asked all my friends who don't immunize, 'Oh, what do you do?' 'Oh, well, we lie. We lie.'"

Lauren understands her friends' strategies, particularly in anticipation of disapproval from doctors. Yet she is uncomfortable with their approach, because she wants doctors to most effectively help her children when they need it, which she believes requires having accurate information about their medical histories. Lauren knows that it would be easier to hide the fact that her children are not immunized, but doesn't feel she can. "It's solely, I just want what's best for my children."

Many parents who reject vaccines believe that in emergency room settings, their children are subjected to extra interventions and unnecessary invasive tests. Although these are presented as necessary to rule out vaccine-preventable illnesses, parents perceive them as punishment for their choices. Expecting this treatment, parents describe their laborious efforts to collect information and prepare. Patricia's experience illustrate this. When her nine-year-old daughter complained for several days that she couldn't sleep and was having difficulty breathing, Patricia, believing she had choked on a piece of carrot the day before, took her to the pediatrician, who sent her for X-rays. When doctors could not see the carrot on the X-ray, she was admitted to the hospital for additional tests and was prescribed antibiotics.

Although her daughter was partially vaccinated in the first few years of life, she had not at that point received a vaccine in over five years. Patricia recalls that the hospital pediatrician, upon learning she was partially unvaccinated, "immediately quarantined her and tested her for pertussis [whooping cough]." Patricia thought this was silly, but since she was pregnant at the time and grateful for the private room the quarantine granted her daughter, she agreed. "I was like, okay, private room, I'm not gonna complain. Go ahead and quarantine us. Whooping cough? Whatever. . . . She choked on a carrot."

Facing suspicion that lack of vaccines led to her daughter contracting pertussis, Patricia recalls the sense of relief when her daughter finally coughed up the carrot shard.

> She finally, after all this, coughed up a sliver this long [*holding her index finger and thumb apart*] and *I* was the crazy person. I was like, "Oh, look. Look!" Thankfully there was a nurse in the room who witnessed the whole thing and knew I didn't just bring it in. Because I was like, "Oh, where's the doctor? I want to show him this! How did he miss this?" And then her oxygen returned to normal immediately and they checked us out. Upon checkout, the doctor says, "We'll, um, we'll let you know what the results of the tests were for the whooping cough."

Stories like these were common among parents who opt out of vaccination but still seek medical care when they feel it is necessary. In each account, the individual doctor who doesn't know them is demonized, described as inflexible and lacking in compassion and common sense. In dismissing them, parents reiterate their role as experts on their children's health, even as they require medical attention from others.

Parents are not the only ones who face disapproval when children are unvaccinated. Pediatricians who have unvaccinated patients also believe that hospital-based pediatricians react negatively to their patients and, in turn, them as providers who facilitate those choices. Kevin, for example, notes, "You're talking on the phone to an emergency room doctor and you let them know that they're unvaccinated, and sometimes you feel a little resentment."

Similarly, Ben has observed negative attitudes toward his patients and their families when they encounter other providers. This was clear to him when he went to see one family whose child was admitted to a local community hospital:

> My patient who was hospitalized—when I spoke to . . . the on-call physician—I know she had given them a really hard time because they don't vaccinate their kid. Now, meanwhile, this is a child who is two and a half

years old, has never been sick once, totally unvaccinated—I guarantee you is healthier than this physician, because—eats organic everything, eats more fruits and vegetables than anyone I know. I mean, just basically got unlucky and got RSV[3] and pneumonia and so got admitted to the hospital, and then the physician gave—actually gave me a hard time about them not being vaccinated.

Ben recalls speaking to the hospitalist, who "said something like, 'You know, maybe you should try to get your patients to vaccinate more.' And I said to her, 'Was this a vaccine-preventable illness?' And she was like, 'No.' So I said, 'What does that have to do with anything, then?'"

In the specific, these experiences illustrate how vaccine status becomes a central concern, even when the current health crisis is unrelated to vaccine-preventable disease. More generally, these interactions show how violation of the norms of vaccine participation are policed, even between professionals.

Refusing Patients Who Refuse Vaccines

Parents who seek out pediatricians who won't mind if their children are deliberately unvaccinated are not always successful. One mother recalls, "I was searching for a doctor that we could use and I called probably fifteen practices and asked, you know, 'Can I bring my child here if they're not vaccinated?' 'No. Absolutely not. What are you thinking?' And things like that, so it's hard to find a doctor that will even take you."

Providers, faced with patients who have come to reject vaccines, are increasingly choosing to expel or exclude these families from their practices. In choosing to do so, they voice two overarching concerns. First, they note that they cannot provide high-quality care when patients and their parents do not trust their expertise. Second, these physicians argue that unvaccinated patients present a risk to other patients—particularly infants—in their practice and waiting rooms and they are unwilling to absorb that risk or place other children in jeopardy.

Many parents in this study describe being explicitly or implicitly made to feel uncomfortable as patients in a practice that inflexibly supports vaccination and refuses to accept parents' own crafted healthcare plans. For example, Patricia recalls seeking out a pediatrician to examine her daughter after she was delivered at home because she had a birthmark-like raised skin discoloration, later diagnosed as a hemangioma (a cluster of capillaries not uncommon in newborns that usually disappear over time without treatment). She recalls of her one appointment with that pediatrician,

> She had some discoloration . . . on one side of her body, so I wanted a pediatrician to look at it, and that was the only thing we brought her in for. And he was—he gave us a lecture on vaccines. . . . He said, "Will she be getting shots at this visit?" I said, "No, we're just here for this right now. He goes, "Well, are you doing"—he asked something about vaccines— and I said, "Well, at this time right now we're not vaccinating right now," and he said, "Oh, well, you probably shouldn't come to this practice then, because all our clients are vaccinated."

In Patricia's story, similar to those that others parents recounted, physicians opt not to treat children for other conditions because of their parents' vaccine choices. As parents recall the encounters, they describe the physicians as inflexible, condescending, and dismissive, seemingly unwilling to meet them where they are. Physicians presumably see these new patients as unlikely to be receptive to a trusting relationship, in light of their sense of resolve against vaccines when they enter. Yet physicians often describe themselves as willing to compromise, not because they respect the parent but because they want to protect the child by any means. Carrie, for example, explains her approach:

> I do also have the philosophy of better some than none. And I am not an exclusionist. Like, I won't say—although there is a small part of me that would love to say—"I don't want to see you anymore if you're not gonna do what I say." But I don't. I try to work with families, because you can't punish the child for the parents' poor decision making. So better to get some vaccines on than none.

The second reason to evict families from medical practices—risk to other patients—brings us to a case that was cited periodically in my research, and returns us to Dr. Bob Sears. A measles outbreak drew national attention, in large part because measles had been declared eradicated from the United States in 2000, but quickly reemerged in 2004. In 2008 eleven children in San Diego became infected; the infant who became the sickest was too young to be vaccinated. Critically ill, he was hospitalized and lost one-third of his body weight before finally recovering. He became infected in the waiting room of his pediatrician, Dr. Bob Sears. Dr. Sears's office is organized like that of many pediatricians. It has a side for well patients and a side for sick patients, a distinction the measles virus failed to observe. Unlike most pediatricians, Dr. Sears endorses an alternative vaccine schedule and estimates that 20 percent of his patients are unvaccinated, while another 20 percent are only partially vaccinated.[4] In an online statement, Sears discussed the outbreak in which his measles-infected patient infected other children in his office:

> I believe our nation can tolerate a certain percentage of unvaccinated children without risking the overall public health in any significant way. Since most children are vaccinated, our nation has enough "herd immunity" to contain outbreaks like this one. However, in the San Diego case, some infants caught measles before they were old enough to even be vaccinated. Fortunately, all cases passed without complications, as is usually the case with measles. So the question is, are unvaccinated parents putting the rest of our children at risk? Maybe a little. But in my opinion parents SHOULD have the right to make health care choices for their children. They should not be forced into vaccinating if they feel strongly against it.[5]

Sears was notably unapologetic about the baby's infection in his office. He acknowledges that it was unfortunate, but holds that the parental rights of those who opt out are of greater importance than the rights of the parents of infants to be safe. The 2014 Disneyland outbreak tells a similar story. Those who were exposed at Disneyland traveled home. Experiencing symptoms, they went to doctors' offices and hospitals, where others were exposed, eventually infecting hundreds. These issues are not unique to measles and arise frequently with more common illnesses like pertussis, which reached a high of more than forty-eight thousand cases (and caused twenty deaths) in 2012.[6]

The pediatrician Sarah Cazan is supportive of parents who reject vaccines, having delayed them for her own children. She is also sympathetic to her colleagues who eject unvaccinated children from their practices. "It's pretty valid. I mean, I had—we—at that private practice that I was in—we had a patient who probably got pertussis in the waiting room." Sarah's sympathy for that policy is reinforced by her memories of that two-month-old baby, hospitalized and struggling to breathe, "gasping, not gasping, turning blue," and her concern about whether the baby would suffer long-term complications.

Many parents would be surprised to know that the American Academy of Pediatrics (AAP) and the Centers for Disease Control and Prevention (CDC) actually discourage doctors from evicting patients from primary care practices. As one CDC publication advises physicians,

> When an infant is due to receive vaccines, nothing is more important than making the time to assess the parents' information needs as well as the role they desire to play in making decisions for their child's health, and then following up with communication that meets their needs. When it comes to communication, you may find that similar information—be it science or anecdote or some mix of the two—works for most parents you see. But keep a watchful eye to be sure that you are connecting with each parent to maintain trust and keep lines of communication open.

The statement continues, "Success may mean that all vaccines are accepted when you recommend them, or that some vaccines are scheduled for another day. If a parent refuses to vaccinate, success may simply mean keeping the door open for future discussions about choosing vaccination."[7]

At the same time, national organizations also advise doctors to bring vaccines up at each appointment and to work to build trust and keep communication lines open. While parents may perceive this as badgering, the AAP advises,

> Health care professionals and parents are bound by the duty to seek medical benefit for and minimize harm to children in their care. When faced with the decision to immunize a child, the welfare of the child should be the primary focus. However, parents and physicians may not always agree on what constitutes the best interest of an individual child. In those situations, physicians may need to tolerate decisions they disagree with

if those decisions are not likely to be harmful to the child. Although decision-making involving the health care of children should be shared between physicians and parents, parental permission must be sought before children receive medical interventions, including immunizations. Parents are free to make choices regarding medical care unless those choices place their child at substantial risk of serious harm.[8]

Barbara Loe Fisher, founder of the NVIC, advises parents to be wary of coercion from doctors who threaten eviction should parents refuse their vaccine recommendations. "If your pediatrician or doctor refuses to provide medical care to you or your child unless you agree to get vaccines you don't want, I strongly encourage you to have the courage to find another doctor." In these ways, the CDC, the AAP, and the NVIC are in agreement on the approach doctors should take in respecting parental choice.

Although the AAP directs physicians to work with parents and to respect parents' concerns, the organization also makes available a strongly worded form that parents who refuse vaccination can be asked to sign should a provider feel it is necessary to document the refusal and their efforts to persuade the parents. The form asks parents to acknowledge that they have read the CDC-issued information, have discussed vaccinations with their child's doctor or nurse, have received answers to all their questions, and understand the possible consequences of rejecting vaccines on schedule, which include the following:

- Contracting the illness the vaccine should prevent (The outcomes of these illnesses may include one or more of the following: certain types of cancer, pneumonia, illness requiring hospitalization, death, brain damage, paralysis, meningitis, seizures, and deafness. Other severe and permanent effects from these vaccine-preventable diseases are possible as well)
- Transmitting the disease to others
- Requiring my child to stay out of child care or school during disease outbreaks

The consent form also asks parents to sign the following statement:

My child's doctor or nurse, the American Academy of Pediatrics, the American Academy of Family Physicians, and the Centers for Disease Control

and Prevention all strongly recommend that the vaccine(s) be given according to recommendations. Nevertheless, I have decided at this time to
decline or defer the vaccine(s) recommended for my child, as indicated
above, by checking the appropriate box under the column titled "Declined."
I know that failure to follow the recommendations about vaccination may en-
danger the health or life of my child and others with which my child might
come into contact.
I know that I may readdress this issue with my child's doctor or nurse at any
time and that I may change my mind and accept vaccination for my child
anytime in the future.
I acknowledge that I have read this document in its entirety and fully understand it.[9]

This form aims to help the 85 percent of pediatricians who report encountering a parent who refuses or delays one or more vaccines and the
54 percent who report encountering a parent who refuses all vaccines.
The form is designed to help document that they have informed parents
that their choices are ill-advised. Yet the wording is alienating to parents
and impedes the other professional goals specified elsewhere of building a relationship of trust and respect between a parent and provider.[10]

Sarah is critical of doctors who use the AAP form. She recognizes
how it might be appealing to some physicians, even as she sees it as dis-
respectful to parents:

> My colleague who is a pediatrician wants to post that—something like
> that letter, "We firmly believe" so that she can *not* have to have that con-
> versation at every well-care [appointment]. And I really think that telling
> a parent that this decision, which is keeping [them] awake at night, is
> so—so not important to me. It's not the way that I care to practice.

Kevin describes his approach in his private practice: "We have a vaccine refusal form that we wrote up, which is less inflammatory than the
AAP's, but I honestly don't even always have them sign that. I sometimes
get—I document in my notes that we talked about the risks and benefits
and that I recommend the vaccines." Worrying that the form can potentially foreclose discussion, Kevin continues, "If I do end up giving it
to them or they get it from someone else, I just say, 'This is just that we

talked about this and this is your decision at this point. You can change it at any time.' But that does take a lot of time."

Parents see the form or documentation about them, even in chart notes, as damaging to the physician-parent relationship. Many understand where the physician practices are coming from, but also explain how hurtful being described as noncompliant can feel. One mother explains,

> So that's a prevailing way of thinking in the medical community, which I kind of understand because of liability, and then they have the problem of if they have told you to do something and you don't do it, and they don't have it documented, . . . [but] they have to put all this awful terminology in your chart like "patient refused to comply with my orders," . . . then when you request your medical records and you see the horrible things that they've written about you, you leave.

Parents, even those not evicted from practices, must decide whether and to what extent they want to continue to wrestle in difficult discussions with their children's providers in hopes of developing a relationship of equals. Most describe this as somewhat futile and give up.

The Right to Opt Out: Perceptions of Personal Belief Exemptions

To access schools, camps, or childcare settings, parents either need documentation from health providers stating that their children have received all recommended vaccines or must find a way to exercise an exemption as permitted by the laws in the state where they live. As parents share information about doctors, parenting, nutrition, and vaccines, they also devise complex strategies to circumvent vaccine requirements while still ensuring their children access to these child-centered activities.

All fifty states offer some form of exemption, even as parents see these exemptions as inadequate. Parents share information online and in person about how to navigate requirements and how to opt out within the framework of exemptions that vary across states. In all states, parents may opt out of vaccination for their children for medical reasons. However, using this requirement is difficult since it often requires documentation from a medical provider that a child is vulnerable to adverse reactions from vaccination. In all but three states (Mississippi, West Virginia, and as of 2016, California), parents can exercise an exemption for religious beliefs that oppose vaccination. Most states require a statement to the school or childcare setting—both public and private—describing the religiously held beliefs. Research suggests that the use of religious exemption does not match data on religious belief or vaccine choice and has increasingly become a tool by which nonreligious parents opt out of vaccination requirements.[11] Parents in about eighteen states may use an exemption based on personal or philosophically held beliefs. Claiming an exemption ranges from a signature on a form, to a signed affidavit or essay, to signatures from pediatricians verifying that parents have been educated about risks of opting out. These requirements vary by state. Because vaccine refusal is relatively uncommon, parents from around the country often share information and offer advice online, which means they sometimes embrace strategies geared toward parents in other states to meet legal and regulatory frameworks that don't apply to them. Nonetheless, this information shapes their perception of state policy.

First, parents resent how little information is offered about the availability of exemptions. Even in states that permit exemptions, parents are hard-pressed to get information about their availability. This is not particularly surprising, considering the strong preference that states have in limiting the size of their unvaccinated population. One mother describes her frustration:

> I work at my son's [Waldorf] school, and we are legally not allowed to discuss the exemption forms if people don't ask for them. . . . I still remember the panic I felt when I got the letter (before I started working there) stating that he would not be admitted if his vaccines weren't up to date. I called, saying, "Isn't there an exemption?" And of course there is, but the thing that pisses me off is that we're not allowed to *say it*! I mean, we can say it after they ask, but not technically before.

Margaret also expresses her frustration with hearing how much parents who want to exercise a personal belief exemption are discouraged from doing so by school personnel who communicate vaccine mandates but not options for exemption. She insists, "The only 'mandatory' requirement for schooling is—is to fill out the no [vaccine] schedule. But they never disseminate that information unless they're pressed. . . . And I kept hearing this from other parents. Parents would say, 'They're telling me my child can't go to school.'"

In an effort to advocate for other families, Margaret, whose own children are young adults who remain entirely unvaccinated, sometimes intervenes with schools.

> And I'd call them up and I'd act ignorant. I'd act like I didn't know anything about it. And, sure enough, they'd say, "Oh, yeah. You have to have vaccines." And I'd say, "Well, no, you don't." And so I think it's really essential that parents become really informed and educated. No matter what decision they make, that's their choice, but choice and our rights to do what we feel is best for our children is essential.

Second, parents—even those who have permitted some vaccinations—laboriously manage information about them for fear of jeopardizing claims to an exemption. Heather's explanation of how she registered her son for kindergarten illustrates this. At that time, her son had had one vaccine, not the full required series. Yet she chose not to disclose this to school personnel.

> According to them, he's had none, . . . [be]cause in this state, you know, we have personal exemption, but the way it was explained to me was that you can't just list one vaccine, because if they've seen that he's had one vaccine [you cannot claim an exemption]. Basically, I have an immunization card that I keep in my records at home, and my school has a different immunization record. Because if you have one vaccine, then they can make the case that, "Oh, you don't really object to vaccines on principle, so you need to do it the way we tell you to do it." And they take the choice away. So as far as they know, he hasn't had any.

Similarly, Anna explained her efforts to get only tetanus for her son without that vaccine being entered in the statewide vaccine registry that records immunizations so schools or childcare settings or other health providers can easily verify vaccine status without requiring parents to submit paperwork.

> Tetanus was the first thing that I wanted to make sure he had because that's what he's most likely at a young age to pick up. But I make sure—the way I did it is I went to the health department, . . . as opposed to a family doc where they have to keep records and submit it to the state. If you go to the health department they give you the card yourself.

Both Anna's and Heather's stories illustrate their commitment to exercising their own preferences for their children's healthcare, alongside a sense of entitlement to use public education resources. It also speaks to a fear of state surveillance. In many states, parents who consent to some vaccines may no longer claim a religious or philosophical exemption, since the state assumes that the belief would apply to all vaccines, not some. In fact, Colorado does allow objection to individual vaccines (which many states do not allow). As one Colorado public health official explains to me, their agency would prefer to have children partially vaccinated rather than completely unvaccinated if parents feel concern about only some vaccines. Yet, as parents share information and read online, they share a perception that the state works against parents and come to see potential risks of disclosing to the state. In keeping "real" vaccine records at home while maintaining control over what information is submitted to the school or state-monitored vaccine registry, parents demonstrate the importance of having freedom of vaccine choice and their fear of having it taken away, even if that is unlikely in their own state.

Conditional Rights to Opt Out: Strategizing Religious Exemptions

Parents frequently discuss the stress of figuring out how to exercise an exemption, particularly in states that are more restrictive. These are often laborious processes, sometimes requiring legal consultation or complex strategies for challenging school personnel. One mother's story on a parenting blog in search of advice is illustrative. In an effort to show her daughter that had gained immunity from her first MMR vaccination and should therefore not be required to seek out others, this mother sought out titer testing to check levels of antibodies in her daughter's blood. While tests showed that her daughter had developed immunity against measles, it also indicated that she lacked immunity to mumps and rubella. Having submitted the paperwork, she desperately reached out online:

> Not thinking, I gave the lab sheet to the school nurse and it had the other test results on it—it showed a negative titer for mumps (I should have blacked this part out). The school district doctor is saying with the knowledge they have from the lab sheet I turned in, that my daughter must get another dose of the mumps since she doesn't have immunity to it. Essentially, it means she needs another dose of the MMR. Do you know any argument I can make that might help me in this situation?

Although she recognizes she may have been able to claim a religious exemption at some point, she fears she jeopardized that: "I don't know if I can even use the religious exemption at this point since I've explained all this to the school nurse and she relayed it to the district doctor."

Facing challenges to claims of religious exemption, parents often encourage each other to find new ways to communicate their objections. One mother advises, "If the MMR mumps uses aborted fetuses or something, you might be able to say it's against your religion. I don't remember which ones do or not, but even being Catholic could allow you to slide out of that one."[12] Another mother at a luncheon I attended encouraged others to claim they have rethought their faith after starting vaccines: "You can always find Jesus."

Parents—overwhelmingly mothers—often advise each other to hire attorneys and consult experts on exemptions. Yet they simultaneously communicate their resentment at having to do so. One mother explains in an online discussion,

> The worry about getting into schools, having to be careful about how we formulate our religious exemption letter, the constant politics regarding consent and schools. Its awful! I feel like I'm walking on eggshells sometimes. . . . I just hope that people can humanize everyone's personal choice and leave it alone.

In these ways, parents align interests over a sense of curtailed freedom. As public health expects individuals to acknowledge their interconnections when it comes to disease risk and community health, parents here experience this as a process by which their own parental choices—informed by their sense of expertise—are limited. As one mother explains in exasperation, "Oh my goodness—so outrageous. there should not even be a legal issue w/vaccines. Either you want it or you don't. Shouldn't have to justify yourself." This online discussion, and others like it, illustrate parents' sense of entitlement to their own choices, free of community question, obligation, or approbation.

A large body of research shows how low-income communities live with heightened surveillance and state scrutiny.[13] For privileged parents, vaccine resistance is one of the few issues that result in the social vitriol and state surveillance that are usually reserved for poor families. Many linked this experience to other losses of privacy and autonomy. For example, Marlene, whose children never received vaccines, explains her resentment of state intervention in families' lives:

> There really is a general attitude to move towards womb to tomb tracking, the national ID tracking and immunization tracking, where all of your data—all of your data about any immunizations—is tracked in a federal system from birth to death, and you know our state legislators were really busy trying to change things.

When I ask her how this happens, she elaborates:

> Well, just continue to put more control in the hands of the government. It's the thought that the people aren't smart enough to take care of themselves, so we need the government to do it for us. And I guess I just believe a lot in individual responsibilities and rights. See, I know I'm responsible for my kids.

Cast in this light, state intervention in vaccine choice, supervision of individual health, and public health monitoring through data collection feel invasive in their lives and violate their views of themselves as solely responsible and best qualified to evaluate what their children need.

State Power and Enforcement of Vaccine Compliance

Schools and childcare settings are the most obvious places where state mandates for vaccines are enforced. Yet the state also has the power to quarantine unvaccinated children—even those whose parents declare exemptions that allow their kids to attend school—when outbreaks occur. Carolyn, a mother of three unvaccinated children, has experienced this government power firsthand. When a measles outbreak was reported at the school where her unvaccinated children attend, county health officials placed them in quarantine, ordering them to stay inside the house and away from others. As is routine with outbreaks of vaccine-preventable illnesses, public health officials commonly quarantine children who are not vaccinated and then offer them prophylactic vaccines. Should they consent to the vaccine, they can return to school. If they do not, they will remain in quarantine. Carolyn recalls being angry. "So what they did is that they lined up everybody and gave everybody more shots and if you didn't get shots, then you were supposed to go home." As Carolyn sees it, the school's response was illogical, and the school officials' effort to line up unvaccinated kids increased rather than decreased the risk of infection. "The crazy thing is then if we're exposed, then everybody else [in line or in the school] is exposed."

Parents who reject vaccines are generally skeptical that prophylactic vaccination (or ring containment, where those surrounding the infected person are strategically vaccinated) works. Carolyn continues, "Even though they got their shot, they're still exposed and they're still passing it around if there's an epidemic. But because we didn't comply and get the shot, we were confined to our house." Carolyn's children were sent home from school immediately; she remembers a teacher expressing sympathy for her position. "They were supposed to go on a field trip the next day and the teacher gives me all the homework and everything and she's like, 'You know what? They're—we're all exposed, so I don't know why you have to stay home.'"

Sharing a sense of indignation and feeling galvanized by the teacher's support, Carolyn opted to attend the field trip in spite of the quarantine order; it did not go well. "So I went to the field trip and there were two nurses that were mothers of the kids in the class, and so they went and called Social Services—or not Social Services, they called the health department to send me home. And when they did, they tacked something on my door that said we're quarantined for a week." As she considers the experience, she feels like the disciplinary response and public health posting were largely symbolic: "They knew themselves that I was not any more contagious than anybody else. It's just, we did not comply."

Parents who experience direct surveillance from public health or child welfare agencies see state action as a means to punish their non-conformity, in an effort to bring them into line. For parents whose non-compliance is punished or examined by the state, these experiences are significant in defining their relationship to the state as an adversarial one. Marlene believes that child protective service agencies might investigate her family; she said defiantly, "I'm willing—my husband and I are willing—to take responsibility for the choices we've made because we believe in what we've learned about the bigger picture [about vaccination]."

The pediatrician Ben Kirkland sees how vaccine resistance represents larger questions about healthcare and the state.

> I think there's a real distrust of the medical system and a real distrust of the government in general. I think that's part of it. . . . I think that people don't feel like it's [the government's] 100 percent looking out for their good, and if it is looking out for their good, it might not be looking out for their individual good, but for the sort of greater good, and that doesn't always make sense to people. So I think there's in a way a healthy dose of skepticism.

In these ways—from limiting access to schools and childcare setting parents have selected for their kids, to managing social disapproval or evictions from pediatric practices, to the possibility of quarantine or CPS investigation—resistance to vaccination highlights the role of state power in daily life. Yet distrust of the state also fuels vaccine refusal.

Circumventing Social and Legal Enforcement

Parents who opt out of vaccination for their children do so in a social and legal context in which their decisions are met with disapproval and even legal sanction. They continue to view themselves as experts on their own children and feel that their primary obligation is to their own children. As such, they sometimes find it surprising when they encounter punitive responses and providers' unwillingness to accommodate their choices. As advocates for their own children who have devoted time and resources to educating themselves on vaccines and making decisions they believe are in their children's best interests, parents often feel misunderstood. Yet collectively, through discussions, forums, and social networks, they challenge this stigma and instead identify an obligation to share what they know with other parents whom they view as unenlightened, or to advocate for other parents like them. This may mean communicating their decisions to others, sharing information about how to best manage legal requirements for school attendance, or suggesting how to navigate legal intervention in their families. As parents with resources, they can also suggest ways to work around providers who are inflexible and might refuse to provide their children care, or to advise each other on how to find physicians who will work with them to find common ground, by which they mean acknowledge their expertise as parents.

Unlike most other health interventions, vaccination is enforced by the state and mandates a certain level of surveillance into family life. Although low-income families are often subjected to state surveillance, this is an unfamiliar experience for those who are white and have education and resources. As privileged parents, they want to live comfortably in their privately held beliefs and among their personally set priorities, while also insisting that their children are entitled to fully participate in educational institutions or organizations that offer children opportunities for social engagement.

As one mother explains succinctly,

> My child's vaccination status is no one's business other than mine and his father's. . . . By state law, I do not have to vaccinate him. And that should not preclude me from ANYTHING. School, medical treatment, or oth-

erwise. And I certainly do not believe that is grounds for CPS knocking on my door.

In viewing the state and its obligations as unreasonable invasion, while simultaneously viewing schools and other childcare settings as optimization opportunities to which they are entitled, parents highlight the role of personal choice and individual investment in their own children. Throughout, these parents seldom express how their personal choice comes at the expense of other children.

Conclusion

What Do We Owe Each Other?

Children who do not receive all their vaccines on the schedule set by federal advisory groups pose a challenge for public health systems. Although this book examines parents who deliberately reject or delay vaccines for their children, the most common reason that children are not fully vaccinated nationally is not vaccine refusal, but missed appointments or lack of access.

One pediatrician describes her publicly insured patients who are undervaccinated: "They might not know the schedule and not know when to come in. Or their [child] has been hospitalized forever so they missed it, or that they're just going—for families who have lots of social issues, or they can't afford to make it here travel-wise." These children remain at increased risk of infection, have higher rates of in-patient admission to hospitals when they become sick—even more than children who are unvaccinated by choice—and may have families least able to afford the time needed to care for sick children.[1]

The parents in this book are not these parents. The parents in this book are the ones who have resources, who never forget about vaccinations because they devote a great deal of time and resources to thinking about them. Yet the children whose parents intentionally refuse vaccinations live in the same communities as the larger group of children who lack access or fall behind because of parental limitations in time, money, access, or information. The undervaccinated, rather than the unvaccinated by choice, are already most vulnerable to health challenges and perhaps become even more so when they share grocery stores, malls, parks, community spaces, or schools with an increasing number of unimmunized children. These different children are inevitably connected as members of communities share risk of disease as well as benefits of immunization, even in ways that are not always visible.

Free Choice and Free-Riding

Parents who refuse vaccines perceive risk to their own children to be measurable and manageable, which makes claims that their children increase risk to other children seem illogical. Despite public claims that an outbreak is only "a plane ride away" as vaccine rates drop below herd immunity levels, the parents in this study continue to see vaccines as an individual choice. One mother insists, "If those kids that are vaccinated are truly protected, what chance—why would you be threatened by my child who is not vaccinated?"

This kind of response—that if you think vaccines work and vaccinate your own children, then unvaccinated children pose no threat—is ubiquitous among parents who reject the logic of public health and instead see vaccines as a technology each parent can freely choose or reject. This view ignores the reality that some children are unvaccinated because they lack access, are medically fragile, or are too young. It also denies our interdependence.

Also hidden is the reality that children who are unvaccinated by choice benefit from others' immunity. Public health officials refer to the "free-rider" phenomenon as one that allows a portion of children to reject vaccines without risk of infection because they are essentially protected by the herd—the large segment of the population that is vaccinated. Parents who opt out are often confronted by those who disapprove of them, who erroneously assume that they are unaware of their role as free-riders, but would assume greater shared responsibility if only they knew. In fact, many of the parents I spoke with (although not all) are aware of their families' status as free-riders, but insist that their responsibility to their own children takes precedence.

Some are upset by the accusations that their children are free-riders, claims that violate their sense of themselves as good people. Consistently, that guilt is assuaged by a belief that they are protecting their children. One mother explains, "I know that if nobody had their children vaccinated, there would be polio and there would be diphtheria and there would be everything else, and I recognize that, but at the same time I *feel* like my children, for whatever reason, [would] have some kind of adverse reaction to vaccines."

Many parents acknowledge that the ability to opt out is a luxury, and recognize that it would be riskier to do so if everyone made the same choice. Yet concern for their children outweighs concerns for herd immunity. One mother explains how she weighed free-riding against shared responsibility:

> I think that ultimately my husband and I felt like we were making a little bit of an elitist decision, meaning that we're banking on the fact that most of the rest of the country is vaccinated. . . . If you believe that there is a potential adverse effect of vaccinations, then you're riding off the fact that everybody else is exposing their kid to those potential adverse effects. So your kid no longer really is at risk. . . . That was the most compelling of the counterarguments we heard, for sure.

There must be a balance between efforts to promote population health, from which we all benefit, and support for the concepts of consent, bodily integrity, and individual choice in healthcare. These issues are complex and representative of a wide array of public health issues, not just vaccines. Yet they are central to understanding when and how we assume risk to support the most vulnerable among us. What do we owe each other? Our privilege to participate in civil society is arguably inextricably linked to our obligation to protect that community, even at some personal potential cost.

Vaccine resistance then represents an individual sense of entitlement to use public resources without shared responsibility to others. As parents claim individual expertise and the right to make their own choices, they do so while continuing to claim that their children are *entitled* to public resources like publicly funded education or use of public spaces like parks, while opting out of public obligation. At heart, the willingness to be free-riders while demanding access to community resources may be one reason why parents who opt out experience high levels of vitriol and disapproval from others.

Expecting resources without contributing to community health represents a certain breach of responsibility. One vaccine policy researcher and pediatrician suggests that there is social significance in these individual choices and supports parents' rights to exercise them. However, she also argues that children who opt out of community health programs like vaccination are not entitled to community participation, including public schools:

> This is a social contract. There are things provided to you and things you have to do. I don't know where that got lost. I think that's a very important thing to understand, whether these people don't perceive or how they don't perceive it applies to them, particularly vis-à-vis public school. Why should kids who are unimmunized be in public school? I have a problem with that. I actually don't have a problem with saying, "You know what? If you're not immunized, you're not going to be in public school. You can homeschool and we'll help you." To me, that's a reasonable statement. Why are you allowed to put other people's kids at risk? I think that it's a complicated situation, but I actually think the whole idea of the social contract is being lost.

The rhetoric of a social contract was common, but not without contention. As one opponent of vaccines announced to a cheering audience of like-minded people at a national meeting in opposition to vaccine mandates, "I don't remember signing a contract!"

Outside the vaccine context, there are few places where our social contract with each other is debated so regularly and openly. We seldom hear reference to social contract when discussing school funding, votes on bonds, taxes, traffic safety, public assistance, fracking, social security, or environmental policy. Even the significant public health programs that limit smoking in community spaces are more often framed as efforts to protect individual rights, rather than an expression of our communal investment in one another's well-being. Yet proponents of vaccines on all sides and ideologies insist we have a social contract that vaccine refusers violate. Even the libertarian-leaning Cato Institute references our social contract:

> There is no reason to be vaccinated against non-communicable diseases if you don't want to. If you believe that your small chance of getting tetanus isn't worth the (very, very) much smaller risk of crippling Guillain-Barré syndrome after the vaccination, that's your business. But vaccination for communicable diseases is part of a social contract that maintains civil society with a general ethic that no one has the right to harm someone

without serious provocation. The fact that someone else may avoid vaccination gives no license to avoidably infect that person, however foolhardy
he or she might be.[2]

Parents most certainly should advocate for their children, but taking advantage of opportunities involves obligations to invest in others'
children too, obligations that are arguably higher for those who have
the best access to high-quality food, healthcare, schools, housing, and
resources. Vaccines highlight the interplay between community risk and
benefit, even as these same extensions of a social contract exist more
broadly.

Building Trust in the Search for Middle Ground

Vaccine resistance is not new and is unlikely to go away. Yet public
health agencies and pediatric providers can build greater trust in vaccine safety and claims of necessity. Their strategies will not change how
privileged parents trust their own expertise over others', but might—for
those who feel uncertain in their decisions and feel their children face
risk with or without vaccines—give them ways to trust public health
more and participate in community immunity. These recommendations
won't resolve distrust of the public sector, but might begin to close the
gap in a polarizing debate.

Stop Marketing Vaccines as Only for Individual Benefit

As shown throughout the book, parents insist that they are experts on
their own children and are best suited to evaluate what their children
need. As consumers, they weigh perceptions of the likelihood of infection, their understanding of the severity of the illness, the risk of vaccines,
and whether they believe that the vaccine will decrease or increase those
risks. Parents consider disease prevalence, vaccines' efficacy, or possible adverse effects of vaccines, including perceived weaknesses in their
children's general health. Parents' insistence that they are best qualified
to make healthcare decisions for their children draws on deep cultural
expectations by which parents generally and mothers specifically are
defined as uniquely responsible for children's health.

Since the early nineteenth century, advertisements to promote the vaccine against diphtheria drew on maternal responsibility and self-interest, rather than community well-being (as smallpox had).[3] The vaccine of course did achieve herd immunity, which is why churches, schools, cities, insurance companies, women's magazines, health departments, and charitable organizations all promoted the vaccine. Yet their effort to persuade women that vaccines were a responsible choice good mothers make has proven durable. Current vaccine campaigns illustrate this, like the CDC's National Infant Immunization Week's slogan, "Love them. Protect them. Immunize them";[4] or the campaign by the national organization Every Child By Two, which advises, "Being a parent is a big responsibility, and the best thing you can do for *your* child's health is to learn the facts so that you can make the best choices" (emphasis added).

Efforts to mobilize vaccination by appealing to parents' love for their children communicates that vaccines are for individual benefit. This ignores the reality that public health systems invest in vaccines and promote them at great cost because they promise *societal*, not just individual, benefits. This frame, for example, undermines claims for vaccines like rubella that largely protect fetuses and pregnant women in the community but provide little individual benefit to young children, and virtually none to boys. Privileged parents who sift through myriad sources of information to feel informed and in control accept the responsibility but don't necessarily reach the conclusions that the pharmaceutical companies or public health agencies believe are self-evident.

Own Uncertainty

Pediatricians, public health officials, and even popular media present a uniform narrative that vaccines are an absolute good.[5] As a result, those who question vaccine safety are dismissed as heretics. This in large part owes to the significant impact vaccines have had in lowering infectious diseases, even eradicating some, and improving community health. Yet medical practitioners know that these interventions do introduce some level of risk: manufacturers have erred in vaccine production and people have been harmed, but even when vaccines are made perfectly, they sometimes don't work or sometimes trigger an adverse reaction. Although much data suggest that parents dramatically overestimate the risks of vaccines, many providers and public health groups might be too eager to dismiss these risks and shortcomings for fear of encouraging parents to opt out.[6] Asserting the dominant narrative that vaccines are always good, we lose the ability to discuss these uncertainties, which, in turn, fuels distrust of authority and a broader misunderstanding of science.

Pediatricians who aim to support parents in making their own choices know they cannot provide sufficient assurances to parents who fear all possibilities. For example, Sarah supports her patients and their families, even when children develop whooping cough or other vaccine-preventable disease, but is clear that she cannot promise parents that everything will always work out. Rather, she acknowledges the uncertainty inevitable in both vaccines and disease and thus wants parents to make their own decisions—in consultation with her—and feel empowered in their choices:

> If your decision has made you fearful, . . . that's a really tough place to be as a parent. To be so in the middle of and surrounded by fear, . . . I can't appease you. I cannot say you're not gonna get exposed to pertussis and you're not gonna get sick. . . . I can also not say to you that I guarantee you shots aren't gonna make you sick—I just can't.

The unknowability of children's lives is a source of anxiety for a large number of middle-class and affluent parents who believe that with careful cultivation, intentional consumption, and laborious attention, their children will thrive.[7] Rather than communicating a sense of certainty that can be earned through consumption or vigilance, we may be better served by acknowledging how specific outcomes are unknowable, even as all risks are not equal.

Stating that some risk is unknowable should not distract from the battery of data that we do know a great deal. The minute risk vaccines present can be interpreted in the context of known risks. This leads to uncomfortable acknowledgment that some diseases have not been seen in decades, but require continued vaccine to stay away, as is the case with polio—though most parents who read extensively already know that—or harder conversations about why parents who do not fear illness or missed days at work should take the vaccine against varicella seriously. Continuing to find ways to acknowledge parents' fears and build toward a sense of what is known, knowable, and beyond prediction may help.

Create Greater Transparency in Vaccine Policy

In the course of this research, I discovered how little is known about how vaccine schedules are set. This leads to the widespread misperception that children receive too many vaccines and concerns about new ones. Although most parents see some vaccines as useful, like the one against tetanus, they perceive others, like influenza or varicella, to be unjustified. Arguments for herd immunity as a reason for increasing vaccination also ring hollow as new vaccines that are largely for individual benefit—like HPV—are proposed for mandates.[8] One state vaccine policy maker acknowledges during our interview that early efforts to require HPV in some states damaged parental trust of all vaccines. Although he supports the widespread use of the vaccine, he argues that states must prioritize easily transmitted infectious diseases in their mandates:

> I believe that contagion should be considered. So, for example, HPV is not contagious in the classroom and should not come to have a school regulation based on a vaccine that would save lives but is not at all related to education. And I think in some ways they [mandates] have been misused as a coercive tool and it's going to come back and have a negative effect by people that are opposed to vaccines.

Parsing out when vaccines should be required is complicated. For those who believe that vaccines are intrinsically good, the more vaccines the better. Disease causes uncertainty and vaccines can prevent that, as terrifying diseases for which there are not vaccines remind us. In the fall of 2014, enterovirus 68 (EV-D68) infected thousands of children throughout the United States, and at least a dozen children died. More perplexing, in Colorado and then around the country, about seventy-five of the children infected between the ages of one and eighteen developed signs of paralysis and limb weakness.[9] Although the CDC is uncertain whether EV-D68 caused the paralysis, the virus belongs to the same family of enteroviruses as polio. Polio too appeared as a mild virus in some and a paralyzing one in others, and like polio, most of the kids who showed signs of paralysis were otherwise healthy. Healthcare workers with whom I spoke from the Children's Hospital of Colorado, the first hospital to describe clusters of paralysis with EV-D68 infection, all describe their sense of disbelief, frustration, and the inexplicability of the variation of symptoms between children—even siblings. "We know how to make vaccines against enteroviruses," one exasperated hospital-based physician mentioned.

There is little doubt the families of affected children would welcome a vaccine that would have protected them from the difficulties they now face. Parents who live in fear of the uncertainty of disease might also embrace a new vaccine. Yet I wonder how the families of the other children—who developed respiratory symptoms that resolved in seven to ten days—would feel about another vaccine against an otherwise in-nocuous disease. Might the calculus look different if they were offered a vaccine against Ebola, a disease that also created panic in the United States in the fall of 2014, despite no domestic transmissions of the virus beyond a few healthcare workers in U.S. hospitals?[10] The U.S. prom-ise to pharmaceutical makers that they are protected from legal claims "related to the manufacturing, testing, development, distribution and administration" of new Ebola vaccines, which will likely also be eligible for expedited approval, will also matter as parents weigh the necessity, safety, and trustworthiness of that vaccine.[11] Parents must be given a clearer understanding of the processes involved in companies' decisions to pursue vaccines against some illnesses over others, to add vaccines to what is seen as an already crowded schedule, to seek long patents on new vaccines that the state might require, or to secure immunity from liability.

Address Profit Incentives

The decisions to pursue vaccines against some diseases but not others reside largely with pharmaceutical companies, which as publicly traded companies, are legally bound to attempt to earn a profit. Several websites that oppose vaccine mandates detail the profit motives that appear to be inextricably linked to vaccine policy. This connection undermines the trustworthiness of vaccines. One vaccine policy researcher and pediatrician recognizes this: "Well, you know, a lot of these problems are created by the fact that we have a market system, the marketplace is responsible for vaccine development and vaccine delivery. That carries inherent problems. Until we want to change that, we're going to have those problems."

Many parents who object to the widespread use of vaccines understand some of how vaccines are made and scheduled and feel distrustful of who makes them and which agencies regulate them to ensure safety. In one simple example, the vaccine researcher and pediatrician Paul Offit is often referred to online as "Paul Profit" since his research led to the creation of the most widely used vaccine against rotavirus, which made him a great deal of money. He is a vocal advocate for vaccination, participates in policy discussions, and speaks out against those who oppose vaccines. He described to me their efforts to dismiss him:

> You're gonna always have that group of people who think there is a big conspiracy. I mean, I think I'm the poster boy for that conspiracy. They see me as simply in it for the money, which is ridiculous. First of all, explain the logic to me. I work twenty-five years in development of a vaccine so I can make money, so I can lie about that, make a vaccine that has the capacity to save two thousand lives a day, so I can make money, so I can lie about vaccine safety so I can hurt children?

Offit recognizes that he is seen as "part of the vaccine industry, or pharmaceutical company, pharmaceutical-doctor complex"; he receives hate mail regularly and threats occasionally. Offit's vaccine is credited with preventing more than 1.5 million emergency room or doctor visits and over $924 million in healthcare costs between 2007 and 2011 in the United States alone.[12] Those who are grateful for lifesaving vaccines respect him and see him as a tireless advocate for public health who puts himself in front of the issue at some personal cost. Offit as an icon in this debate provides one example of how challenging it is to pull apart for-profit vaccine development, expertise, and parental distrust.

That a handful of for-profit pharmaceutical companies manufacture all the country's vaccines (and cannot be sued in state or federal court because of liability protection granted by Congress in 1986) drives suspicions. Despite vaccines' place in the marketplace, the relative profit-ability of vaccines is subject to debate. One researcher explains to me, "Vaccines are not big money makers, for an obvious reason. They're something you take once for a few times in your lifetime. You know, they're not like lipid-lowering agents or neurological drugs."

Offit too insists that vaccines represent a small portion of profits to pharma. Comparing the vaccine against rotavirus, which is still patent-protected, to other pharmaceutical products, he explains,

> Rotavirus makes about $500 million a year roughly. . . . That's not much money. Lipitor is a $13 billion a year product, that is one of several lipid-lowering agents. When you're taking a drug every day and you have an adult population that's taking it every day, that's huge, as compared to—I mean there's 300 million people in this country, there's a birth cohort of 3.5 million people. That's nothing.

Many public health advocates argue that the limited profitability is why so few companies manufacture vaccines. One ACIP member com-pares vaccines, which frequently face shortages, to other products that serve no public health goal, like products to treat hair loss:

> If Propecia ever went down because of a manufacturing problem, we would not have a potency product shortage, or a hair loss product short-age, because the infrastructure there is solid. But look what happens with vaccines. At the end of every ACIP [meeting], we go through vaccine shortages, because there's at most two companies that make any vaccine. Some companies are just one. . . . If it was such a great market, where are the other companies?

Vaccines represent about 10 percent of pharmaceutical company revenue, which may be one of the reasons few companies manufacture most vaccines. Yet older vaccines provide stable income from products that require little research, development, or marketing, and are legally mandated to be consumed, all of which makes parents skeptical. Critics of vaccines search the motives of manufacturers for signs of trustworthi-ness, with pharmaceutical companies often coming up short. Identifying how to address these concerns more directly and with more transparency would help to allay fears about vaccine safety, even as they are unlikely to entirely solve them.

Earn Trust in Regulators

Members of the ACIP design vaccine schedules; then, often with the endorsement of national medical organizations, states adopt those recommendations and enforce them through school attendance. Whether parents see vaccine schedules as reliable is often tied to perceptions of the members who create recommendations. One factor that undermines trust is the revolving door between government and industry.

The concept of a revolving door, by which members of a regulated industry subsequently join regulatory agencies, or regulators leave and join a regulated industry, is not new and has been discussed for more than fifty years.[13] In 2005 the Revolving Door Working Group, comprising members of trade organizations, nonprofits, consumer advocacy groups, and government accountability groups, found that the revolving door "increases the likelihood that those making policies are sympathetic to the needs of business—either because they come from that world or they plan to move to the private sector after finishing a stint with government."[14]

The revolving door is one way of explaining how regulations fail and how widespread conflicts of interest may go unchecked. This is yet another source of parents' distrust of vaccine safety. For example, the ACIP includes researchers who have conducted basic research that has created vaccines, been paid to run clinical trials to license vaccines, or consulted for pharmaceutical companies. Even when members of the committee have an identifiable financial interest in the vaccine under review and are not allowed to vote, they may still participate in—and arguably influence—discussion.[15] Pharmaceutical companies also hire former government officials without time between public service and private contract. Although on the surface, this seems reasonable, it allows parents to extrapolate that there had already been a close relationship between the parties who might otherwise be adversaries. Julie Gerberding provides one clear example.

An infectious disease specialist, Dr. Gerberding joined the CDC in 1998 and became acting director in 2001, then permanent director in 2002. In this role, she "led the agency during more than 40 emergency response initiatives for health crises including anthrax bioterrorism, food-borne disease outbreaks, and natural disasters, and advised governments around the world on urgent public health issues such as SARS, AIDS, and obesity."[16] She is well respected and has been honored with numerous awards, ranging from *Time* magazine's 100 Most Influential People in the World to a government award for distinguished service. In 2009 Gerberding left the CDC and became president of Merck's vaccine division. She is simultaneously a member of the Institute of Medicine (IOM), the health arm of the National Academy of Sciences, which is an independent organization, charged with advising the government and private sector on scientific knowledge (including vaccine safety). Her IOM profile describes her accomplishments at Merck, which include overseeing "Merck's current portfolio of vaccines, planning for the introduction of vaccines from the company's pipeline, and accelerating efforts to broaden access to Merck's vaccines around the world."[17]

Gerberding's move from one of the most powerful governmental positions in the country for health policy and public health regulation to Merck, one of the largest vaccine manufacturers in the world, does little to assure parents who already distrust vaccines that the safety of vaccines is appropriately evaluated, monitored, and enforced—or that calls for more vaccines in response to, say, outbreaks, disasters, or bioterrorism are reasonable or impartial.

This close relationship goes far beyond vaccine policy but is illustrative of the broader entanglement of for-profit corporations and the state. U.S. Supreme Court decisions like *Citizens United v. Federal Election Commission* (2010), which recognized First Amendment free speech rights of corporations; or *Burwell v. Hobby Lobby* (2014), which constitutionally protected the religious beliefs of privately held for-profit corporations, including the right to block healthcare coverage for individual employees who wish to use contraceptives as part of their health insurance; or the 2015 decision *Michigan v. Environmental Protection Agency* (2015), which requires the EPA to consider costs to companies before regulating toxic emissions, further erode individual trust that the government has placed individuals' needs above those of corporations. Parents' anxieties about the seeming proliferation of chemicals and lack of environmental regulation of toxins also reflect this. The increasing number of government and corporate partnerships, including the FDA's "pay-to-play" model, which requires pharmaceutical companies to financially support the agencies that regulate them, undermines faith in public institutions charged with ensuring public safety. In these ways, parents who on one hand embrace their roles as neoliberal consumers—committed to individual choice—also express distrust in neoliberal state policies that have eroded consumer protection and regulation.

Eradicate the Culture of Mother Blaming

There is no way to examine these meticulous and laborious healthcare decisions without considering how they are situated in a culture in which mothers are presumed to be responsible for children's well-being and blamed for children's failures. Not surprisingly, these mothers take this to heart. They reconfigure professional lives to practice what they think is good mothering and to be available to intensively invest in their children—be it with nutrition, education, or healthcare. Throughout, they work to define themselves as good mothers in contrast to those who fail to invest similarly in their children; the time and resources employed remain invisible.

The norms dictating that mothers should question more, ask more, and invest more become observable as mothers speak of regret. When they recall following expert advice rather than their own sense of intuition, they express remorse. For example, one mother who delayed vaccines explained her sense of failure: "You know, as a mother, I really wish I would have taken my instincts more seriously at the beginning, because I think actually going to alternative health [providers] would have been a benefit to anybody." Statements like these—from parents whose kids fared well with the care they did receive—show how mothers evaluate their success by examining the *process* of reaching decisions and their relative sense of control. This makes sense in light of how women also evaluate the quality and success of childbirth experiences in terms of their sense of control, their perceived ability to exercise what they described as their natural wisdom during the birth experience, and their ability to limit medical interventions.[18] With vaccine resistance, we see that these pressures on mothers are boundless.

Mothers understand the significance of decisions for their children and feel responsible for making good ones, messages that have been communicated in U.S. health promotion campaigns, parenting magazines, and social interactions for decades. They are willing to work hard to step away from the herd and are proud of their ability to do so. One mother left a demanding job she felt was damaging to her health and well-being to instead focus on her child. She sees herself as having freed herself from social pressures that pushed her into a toxic workplace, as well as those that expect parents to follow vaccine recommendations, and now aims to set her own path:

> I still have judgments about just doing stuff blindly, but I don't have any bottom-line decision about whether it is better to immunize your kids. . . . I don't know, but that is the choice that I made. I don't have any judgment other than the judgment against stupidity and people just, like, do it because everybody else does. What everybody else does really isn't working for the world at large, at least within this country of ours.

Mothers who refuse vaccines rely on a complex combination of information, intuition, and relative confidence in their own natural ability as mothers to make good decisions for their children. They do not always tout their way as best, but reiterate the individualist nature of parental decisions—and outcomes. As one mother explains, "Just to blindly follow or not follow doesn't seem wise to me, because ultimately I would be responsible."

Mothers who reject vaccine recommendations and challenge medical experts are most likely to have resources on which to draw. The gendered work of mothering requires women to actively strategize in support of their own children, but not necessarily all children, sometimes embracing and other times rejecting expert advice. They do so on their own terms, largely without fear of state intervention in their families. This is not to say they do not experience social disapproval or challenges in interactions with healthcare providers or schools. However, these unpleasant interactions carry limited consequences for them. What is clear is that as mothers face social vitriol for opting out of public health, they also face criticism for other outcomes, including disabilities they fear their children could develop, learning disabilities that could manifest, or behavioral problems schools will ask them to address. Shifting the cultural rhetoric so mothers are empowered to make informed decisions for their children while not assigning them all the blame for possible outcomes might create a kinder landscape for all mothers, which in turn might allow mothers to trust others with their children—and in turn, to share responsibility for others.

Ensure Reciprocity for the Herd

As discussed, parents who prioritize individual choice do so as free-riders. They can feel relatively secure opting out of vaccines in a community where a high portion of children are vaccinated and disease prevalence is relatively low. These parents free-ride off of others' immunity and reject demands that they have an obligation to others. As one pediatrician explains, "I always tell people, too, especially with newborns, it really does take a village. You need help, you have to reach out and get help. The flip side of that is, you've got to protect that village. You need to help with that village." Vaccine-refusing parents do not express a sense of obligation to others. This may reflect larger ideologies that support individualist parenting, isolate families from each other, and create communities where the proverbial herd does little for the individuals, too.

To conceptualize vaccines as a social obligation or requirement further erases individual choice. As children and their families increasingly face a growing number of generic bureaucracies, they feel constrained.[19] Government programs—including but not only for vaccine mandates—were enacted to ensure a minimal level of care for all families. Counterintuitively, these same programs may shape relationships among unequals, coercing compliance for some, while broadening choice for others. Colorado's enforcement policies illustrate this: despite liberal access to personal belief exemptions, families who receive public assistance may be required by federal agencies to demonstrate compliance with current recommended vaccines to maintain eligibility and avoid sanctions.[20] Outside the vaccine context, we can see how families who receive public assistance face ridicule from those who reject the logic that we should support the most vulnerable among us, even with food.

They instead tout the importance of individualism or express resentment that the state helps some families while doing little for theirs.

None of the participants of this study were receiving public assistance at the time we met. However, they share a broader view that more rigid requirements and increased bureaucracy serve organizational interests more than those of the people who seek care. This inflexibility—a one-size-fits-all approach—is seen as eliminating possibilities for more fluid and reciprocal relationships where individual preferences, goals, and needs are taken into consideration. The growth, for example, of charter schools, or school choice processes, which were also intended to create justice for children in failing schools, are disproportionately used by white affluent families to individualize their children's education.[21] We are left with a challenge: social equity programs usually come with expectations for social participation, yet choice remains most available to those with the resources to opt out when they so choose, while still claiming public resources they want.

In these ways, vaccine choices represent parents' desires to carve their own preferences, away from the pack. This matters because they see the pack as failing individual families. Vaccine resistance emerges from broader distrust of the public sector and a sense that those charged with ensuring public safety and individual liberty fail to do so. This is a complex balance. Individuals want the ability to express unfettered preference, while also ensuring that each of their options is safe, reliable, affordable, and authentic. The latter requires regulation, while the former is often positioned as best facilitated by lack of regulation—and a prioritization of individual choice.

The most passionate opponents of vaccine mandates claim the importance of individual choice. Challenging medical recommendations and state insistence on vaccines, the NVIC founder, Barbara Loe Fisher, insists that individual preference is key:

> I do not tell anyone what risks to take and never will. The right and responsibility for making a risk decision belongs to the person taking the risk. When you become informed and think rationally about a risk you or your child will take—and then follow your conscience—you own that decision. And when you own a decision, you can defend it. And once you

can defend it, you will be ready to do whatever it takes to fight for your freedom to make it, no matter who tries to prevent you from doing that.[22]

For those who focus on the centrality of individual liberty, collective responsibilities seem irrelevant. These views insist on individual rights and responsibilities, but also reflect the social reality that families in the United States do not perceive community support to be improving their lives. Middle-income families see higher levels of economic downturns, and even when they participate in social institutions like public schools, they continue to see demands for more private investment.[23] In short, it is difficult for families to identify how the herd is supporting their families, even as they are asked to accept risk for the benefit of others. Vaccine requirements in the 1960s and 1970s were aimed to create access as part of the War on Poverty and Great Society programs. They aimed to equalize access to health for all children. Yet they have over time become perceived as a way the state requires public participation without also providing support that increases the well-being of all families. Gaining trust from families so they will feel responsible for protecting the herd requires supporting them so they perceive that the herd is helping them too.

Vaccine Resistance in Perspective

Vaccine resistance, practiced most commonly by those with the greatest access to resources and education, raises fundamental questions about individual choice, bodily integrity, community responsibility, and individuals' relationship to the state. These important questions are bigger than vaccine choice. However, increasingly we see parents who reject vaccines or rework medical knowledge to meet their own preferences presented as one side of a two-sided debate, even as they are significantly lopsided positions, with many more than two sides. As healthcare providers, parenting blogs, and popular media call for greater dialogue about vaccines, it is easy to lose sight of the reality that most parents want vaccines and feel grateful that they are available. As one pediatrician explains, "I would say that the large majority of our patients come in and say thank you very much for the vaccinations."[24]

Many parenting blogs have arisen in the last few years in support of vaccination, including Voices for Vaccines, Informed Parents of Vaccinated Children, Families Fighting Flu, and Shot of Prevention, which is cohosted by a mother who lost her child to pertussis. These and other sites, including those of government and advocacy organizations, include first-person narratives of parents whose children have been harmed by vaccine-preventable disease, who have changed their views on vaccines, or who share why they choose to vaccinate.[25] They tell the stories of parents who made the wrong choice and lost their child, or came to see the light and accepted vaccines. Yet many of these also include a desire to protect all children, to do the right thing, or to avoid infection with diseases previous generations worked hard to defeat. Although individual benefit plays some role, there is a clear effort to acknowledge community responsibility. There are other signs that community responsibility may increasingly become a part of vaccine discussion. One 2014 study found that more than 80 percent of parents believe that preschool children should be current on their vaccinations, with 74 percent saying they would consider removing their children from a care facility in which 25 percent or more children were unvaccinated.[26] These views represent concerns for one's own children, but also new institutional pressures to protect all children. Laws passed in California and Vermont in 2015 to limit personal belief exemptions may also suggest that the tides are turning.

In the United States, at least 80 percent of new parents intend to fully vaccinate their children, and many follow the ACIP schedule.[27] Even among those parents, however, as many as 25 percent express concerns about vaccine safety.[28] Something happens as parents learn more about vaccines. My findings suggest that much of this emerges from larger cultural definitions of what it means to be a good parent, to fully invest in one's own child, and to feel as though risk is controllable through vigilance, information gathering, and desire.

Although opting out remains an elite phenomenon, these broader questions of trust, community, individuality, and shared responsibility are not. In the course of conducting this research, I explored the corners of the debate—the one that holds vaccine-injured children and the other than holds children killed or disabled by vaccine-preventable illness. I see parents' fear of the uncertainties that surround children, and I sometimes share them. I also recognize the pressures on parents to anticipate all possible outcomes and aim to control for them. As we share schools, communities, resources, and risk, infectious disease cannot remain a private concern, nor can we rely on individual resources to protect our own children. We can do better and deliver higher-quality public health worthy of our collective trust, but in the end, we must find ways to protect each other's children and support everyone's family.

Billy—like almost all the parents in this study—was generous with his time. He invited me into his immaculate home, in which angel statues and lace doilies in almost every room illustrate the care he lavishes on his home and family, which includes his disabled teen son, elementary-aged daughter, and wife, who works full-time. His son, Christian, consumes most of Billy's time and energy, as he lives in a minimally conscious state, showing some evidence of awareness of his environment, seemingly enjoying an electric fish tank, for example, but without the ability to interact.[1] When I came over to interview Billy, we began by watching videos of his son as a healthy nine-month-old baby, spinning and bouncing in a doorway hanging bouncer, much like the one my own kids had loved at the same age. We talked for several hours altogether—about Billy's family, his background, his relationship with his wife. He told me how his son had developed a seizure disorder as a toddler and over several years of intractable seizures, was left without any ability for voluntary movement or communication. Only years later did a neurologist suggest that Christian's condition may have been caused by the now-discontinued DPT vaccine.

Driving home from Billy's house, I was distracted by the details of his story. I was about to take my own then nine-month-old baby to his pediatrician for the same round of vaccines Billy identified as possibly causing his child's seizures, even as the suspected vaccine had been reformulated years ago because of safety concerns. With my two older children, I had never questioned whether to consent to the federally recommended vaccine schedule. Yet Billy's experience and my visceral understanding of his sadness and regret as a parent gave me pause.

Studying at Eye Level

My ability to empathize with Billy as a parent making the same choices is but one way that I was similarly situated to the participants of my study. Most of these parents were around my age, of my race, and live in similarly middle-class worlds; most were college-educated and white, like me. As I listened to parents describe their process of rejecting vaccination or regretting their prior consent to vaccines, I usually understood their feelings of vulnerability or guilt in watching a happy baby burst into tears and then glance up, bottom lip quivering, with a look that communicates shock and betrayal. I understood how much harder commission is than omission—to have solicited a potential risk (of an adverse reaction), rather than passively accepting unknown risk (in this case, the risk of infection). Unlike these parents, I do not challenge vaccine recommendations and do not regret having fully vaccinated my three children. Throughout this study, I was both an insider and outsider to these social worlds.[2] This position raised new issues for me about what it means to "study across," or at eye-level, questions with which I grappled throughout the study.

This position was also salient for the participants. Many followed up by e-mail after our interview, called to check in, or communicated their goals for my work to me. Some made clear during interviews and e-mails that they had Googled me, read my articles, or checked my first book out of the library to evaluate my fairness in representing participants' positions. As I have elaborated elsewhere, parents appeared to understand how researchers have the power to represent them and felt empowered to provide input not just on my efforts to capture their stories, but on how they would like to see me use the data as well.[3]

Studying Vaccine Policy, Practice, and Preference

I came to study vaccine resistance by following a path that was full of twists and turns. My first book, *Fixing Families: Parents, Power, and the Child Welfare System*, examined the experiences of parents and the expectations of the system charged with protecting children and rehabilitating families.[4] After more than five years of following drug-addicted parents through the bureaucratic hoops that would more often mystify than help them regain custody of their children, I was tired. I searched for a new project topic that would allow me to continue to examine how families navigate state policy. In 2003, while I was a postdoctoral fellow in health policy at the University of California, San Francisco, I glanced at the front page of the *New York Times* to see then-president George Bush receiving a vaccine against smallpox, a long-eradicated disease that his administration theorized could be used in bioterrorism.

In the months leading up to this photo, vaccines were a hot topic at my house as well. My husband, Dave, was completing his residency in pediatrics, and he and several of my friends at the medical campus where I worked were asked to get the new smallpox vaccine because they were likely first responders in these hypothetical bioterrorist attacks, but were too young to have been vaccinated against it as children. Dave and I discussed whether he could safely be vaccinated without shedding live virus near our children and questioned how safe the vaccine was.

Others' questions of vaccine safety also filled out home, as Dave frequently saw children admitted to the hospital with acute episodes of vaccine-preventable illnesses. Their parents always seemed to him to be surprised by how sick their children had become, adding to his frustration. One particularly memorable day, he worked later than usual. He was struggling to call the state poison control office to mobilize the shipment of enough antitoxin from various locations to treat a boy who had been airlifted to the children's hospital with full-blown tetanus: lockjaw and spinal curvature caused by the neurotoxins released into his bloodstream by the bacteria found in soil all around him. Tetanus is rare due to high vaccine rates, and antitoxin, therefore, is hard to procure and very expensive. As Dave relayed the tragedy to me, he explained with disbelief, the child's father "just kept saying that he really thought tetanus had been eradicated."

The hypothetical risks of bioterrorism that evolved daily (from calls for duct tape on windows to pronouncements of vaccines for all early responders in disasters), my front-row seat observing pediatric trainees' experiences at a publicly funded children's hospital, and my own experience of navigating vaccines for my children (then an infant and a three-year-old) in a region with high levels of vaccine resistance collectively led me to this research and provided me an important viewpoint from which to observe this issue.

In the summer of 2003 I enrolled in an intensive course that provided training in clinical research, including research design, grant writing, institutional negotiations, and professional development. For the course I was assigned to a workgroup consisting mostly of U.S.-

trained physicians and a few other clinicians. The group included a Thai psychologist working on HIV and AIDS outreach in Bangkok, and two Ugandan physicians who were also affiliated with the university's AIDS center. Our group leader, a biostatistician, tried to thoughtfully provide feedback, even as my qualitative approaches challenged him. Each week, we presented our research topics to each other and looked for suggestions. Mine was uniquely and consistently met with confusion, not only because I am a sociologist who collects qualitative data, but also because the topic made little sense to my summer colleagues. As one of the Ugandan physicians would announce with a furrowed brow, "I do not understand. They have the vaccines but they do not want them?" My affirmative answer would yield an additional confused look, with the phrase "I do not understand" repeated again and again. As I sat in a lecture hall with trays of catered breakfasts never seen in the halls of sociology, provided generously by the pharmaceutical companies who sponsored the course, I was aware of the worlds I straddled.

By 2004, I had accepted a job in Colorado, a state with the lowest vaccine rates in the country, owing in large part to its permissive framework for vaccine refusal. Although I intended to begin data collection for this project as soon as I unloaded the moving truck, in fact it was not until 2007, shortly after the birth of my third child, that I earnestly launched this study. I collected data over seven years, following the questions of vaccine resistance and choice everywhere they went.

Data Collection

This book draws on interviews with parents, healthcare providers, researchers, attorneys, policy makers, and advocates, as well as ethnographic observations and content analysis. Collected between 2007 and 2014, these data represent the multiple perspectives on a deeply divisive issue. Data from parents and most of the healthcare providers are from Colorado. Other data, from researchers, policy makers, attorneys, and authors, or from online discussions, draw from conversations that cross state lines or that shape national policy. When possible, I aim in the preceding pages to place data in their institutional and procedural context, identifying how these views fit within larger regulatory frameworks.

Interviewing Parents

I began by reaching out to parents who reject vaccines, but quickly discovered that operationalizing this group was not a straightforward task. Epidemiological data typically treat parental rejection of vaccines as categorical, but I found that this is not a group with clearly delineated lines of membership or absolute behavior. Parents constantly reassess the necessity of vaccines for their children, based on shifting perceptions of need and risk. They also consider each child in the family differently, at different ages (see table of parent participants). So rather than approaching vaccine decisions as an all-or-nothing proposition, I instead included parents who reject some or all vaccines or who consent to vaccines on a schedule of their own design. In doing so, I explore how parents challenge expert advice and substitute their own judgment instead. Eighteen participants had at least one child who has not received any vaccines, or no more than one vaccine.[5] Nine chose select vaccines for their children, opting out of a significant portion, and seven gave all vaccines but on a schedule of their own devising, which included decoupling vaccines usually given in combination, delaying consent, or spacing vaccines differently than recommended. Notably, parents may consent to vaccinate one child but not others, because they began questioning vaccines after starting a traditional vaccine schedule, their children had another health condition they feared made them vulnerable to adverse reactions, or they considered their sons to be at higher risk or needing vaccines less than their daughters. They also might have selected vaccines they perceived as protecting against a serious risk while rejecting others. There were no consistent patterns among parents who rejected all vaccines and those who consented to some. They engage in the same processes of assessing risk and benefit from an individualized perspective and sometimes move among categories, based on experience, research, or perceived needs of each child.

Parents were recruited through what I think of as an "inconvenience sample," since they were hard to locate and not always interested in participating in research. I sent invitations by e-mail to colleagues, friends, and acquaintances, as well as listservs and online groups for homeschooling, natural living, natural and home birth, extended breastfeeding, autism support, chickenpox parties, or vaccine education. Some participants were referred through others who were familiar with my research. At times, I brought whatever book I was currently reading on vaccine history or policy with me to children's birthday parties and swim lessons, in hopes that a bored parent nearby would notice, ask, and offer to participate. Accessing the social worlds of these parents was easier because I was already there. Yet, as savvy consumers of science, they were not necessarily eager to participate.

Although snowball sampling is an important tool in qualitative research, few parents referred other parents to me, explaining that they did not want their friends to know they had participated in research, even as their friends knew of their choice to refuse vaccines. Participants reside in Colorado, but live in or near different regions of the state, including Denver, Colorado Springs, and Boulder, and the outlying suburbs around these cities. Some identify as politically or religiously conservative, while others express leftist views. These did not meaningfully shape their views, illustrating how vaccine questions are located at the places where left meets right.

I worked to recruit both mothers and fathers, though it became clear early on that children's healthcare decisions remain largely maternal terrain. Overwhelmingly, women claimed expertise and responsibility for this aspect of their children's lives, underscoring how vaccine choices are gendered. Of the thirty-four parents I interviewed, five were fathers. All but one parent was white, which reflects the reality that vaccine refusal is more prevalent among white families.[6] All but one parent identified as heterosexual. Parents had varying degrees of religiosity, but only the parents who were Christian Scientists said that religion informed their decision to reject vaccines. Some who identified as Evangelical Christian referenced ways vaccines violated their understanding of the Bible, but these were not their primary reasons for rejecting vaccines. Parents who worked for wages tended to work in elite careers or to have jobs with high levels of flexibility. This latter category included parents who run family-owned businesses or were professionals with limited work hours and great autonomy, including massage therapist, yoga instructor, artist, birth coach, and writer. There were also large numbers of parents who did not work for wages. Parents ranged in age from twenty-six to sixty, though most were in their thirties and forties. Only two parents did not have minor children at home. The diversity in ages means that I have captured parents' narratives of their vaccine choices, not necessarily as they are making them, but as they have made sense of them. Personal belief exemptions have been available in Colorado since 1989, so all parents had access to those exemptions while living in the state. The schedule of recommended vaccines set forth by the federal government has changed slightly over time, which means that physicians have offered parents an increasing number of vaccines as new ones became recommended; however, those required by law for school attendance have changed only slightly during these children's lives.[7]

Parents do not necessarily identify as activists on this issue, with only one mother and three fathers reporting participation in efforts to oppose vaccine mandates, going out of their way to convince others (outside their social network) not to vaccinate, or participating in advocacy organizations, lobbying efforts, or organized events. All others consider vaccines to be a personal choice for individual parents to make on behalf of their own children. Four parents (Billy, Barb, Ruby, and Tracy) believe that their children were harmed by vaccination. In all four cases, they did not apply to the Vaccine Injury Compensation Program, so their claims of vaccine injury were not substantiated by a court, nor by medical experts. However, their observations of symptoms they attribute to vaccination—including the onset of seizures, autism, fainting, prolonged pupil dilation, and loss of concentration—profoundly shaped their concerns and inspired them to reject vaccines for their other children. Other parents fear possible serious adverse reactions, but their children do not have a history of them.

Interviews lasted between one and four hours and were recorded and transcribed verbatim. Interviews explored parents' background, education, relationships, pregnancy and birth experiences, choices about their children's healthcare, and broader perceptions of and experiences with vaccination and healthcare systems. I coded and analyzed transcripts thematically, employing what the sociologist Kathy Charmaz calls "constructivist grounded theory," where data are collected and analyzed "to learn participants' implicit meanings of their experiences to build a conceptual analysis of them."[8] All names of parents are pseudonyms.

Interviewing Healthcare Providers

I interviewed healthcare providers to understand their experiences with parents in their clinical practices. I specifically sought out pediatricians who provide primary care, since vaccines and discussions of them constitute a large part of their practice. I purposively sampled physicians who are known by parents to be "vaccine-flexible," who are involved in vaccine policy locally or nationally, or who provide care to low-income families to see how their experiences differ from those who provide care to higher-income families. Complementary healthcare providers loomed large in parents' stories of vaccine decision making, and as such, I interviewed several chiropractors who oppose the use of vaccines, a naturopathic doctor who participates in community educational events about vaccines, and a self-described energy healer who describes part of her practice as healing vaccine injuries. Several of these healthcare providers—both pediatricians and complementary providers—also discussed at length their own decisions to delay or reject vaccines for their own children. Therefore I discuss five of the fifteen healthcare providers also as parents who made decisions that differed from the ACIP-recommended schedule.

Interviewing Key Informants

Vaccine controversies travel beyond the boundaries of the state; I followed these questions nationally. I interviewed physicians and researchers involved in setting the national debate, which included serving as national advisory committee members, authors, vaccine researchers, or state advisors.

Additionally, I draw on interviews with others who shape vaccine policy and practice. This includes eleven attorneys who work in the National Vaccine Injury Compensation Program representing parents or working as special masters adjudicating cases, which provided insight into how actual injuries appear, what patterns exist, and how the compensation system supports families. This system has fewer than a hundred attorneys nationally and only eight special masters who hear every case.

Other interviews with the head of a local autism support group, members of the state health department, and members of organizations that oppose vaccine mandates fleshed out the context in which these controversies are analyzed. These interviews inform my analysis, but I draw on them less often than my interviews with parents and providers.

Observing Vaccine Choices: Ethnographic Observation and Content Analysis

In my efforts to understand how questions about vaccines move through different social spaces, I looked for places to observe vaccine discussions. Over several years I attended annual meetings of national organizations that oppose vaccine mandates or support natural living (which includes avoiding vaccination). I attended sessions, had lunch with parents, observed casual conversations, and spoke with organizers, presenters, and attendees. I also attended several different community educational events in different Colorado cities held by pediatricians for parents about vaccines. In these sessions, a pediatrician, naturopath, or chiropractor presents information about vaccine safety and necessity as they understand it, and parents listen, ask questions, and discuss concerns.

In addition to in-person observation, I observed and analyzed online discussions about vaccine choice. These came from listservs, blogs, online discussions on social media sites, and online posts. I never posted questions, nor did I participate in these forums. These discussions provided valuable insight into how parents who do not attend meetings talk to other parents about their concerns, strategies, and goals.

To understand more of the contours of regulation and expert knowledge, I sought out places where vaccines are discussed by elites. To understand medical knowledge, I attended lectures and Grand Rounds presentations at the local children's hospital about childhood vaccination. In doing so, I could observe how physicians talk to each other about parents who don't vaccinate, how they define vaccine safety, necessity, and treatment of vaccine-preventable diseases, and what information pediatric trainees receive.

The Institute of Medicine (IOM) has written several reports on vaccine safety and is touted as a neutral arbiter of expert knowledge. As such, I attended a full-day meeting at the IOM about vaccine safety to see how IOM members interact, how they discuss their work formally and in informal discussions over their ninety-minute catered lunch break or in hallways, and how staff view the IOM's work, which I learned during casual conversations with them. I also listened in on national advisory committee meetings that allow observers to call in but not participate in the discussion and analyzed their documents. In the Vaccine Injury Compensation Program, I watched court hearings where expert witnesses, almost always physicians or medical researchers, testify about the relationship between a disability and the likelihood that it was caused by a vaccine; I also spent time with attorneys in their practices. In all, I have not represented the entire universe of vaccine decisions, but have tried to follow the question everywhere it went to present as many perspectives as I can.

Analytical Choices

In studying contested meanings of health, illness, and vaccines, I am writing from the spaces between parents' perceptions and the meanings favored in official circles. Throughout, I often draw on formal definitions from federal agencies and groups like the Centers for Disease Control and Prevention (CDC), the National Institutes of Health (NIH), and the IOM. There are many participants in my study who would question that choice. A meaningful discussion of points of disagreement requires a common set of facts. Thus, I have accepted that while government agencies have a perspective, they represent public health goals and carry the legitimate authority of peer-reviewed science in their data and figures. I choose to use their information and terms. I have when possible triangulated data and figures from multiple sources, but I do accept CDC infection rates and NIH definitions of disease, for example, as reasonable representations of illness and incidence. A subset of parents who refuse vaccines also reject the validity of these sources and provide other studies they find to be more credible. When possible, I trace the citations and studies that purportedly challenge official science, but often find these claims to be unsupported by data. I also found that articles citing studies that supported claims of the dangers of vaccines or superior health of unvaccinated children cited other secondary sources that cited more secondary sources, but seldom linked to contemporary scientific peer-reviewed studies, which rendered these claims less credible. I accept that facts are contested, but also find some to be more credible than others. My acceptance of official organizations and norms of scientific inquiry marks a certain unbridgeable distance from which I reach out to parents, hear their stories, and present their views.

These differences in understanding of scientific method, research, and knowledge production are visible in Billy's story above. Billy has come to feel certain that his son was harmed by vaccines. He receives support for this view. His son's story and picture were displayed on the memorial bulletin board at an NVIC meeting, and several participants who are passionate in their opposition to vaccines referenced his family in our discussions. Yet no physician can tell him with certainty whether the DPT vaccine caused his son's seizures, in part because seizure disorders often develop without explanation. No official organization counts his son as a child who suffered a deleterious adverse reaction from a vaccine. Despite more than a decade of consultations, Billy will never receive any validation that his son's condition was definitively caused by a vaccine. This does not detract from his certainty that it was. In my analysis, I work to present both parents' perceptions and the places where their understandings are disconnected from expert knowledge.

Representing Participants

I reference all parents and most providers by pseudonyms. There are two participants I personally interviewed that I reference by their real names because they are important and divisive figures in the vaccine debate: Bob Sears, author of the best-selling *Vaccine Book*, which created what is colloquially known as the Sears schedule, and Paul Offit, the creator of a vaccine against rotavirus, who is a public advocate for vaccination. When I reference public lectures, education events, writings, or trainings, I use the real names of the presenters, since these public events are publicly available.

At times, I made small insubstantial corrections to parents' speech, removing extra utterances like "um," "like," or "you know." I did this because the parents who reject expert advice are generally and erroneously portrayed as ignorant. Throughout the book, I did not want these speech details to detract from their ideas. I did not change any other words from their interviews.

Finally, I did not accept any funding for this research beyond faculty development funds from the University of Denver, where I was employed during much of this research. Doing so, I feared, might create the perception that I was not neutral in examining this issue. I hope I have succeeded in presenting all sides of this emotionally laden issue with respect. I accept that many participants will not agree with my analysis, but I aspire for them to feel that I represented them fairly.

Parent Participants

Pseudonym	Age	Relationship status	Number of children	Employment	Education
At least one child received none or only one of the recommended vaccines[a] (n = 18)					
Tara Milon	39	Married	1	Lay healer	MA
Molly Jones	35	Divorced/ repartnered	3	Doula	Some college
Carolyn Kalman	47	Married	3	Homemaker	BA
Janine Bouche	35	Separated	1	Sales	BA
Lauren Tate	32	Married	4	Homemaker	Some college
Anna Chase	31	Married	2	Acupuncturist	BA
Marlene Bryant	47	Married	4	Homemaker/ family business	High school
Patricia Etter	42	Married	8	Homemaker	High school
Elizabeth Nowak	35	Married	2	Principal	MA
Paula Parenti	55	Divorced	4	Part-time administrative	Some college
Gabriela Luce	32	Married	1	Homemaker	Some college
Margaret Spencer	54	Married	2	Family business	Some college
Ruby Caine	36	Married	2	Yoga instructor	Some college
Jackie Russell	60	Married	3	Volunteer	BA
Billy Folsom	43	Married	2	Homemaker	High school
Ken Strauss	32	Married	2	Computer programmer	Some college
Jake Kalman	46	Married	3	Chiropractor	Doctorate
Tom Sanders	52	Married	4	Chiropractor	Doctorate

Parent Participants (*cont.*)

Pseudonym	Age	Relation-ship status	Number of children	Employ-ment	Education
Children received some recommended vaccines (*n* = 9)					
Leanne Boggess	32	Married	4	Homemaker	BA
Gina Paquin	38	Divorced	1	Secretary	BA
Heather Moss	32	Married	2	Homemaker/ birth coach	MA
Steph O'Neill	33	Married	1	Part-time administra-tive	BA
Astrid Villa	41	Married	1	Full-time administra-tive	MA
Katie Reynolds	41	Married	2	Homemaker/ freelance writer	MA
Sarah Cazan	37	Married	2	Physician	Doctorate
Barb Schoenhorn	45	Married	2	Homemaker/ author	Some college
Ben Kirkland	38	Married	2	Physician	Doctorate
Children received all on personalized schedule (*n* = 7)					
Solange Khan	45	Married	3	Homemaker/ musician	BA
Tammy Shaffer	34	Married	1	Homemaker	BA
Jane Silver	42	Married	1	Physician	Doctorate
Kristin Mann	40	Married	2	Homemaker/ artist	BA
Melissa Pallamore	30	Married	1	Full-time administra-tive	MA
Lindsey Easter	26	Married	1	Homemaker	Some college
Tracy Teller	37	Married	3	Bus driver	High school

[a] Some families opted for the tetanus vaccine, but not others. Notably, there is not herd immunity protection against tetanus.

APPENDIX B: VACCINE SCHEDULE

Figure 1. Recommended immunization schedule for persons aged 0 through 18 years – United States, 2015.

(FOR THOSE WHO FALL BEHIND OR START LATE, SEE THE CATCH-UP SCHEDULE [FIGURE 2]).

These recommendations must be read with the footnotes that follow. For those who fall behind or start late, provide catch-up vaccination at the earliest opportunity as indicated by the green bars in Figure 1. To determine minimum intervals between doses, see the catch-up schedule (Figure 2). School entry and adolescent vaccine age groups are shaded.

This schedule includes recommendations in effect as of January 1, 2015. Any dose not administered at the recommended age should be administered at a subsequent visit, when indicated and feasible. The use of a combination vaccine generally is preferred over separate injections of its equivalent component vaccines. Vaccination providers should consult the relevant Advisory Committee on Immunization Practices (ACIP) statement for detailed recommendations, available online at http://www.cdc.gov/vaccines/hcp/acip-recs/index.html. Clinically significant adverse events that follow vaccination should be reported to the Vaccine Adverse Event Reporting System (VAERS) online (http://www.vaers.hhs.gov) or by telephone (800-822-7967). Suspected cases of vaccine-preventable diseases should be reported to the state or local health department. Additional information, including precautions and contraindications for vaccination, is available from CDC online (http://www.cdc.gov/vaccines/recs/vac-admin/contraindications.htm) or by telephone (800-CDC-INFO [800-232-4636]).

This schedule is approved by the Advisory Committee on Immunization Practices (http://www.cdc.gov/vaccines/acip), the American Academy of Pediatrics (http://www.aap.org), the American Academy of Family Physicians (http://www.aafp.org), and the American College of Obstetricians and Gynecologists (http://www.acog.org).

NOTE: The above recommendations must be read along with the footnotes of this schedule.

"Recommended immunization schedule for persons aged 0 through 18 years—United States, 2015." Centers for Disease Control and Prevention, http://www.cdc.gov/vaccines/schedules/downloads/child/0–18yrs-schedule.pdf.

NOTES

INTRODUCTION

1 Jacks, "To the Parent of the Unvaccinated Child."
2 Associated Press, "Measles Outbreak."
3 Cohen and Goldschmidt, "Arizona Measles Exposure."
4 The majority of those who contracted measles were unvaccinated. See CDC, "2015 Measles Cases in the U.S."
5 Cohen and Goldschmidt, "Arizona Measles Exposure."
6 U.S. Senate, *Testimony of Dr. Timothy Jacks.*
7 Heimer, "Meet Megan."
8 Heimer, "To the Parent of the Immunocompromised Child."
9 McCoy, "Amid Measles Outbreak."
10 Cohen and Goldschmidt, "Arizona Measles Exposure."
11 Starr, *Social Transformation of American Medicine,* 4.
12 In the 1970s, vaccines against tetanus, diphtheria, pertussis (whooping cough), polio, measles, mumps, and rubella were recommended. In 2014 recommended vaccines still include vaccines against diphtheria, tetanus, and pertussis (combined DTaP vaccine), polio (inactivated vaccine), measles, mumps, and rubella (combined MMR vaccine), and now also include hepatitis B, rotavirus, Hib (haemophilus influenzae b), pneumococcal, influenza, varicella (chickenpox), hepatitis A, and meningococcal (certain high-risk groups only). There are various combination shots, with the rotavirus vaccine being oral, so the number of actual injections can vary. Children's Hospital of Philadelphia, "History of Vaccine Schedule." See also College of Physicians of Philadelphia, "Development of the Immunization Schedule."
13 Department of Health and Human Services, "Immunization and Infectious Diseases."
14 Federal goals define key vaccines as ≥1 dose measles, mumps, rubella vaccine (MMR) (91.6%), ≥3 doses of hepatitis B vaccine (HepB) (91.1%), ≥3 doses of poliovirus vaccine (93.9%), and ≥1 dose of varicella vaccine (90.8%). See CDC, "National, State, and Local Area Vaccination Coverage."
15 Omer et al., "Nonmedical Exemptions to School Immunization"; Orenstein and Hinman, "Immunization System in the United States."
16 CDC, "Frequently Asked Questions."
17 Gellin and Schaffner, "Risk of Vaccination."

18 Kennedy, Basket, and Sheedy, "Vaccine Attitudes."

19 Benin et al., "Qualitative Analysis of Mothers' Decision-Making"; Pieter, Chow-dhury, and Ramos-Jimenez, "Patterns of Vaccination Acceptance"; Casiday, "Children's Health and the Social Theory of Risk."

20 Offit, "Why Are Pharmaceutical Companies Gradually Abandoning Vaccines?"; Prifti, "Vaccine Industry"; Kaddar, "Global Vaccine Market Features."

21 Truong, "Pediatric Vaccine Stockpiling Problem"; Collier, "No End in Sight for Adult Hepatitis B Vaccine Shortage"; Lee et al., "Benefits to All"; Boulis, Goold, and Ubel, "Responding to the Immunoglobulin Shortage."

22 Nesi, *Poison Pills*; Mintz and Liu, "China's Heparin Revisited"; Powell, "Heparin's Deadly Side Effects"; Harris and Wilson, "Glaxo to Pay $750 Million"; Frizell, "Tylenol Maker Admits to Selling Liquid Medicine Contaminated with Metal."

23 Gagne and Choudhry, "How Many 'Me-Too' Drugs"; Carpenter, "Can Expedited FDA Drug Approval"; Tomljenovic and Shaw, "Too Fast or Not Too Fast."

24 Volmink and Garner, "Directly Observed Therapy for Treating Tuberculosis"; Baldwin, *Contagion and the State in Europe*, 93–97; Freeman and Frierson, "Court-Mandated, Long-Acting Antipsychotic Medication"; St. Lawrence et al., "STD Screening."

25 Data draw from post-1994 vaccine schedules, excluding influenza and hepatitis A. See CDC, "Benefits from Immunization."

26 Individual immune systems have some variation, so occasionally a person's immune system will not generate an immune response. See College of Physicians of Philadelphia, "Top 20 Questions about Vaccination."

27 CDC, "Advisory Committee on Immunization Practices (ACIP)."

28 Dempsey et al., "Alternative Vaccination Schedule."

29 See 23andMe.com or Ancestry.com as examples. Although the promise of using genetic-level information to tailor drugs or cancer treatments is exciting to envision, in reality these technologies are far from reaching the market, are of questionable interest to for-profit corporations, raise new issues of safety and testing, and rely on physicians unlikely to be able to interpret genetic information or unwilling to classify patients. Hedgecoe, *Politics of Personalised Medicine*; Hunt and Kreiner, "Pharmacogenetics in Primary Care." See also Roberts, *Fatal Invention*, 147–225.

30 Clarke et al., "Biomedicalization."

31 Juffer, "Dirty Diapers and the New Organic Intellectual"; Wilkins, "Affective Practices and Neoliberal Fantasies"; Murphy, "Risk, Responsibility, and Rhetoric."

32 Rose and Novas, "Biological Citizenship," 441; Crawford, "Healthism."

33 Fenton et al., "Cost of Satisfaction."

34 This occurs in other sectors too. See, for example, Wilkins, "Affective Practices and Neoliberal Fantasies."

35 Buck v. Bell.

36 National Conference of State Legislatures, "States with Religious and Philosophical Exemptions." California and Vermont had personal belief exemptions, but

because of legislation passed in 2015, Vermont will recognize only religious and medical exemptions and California will recognize only medical ones. Missouri's personal belief exemption applies only to daycare, preschool, and nursery school.

37 Booth, "Colorado Parents." As of 2011, Colorado was second only to Alaska in per capita usage.

38 Omer et al., "Geographic Clustering of Nonmedical Exemptions"; Smith, Chu, and Barker, "Children Who Have Received No Vaccines"; Wei et al., "Identification and Characteristics of Vaccine Refusers."

39 Cheal, *Family and the State of Theory*, 83.

40 General Accounting Office, "Report to Congressional Requesters."

41 Apple, *Perfect Motherhood*, 2.

42 Litt, *Medicalized Motherhood*.

43 Apple, *Perfect Motherhood*, 133.

44 Soet, Dudley, and Dilorio, "Effects of Ethnicity and Perceived Power."

45 Taylor and Leitz, "Emotions and Identity."

46 Morgen, *Into Our Own Hands*.

47 Solinger, *Beggars and Choosers*, 5.

48 Berlin, *Liberty*; Roberts, *Killing the Black Body*.

49 Lareau, *Unequal Childhoods*.

50 Salganicoff, Ranji, and Wyn, "Women and Healthcare."

51 Avishai, "Managing the Lactating Body"; Hays, *Cultural Contradictions of Motherhood*.

52 Elliott, Powell, and Brenton, "Being a Good Mom"; McQuillan et al., "Importance of Motherhood."

53 Bryant et al., "Caesarean Birth," 1199.

54 Silverman, *Understanding Autism*; Scott, "'I Feel as If I Am the One Who Is Disabled'"; Kaufman, "Regarding the Rise in Autism"; Blum, "Mother-Blame"; Singh, "Doing Their Jobs."

55 Bobel, for example, found that the women she termed "natural mothers," who reject mainstream parenting advice and commercialism in favor of natural and instinctual mothering practices, believed that they "wrested control of their personal lives away from institutions and experts and others who claim to 'know best' and returned it to the site of the individual family." *Paradox of Natural Mothering*, 26. As another example, see Lois, *Home Is Where the School Is*. On breastfeeding as an elite practice, see Avishai, "Managing the Lactating Body"; and Reich, "Public Mothers and Private Practices."

CHAPTER 1. THE PUBLIC HISTORY OF VACCINES

1 Colgrove, "Immunity for the People," 249.

2 Riedel, "Edward Jenner."

3 Jenner House and Museum, "What Is Small Pox?"

4 Riedel, "Edward Jenner."

5 Ibid.

6 This story and others like it illustrate the lack of ethical standards regarding medical research at the time.

7 Riedel, "Edward Jenner."

8 Lakhani, "Early Clinical Pathologists," 757.

9 Jefferson, letter to "The Rev. Doctr. G. C. Jenner," Monticello, May 14, 1806; College of Physicians of Philadelphia, "History of Vaccines Timeline."

10 Johnson, *Ghost Map*.

11 Hodge and Gostin, "School Vaccination Requirements."

12 Ibid; see also Yale Law Journal, "Police Power."

13 The state also accommodated privileged girls, whose smallpox scars were hidden to protect their beauty by supplying "its three female doctors to verify protection among the daughters of the well-to-do." Colgrove, *State of Immunity*.

14 Hodge and Gostin, "School Vaccination Requirements."

15 Stern and Markel, "History of Vaccines and Immunization," 617–18.

16 Colgrove, *State of Immunity*.

17 Chap. 75, § 137.

18 Quoted in Hodge and Gostin, "School Vaccination Requirements."

19 Quoted in Parmet, Goodman, and Farber, "Individual Rights versus the Public's Health."

20 Jacobson v. Massachusetts.

21 Ibid., 197.

22 Hodge and Gostin, "School Vaccination Requirements."

23 There are exceptions to this trend. *Lochner v. New York* (1905) rejected a law to protect workers from excessive hours, ruling that it interfered with the right of liberty and individual contract. Of course, *Muller v. Oregon* (1908) holds that work restrictions for women were constitutional.

24 Apple, *Perfect Motherhood*; Trattner, *From Poor Law to Welfare State*.

25 Colgrove, *State of Immunity*, 49.

26 Willrich, *Pox: An American History*.

27 Colgrove, *State of Immunity*.

28 Ibid.

29 Baker, "Immunization and the American Way."

30 CDC, "Diphtheria."

31 Baker, "Immunization and the American Way."

32 Ibid.

33 Colgrove, *State of Immunity*, 83.

34 Baker, "Immunization and the American Way"; ibid.

35 Baker, "Immunization and the American Way," 200.

36 Colgrove, *State of Immunity*, 87; Mullin, "Recent Advances in the Control of Diphtheria."

37 DeHovitz, "1901 St Louis Incident."

38 Colgrove, *State of Immunity*, 152.

39 Baker, "Immunization and the American Way"; Colgrove, *State of Immunity*, 90–92.

40 Allen, *Vaccine*.
41 For a discussion of the rates and limits of medical intervention and life expectancy changes, see McKinlay and McKinlay, "Questionable Contribution of Medical Measures."
42 Heller, *Vaccine Narrative*.
43 Starr, *Social Transformation of American Medicine*.
44 Heller, *Vaccine Narrative*.
45 Colgrove, *State of Immunity*, 90.
46 Quoted in Colgrove, *State of Immunity*, 95.
47 Ibid.; Apple, *Perfect Motherhood*.
48 Quoted in Colgrove, *State of Immunity*, 98.
49 Lemons, "Sheppard-Towner Act"; Meckel, *Save the Babies*,104–19.
50 Sheppard–Towner Maternity and Infancy Act (1921).
51 Barker, "Women Physicians."
52 Starr, *Social Transformation of American Medicine*, 232.
53 Allen, *Vaccine*, 267.
54 Colgrove, *State of Immunity*, 111; Cherry, "Historical Review of Pertussis."
55 Baker, "Immunization and the American Way."
56 Colgrove, *State of Immunity*, 111–13; Allen, *Vaccine*, 268.
57 Allen, *Vaccine*, 268–70, 379.
58 Baker, "Immunization and the American Way."
59 Ibid.
60 Colgrove, *State of Immunity*, 115–17.
61 Oshinsky, *Polio: An American Story*, 239.
62 Colgrove, *State of Immunity*; Apple, *Perfect Motherhood*.
63 Colgrove, *State of Immunity*, 116; Baker, "Immunization and the American Way."
64 Oshinsky, *Polio: An American Story*, 130–35.
65 Koprowski, "First Decade (1950–1960) of Studies"; Oshinsky, *Polio: An American Story*, 135–36.
66 Baker, "Immunization and the American Way."
67 Oshinsky, *Polio: An American Story*.
68 Quoted in Baker, "Immunization and the American Way," 204.
69 Ibid.
70 Quoted in Oshinsky, *Polio: An American Story*, 211.
71 Blume, "Lock In, the State and Vaccine Development"; Oshinsky, *Polio: An American Story*, 200.
72 Colgrove, *State of Immunity*, 118–22.
73 Oshinsky, *Polio: An American Story*, 7.
74 Colgrove, *State of Immunity*, 122.
75 Offit, "Cutter Incident," 1411.
76 Blume, "Lock In, the State and Vaccine Development."
77 Colgrove, *State of Immunity*, 129–33.

78 Blume, "Lock In, the State and Vaccine Development."

79 Nkowane et al., "Vaccine-Associated Paralytic Poliomyelitis."

80 Colgrove, *State of Immunity*, 189.

81 Hinman et al., "Live or Inactivated Poliomyelitis Vaccine."

82 Colgrove, *State of Immunity*.

83 Quoted in Conis, *Vaccine Nation*, 47.

84 Ibid., 37; CDC, "Achievements in Public Health."

85 Measles complications can be serious. Six to 20 percent of the people who get the disease will get an ear infection, diarrhea, or even pneumonia. One in 1,000 people with measles will develop inflammation of the brain, or will die. CDC, "Measles (Rubeola)."

86 CDC, "Rubella: Epidemiology and Prevention."

87 Heller, *Vaccine Narrative*, 65.

88 Ibid.; Reagan, *Dangerous Pregnancies*.

89 Quoted in Colgrove, *State of Immunity*, 153.

90 Ibid., 151.

91 Ibid., 157.

92 Ibid., 160.

93 Ibid., 174.

94 Ibid., 177.

95 Quoted in Conis, *Vaccine Nation*, 81.

96 Colgrove, *State of Immunity*, 177–79.

97 Reiss, "Thou Shalt Not Take the Name."

98 Sencer and Millar, "Reflections on the 1976 Swine Flu Vaccination Program."

99 Quoted in ibid., 30.

100 Colgrove, *State of Immunity,* 193–94.

101 Sencer and Millar, "Reflections on the 1976 Swine Flu Vaccination Program," 31.

102 Colgrove, *State of Immunity,* 195–96.

103 Roan, "Swine Flu 'Debacle' of 1976."

104 Colgrove, *State of Immunity*, 195.

105 Ibid., 196.

106 Ibid., 199.

107 Ibid.

108 Wright v. DeWitt Sch. Dist., 385 S.W.2d 644 (Ark. 1965).

109 Allen, *Vaccine*, 271–76.

110 Cherry, "Historical Review of Pertussis"; Barlow et al., "Risk of Seizures."

111 Fulginiti, "New Pertussis Vaccine."

112 Offit, "Cutter Incident, 50 Years Later."

113 Colgrove, *State of Immunity,* 208.

114 Ibid., 209.

115 Ibid., 211.

116 Allen, *Vaccine*, 254–55.

117 Colgrove, *State of Immunity*, 212.

118 Ibid.

119 Scott, "National Childhood Injury Act."

120 Colgrove, *State of Immunity*, 214–15.

121 Mariner, "National Vaccine Injury Compensation Program."

122 Colgrove, *State of Immunity*, 219.

123 Ibid., 229.

124 Epstein, *Impure Science*; Morgen, *Into Our Own Hands*; Davis, *The Making of "Our Bodies, Ourselves."*

125 Largent, *Vaccine: The Debate in Modern America*, 74–82.

126 The physician John Waterhouse was given some of Jenner's vaccine, and insisted on widespread vaccination. Unlike Jenner, he initially saw vaccination as an opportunity for profit; he was unsuccessful in his attempts to hold a monopoly on the vaccine in America.

CHAPTER 2. PARENTS AS EXPERTS

1 McCarthy, *Mother Warriors*, 3–9.

2 Lupton, "Risk as Moral Danger," 463.

3 Lareau, *Unequal Childhoods*, 8; Nelson, *Parenting Out of Control*.

4 Allen, *Vaccine*, 16.

5 Canterbury v. Spence.

6 Blum, "Mother-Blame in the Prozac Nation"; Singh, "Doing Their Jobs."

7 National Vaccine Information Center (www.nvic.org) and the Vaccination Risk Awareness Network (http://vran.org).

8 Heller, "Social Meanings of Vaccines," 8.

9 Ibid., 9.

10 Ibid., 23.

11 Rosenstock, "Why People Use Health Services."

12 Conrad, "Meaning of Medications."

13 CDC, "Polio Vaccine." There have been more recent cases of imported vaccine-acquired polio that came from the oral polio vaccine. See, for example, Alexander et al., "Transmission of Imported Vaccine-Derived Poliovirus."

14 She may be confusing German measles (more damaging to fetuses than measles) and measles (which is also an issue and can cause miscarriage); CDC, "Measles (Rubeola)."

15 CDC, "About Tetanus."

16 See appendix B for the current vaccine schedule.

17 CDC, "Tetanus: For Clinicians."

18 CDC, "Possible Side Effects of Vaccines."

19 The history of this vaccine is described in chapter 2.

20 The measles-mumps-rubella (MMR) vaccine is produced with eggs, but is generally considered safe for children with egg allergies. More risky vaccines include seasonal flu vaccine and others not regularly offered to children, including those against yellow fever and rabies. See Mayo Clinic, "Egg Allergy."

21 Freed et al., "Parental Vaccine Safety Concerns"; Hilton, Petticrew, and Hunt, "'Combined Vaccines'"; Heininger, "Internet-Based Survey"; Kennedy et al., "Confidence about Vaccines."

22 Dempsey et al., "Alternative Vaccination Schedule Preferences."

23 Offit et al., "Addressing Parents' Concerns."

24 Occasionally, Paula references hep B and Hib interchangeably. After speaking to many physicians, I am convinced she meant Hib, which, as older doctors particularly remember, was a common cause of invasive bacterial disease that could be devastating.

25 She is most likely referencing the discredited and retracted study of Andrew Wakefield, cited as Wakefield et al., "Retracted." For a discussion of the issue, see also Kirkland, "Credibility Battles."

CHAPTER 3. VACCINES AS UNNATURAL INTERVENTION

1 Pope, "Six Reasons to Say No."

2 Bobel, *Paradox of Natural Mothering*, 128.

3 Offit et al., "Addressing Parents' Concerns," 125.

4 Copelton, "'You Are What You Eat.'"

5 Mooney, "Babies Are Getting Brain Bleeds."

6 Schulte et al., "Rise in Late Onset Vitamin K Deficiency Bleeding"; Volpe, "Intracranial Hemorrhage."

7 Hancock, "Vitamin K."

8 PubMed Health, "Hepatitis B."

9 National Network for Immunization Information, "Hepatitis B."

10 CDC, "Viral Hepatitis: Statistics and Surveillance."

11 World Health Organization, "Global Alert and Response: Hepatitis B."

12 Immunization Action Coalition, "Hepatitis B Shots Are Recommended."

13 CDC, "Viral Hepatitis: Statistics and Surveillance"; WHO, "Hepatitis B."

14 Mercola, "Flu Vaccine."

15 Children's Hospital of Philadelphia (CHOP), "How Are Vaccines Made?"

16 CHOP, "General Vaccine Safety Concerns."

17 CDC, "Chicken Pox (Varicella)."

18 Immunize for Public Health, "Varicella (Chickenpox)."

19 Ibid.

20 Chaves et al., "Loss of Vaccine-Induced Immunity."

21 Immunization Action Coalition, "State Information."

22 Freedman, "Mailing 'Chickenpox Lollipops.'"

23 American Academy of Pediatrics, "Chicken Pox Immunity."

24 Hales et al., "Examination of Links"; Reynolds et al., "Impact of the Varicella Vaccination Program."

25 Allen, "Shingles & Chickenpox."

26 Mercola, "Chickenpox (Varicella) Vaccine," emphasis in original.

27 Immunize Colorado, "Fact or Fiction?"

CHAPTER 4. THE LIMITS OF TRUST IN BIG PHARMA

1 Fisher, "Vaccines."
2 CHOP, "Too Many Vaccines?"
3 Offit et al., "Addressing Parents' Concerns," 127.
4 Viruses and bacteria are grown on tissue and isolated to develop new vaccines. Depending on the vaccine and era of research, this may have included, for example, tissue from monkeys, rabbits, or human fetuses. Some argue that the DNA from those initial cell lines still remains in vaccines today, though parents sometimes misunderstand and mistakenly assume that each batch of vaccine manufacturing requires those tissues. See Offit, *Vaccinated: One Man's Quest,* 40–43.
5 See, for example, Refutations to Anti-Vaccine Memes, "Vaccine Ingredients: Formaldehyde."
6 Autism Speaks, "Jenny McCarthy and Jim Carrey Lead 'Green Our Vaccines' Rally."
7 McCarthy, "Green Our Vaccines Rally."
8 MacKendrick, "More Work for Mother."
9 van der Pol et al., "Efficacy of Proton-Pump Inhibitors"; "Acid Reflux Meds on Rise."
10 Baker, "Mercury, Vaccines, and Autism."
11 21 CFR 610.15(a); Food and Drug Administration, "Thimerosal in Vaccines."
12 Branches et al., "Price of Gold."
13 FDA, "Thimerosal in Vaccines"; Harada, "Minamata Disease."
14 Bakir et al., "Methylmercury Poisoning"; Rustam and Hamdi, "Methyl Mercury Poisoning."
15 Grandjean et al., "Cognitive Deficit."
16 Amin-Zaki et al., "Intra-Uterine Methylmercury."
17 National Academies of Science, *Toxicological Effects of Methylmercury.*
18 FDA, "Thimerosal in Vaccines."
19 The May 2013 DSM-5 merged all autism disorders into one umbrella diagnosis of ASD.
20 CDC, "Autism Spectrum Disorder"; Weintraub, "Prevalence Puzzle."
21 CDC, "Autism Spectrum Disorder"; Silverman, *Understanding Autism*; Weintraub, "Prevalence Puzzle"; Cheslack-Postava, Liu, and Bearman, "Closely Spaced Pregnancies"; Fountain, King, and Bearman, "Age of Diagnosis"; King and Bearman, "Diagnostic Change"; Liu, King, and Bearman, "Social Influence and the Autism Epidemic."
22 Kirkland, "Legitimacy of Vaccine Critics"; Silverman, *Understanding Autism*; Stehr-Green et al., "Autism and Thimerosal-Containing Vaccines"; Weintraub, "Prevalence Puzzle."
23 Allen, *Vaccine, 302, 329*; Baker, "Mercury, Vaccines, and Autism."
24 Baker, "Mercury, Vaccines, and Autism"; Kirby, *Evidence of Harm.*

25 Pichichero et al., "Mercury Levels in Newborns."

26 CDC, "Joint Statement."

27 IOM, "About the Institute of Medicine."

28 Stratton, Gable, and McCormick, *Immunization Safety Review*, 1.

29 Just the Vax, "Still No Independent Confirmation."

30 Dachel, "Moms in Charge Presents."

31 FDA, "Vaccines, Blood & Biologics."

32 Ibid.

33 Fulton, "Bioterrorism Bill."

34 Ibid.

35 Wechsler, "Congress Expands Drug Safety Surveillance."

36 Health Resources and Services Administration, "Countermeasures Injury Compensation."

37 DeWeerdt, "Vaccines: An Age-Old Problem"; Markel, "April 12, 1955."

38 See chapter 2 for longer discussion of the Cutter Incident. See also Offit, "Cutter Incident, 50 Years Later."

39 Watkins, "Rotarix Rotavirus Vaccine Contaminated."

40 Limbach, "Merck Recalls Gardasil."

41 FDA, "Inspections, Compliance, Enforcement."

42 Dennehy, "Rotavirus Vaccines"; Vesikari, "Rotavirus Vaccines."

43 Dennehy, "Rotavirus Vaccines." Risks of complication and death are not equally distributed globally. In the United States, where children have ready access to intravenous fluids for hydration, deaths are extraordinarily rare.

44 CDC, "Rotashield" (Rotavirus) Vaccine and Intussusception."

45 Rennels, "Rotavirus Vaccine Story," 123.

46 CDC, "Rotashield" (Rotavirus) Vaccine and Intussusception."

47 There is a debate over whether Rotashield was still better than nothing in the countries with the highest infant mortality from rotavirus. Nonetheless, it was removed from the global market, even as it remained licensed abroad.

48 CDC, "Rotashield" (Rotavirus) Vaccine and Intussusception"; CDC, "Rotavirus Vaccine (Rotashield®) and Intussusception: Historical Information."

49 It is worth acknowledging that increased rates of intussusception have plagued later rotavirus vaccines as well. See Yih et al., "Intussusception Risk."

50 Trouiller et al., "Drug Development for Neglected Diseases"; Ma et al., "Global Tuberculosis Drug Development Pipeline."

51 Business Wire, "National Vaccine Information Center."

CHAPTER 5. WHO CALLS THE SHOTS?

1 Fox, "Teen's Death Shows How Flu Can Kill." See also the Booth family profile at FamiliesFightingFlu.org.

2 Becker et al., *Boys in White*.

3 Hochschild, "Emotion Work"; Pierce, *Gender Trials*.

4 Halpern, *American Pediatrics*.

5 Committee on Hospital Care and Institute for Patient- and Family-Centered Care, "Patient- and Family-Centered Care."

6 Committee on Community Health Services, "Pediatrician's Role in Community Pediatrics."

7 Kao et al., "Relationship between Method of Physician Payment and Patient Trust." Patients who are satisfied may also use more well-care. See Fenton et al., "Cost of Satisfaction."

8 They have more recently, like all pediatric practices, changed to all thimerasol-free vaccines as well.

9 Nichol et al., "Effectiveness of Influenza Vaccine."

10 Kolata, *Flu: The Story of the Great Influenza Pandemic*; Barry, *The Great Influenza*.

11 WHO, "Influenza (Seasonal)."

12 CDC, "Estimating Seasonal Influenza-Associated Deaths."

13 CDC, "Estimates of Deaths Associated with Seasonal Influenza."

14 Molinari et al., "Annual Impact of Seasonal Influenza."

15 Poehling et al., "Underrecognized Burden of Influenza."

16 Fairbrother et al., "High Costs of Influenza."

17 Nichol, Mallon, and Mendelman, "Cost Benefit of Influenza Vaccination"; Wilde et al., "Effectiveness of Influenza Vaccine"; Demicheli et al., "Vaccines for Preventing Influenza in Healthy Adults."

18 Fisher, "Influenza Deaths."

19 See also FamiliesFightingFlu.org for other stories of parents who lost children in flu-related deaths.

20 CDC, "CDC Reports About 90 Percent of Children."

21 Meharry et al., "Reasons Why Women Accept or Reject"; Brown et al., "Omission Bias and Vaccine Rejection."

22 Greenwood, "Curing the Common Cold."

23 Fisher, "Influenza Deaths."

CHAPTER 6. THE SLOW VAX MOVEMENT

1 Olmsted, "Weekly Wrap."

2 Smith et al., "Association between Intentional Delay"; Robison, Groom, and Young, "Frequency of Alternative Immunization."

3 CDC, "Advisory Committee on Immunization Practices."

4 The Affordable Care Act may eliminate some of these costs for preventative care.

5 Immunization Action Coalition, "Ask the Experts."

6 Offit et al., "Addressing Parents' Concerns"; Hilton, Petticrew, and Hunt, "'Combined Vaccines'"; CDC, "Frequently Asked Questions."

7 Kids Play Safe, http://kidsplaysafe.net/results.php.

8 Colorado Department of Public Health and the Environment, "Youngest Children Are at Greatest Risk."

9 American Academy of Pediatrics, *Red Book*.

10 Sears, "CNN.com & Dr. Bob," citing story from Cohen, "Should I Vaccinate My Baby?"
11 Tenpenny, "Order Vaccine Titer Tests."
12 Titer levels from passive immunity can interfere with the success of some vaccines like measles, while stress and other conditions can also interfere with immune response. See, for example, Markowitz et al., "Changing Levels of Measles Antibody Titers"; Miller et al., "Psychological Stress and Antibody Response"; Albrecht et al., "Persistence of Maternal Antibody."
13 American Academy of Pediatrics, *Red Book*, 449.
14 Pediatrics Digest Summary, "Timely versus Delayed Early Childhood Vaccination."
15 Smith and Woods, "On-Time Vaccine Receipt."
16 Sears, *Vaccine Book*, xii, xvi.
17 Ibid., xiii.
18 Ibid., xiv.
19 Petousis-Harris et al., "Family Physician Perspectives"; Haber, Malow, and Zimet, "HPV Vaccine Mandate Controversy."
20 Palevsky, "About Dr. Palvesky."
21 Anderson, "Empowering Patients"; Kivits, "Researching the 'Informed Patient'"; Lareau, *Unequal Childhoods*.
22 Wightman et al., "Washington State Pediatricians' Attitudes."
23 American Academy of Pediatrics, "Immunization Training Guide."
24 Ibid.
25 O'Leary et al., "Vaccine Financing."
26 Robison, Groom, and Young, "Frequency of Alternative Immunization"; Smith et al., "Association between Intentional Delay"; Nadeau et al., "Vaccinating My Way"; Buttenheim et al., "MMR Vaccination Status."

CHAPTER 7. FINDING NATURAL SOLUTIONS
1 DeVault, *Feeding the Family*; Bowen, Elliott, and Brenton, "The Joy of Cooking?"
2 AAP, "Breastfeeding Benefits Your Baby's Immune System."
3 Wolf, "Is Breast Really Best?"
4 Avishai, "Managing the Lactating Body"; Blum, *At the Breast*.
5 Copelton, "'You Are What You Eat'"; Waggoner, "Expanding the Reproductive Body."
6 See Sears, "Attachment Parenting Babies"; and Attachment Parenting International, "API's Eight Principles."
7 Epstein, *Impure Science*; Brandt, *No Magic Bullet*.
8 Reagan, *Dangerous Pregnancies*, 2.
9 Omer et al., "Vaccine Refusal"; Salmon et al., "Health Consequences of Religious and Philosophical Exemptions"; Sugerman et al., "Measles Outbreak."
10 See, for example, Pan American Health Organization, "Measles and Rubella."
11 On gated communities, see Dinzey-Flores, *Locked In, Locked Out*. On imagined communities, see Anderson, *Imagined Communities*.

12 Casper and Carpenter, "Sex, Drugs, and Politics"; Colgrove, *State of Immunity*.

CHAPTER 8. VACCINE LIBERTY

1 Wakefield, "Dr. Andrew Wakefield, Health Freedom Rally."
2 Goffman, *Stigma*.
3 Respiratory syncytial virus (RSV) is a common virus that leads to mild cold-like symptoms in older children and can be more serious in younger children, especially infants.
4 Steinhauer, "Public Health Risk."
5 Sears, "Dr. Bob Sears Offers Advice."
6 CDC, "Pertussis Outbreak Trends."
7 CDC, "Talking with Parents."
8 Diekema and Committee on Bioethics, "Responding to Parental Refusals."
9 American Academy of Pediatrics, "Documenting Parental Refusal."
10 Ibid.
11 Reiss, "Thou Shalt Not Take the Name of the Lord."
12 Because some early vaccines were developed using fetal tissue to grow the initial virus for isolation, some fetal DNA remains in the vaccine.
13 See, for example, Gilliom, *Overseers of the Poor*; Reich, *Fixing Families*; Flavin, *Our Bodies, Our Crimes*; Stuart, "From 'Rabble Management.'"

CONCLUSION

1 Glanz et al., "Population-Based Cohort Study."
2 Michaels, "Vaccination and the Social Contract."
3 Colgrove, *State of Immunity*, 90.
4 CDC, "National Infant Immunization Week."
5 Heller, *Vaccine Narrative*.
6 Gust et al., "Parents with Doubts"; Gust et al., "Underimmunization among Children"; Byington, "Vaccines."
7 See, for example, Lareau, *Unequal Childhoods*; Ungar, "Overprotective Parenting"; Nelson, *Parenting Out of Control*; Lee, MacVarish, and Bristow, "Risk, Health and Parenting Culture."
8 Haber, Malow, and Zimet, "HPV Vaccine Mandate Controversy"; Brisson et al., "Incremental Impact of Adding Boys."
9 Szabo, "Unexplained, Polio-Like Illness"; CDC, "Enterovirus D68."
10 CDC, "Cases of Ebola."
11 Reuters, "U.S. Firms to Be Given Special Dispensation."
12 Leshem et al., "Rotavirus Vaccines."
13 Gormley, "Test of the Revolving Door Hypothesis."
14 Revolving Door Working Group, "A Matter of Trust"; Meghani and Kuzma, "'Revolving Door' between Regulatory Agencies and Industry."
15 U.S. House of Representatives, "Conflicts of Interest."
16 Institute of Medicine, "Member Profiles: Julie Gerberding."

17 Ibid.
18 Brubaker and Dillaway, "Medicalization"; Malacrida and Boulton, "Best Laid Plans?"
19 Lareau and Lopes Muñoz, "'You're Not Going to Call the Shots.'"
20 General Accounting Office, "Report to Congressional Requesters."
21 Welner, "Dirty Dozen"; Orfield and Frankenberg, *Educational Delusions?* Notably, charter schools (and private schools) have much lower rates of vaccination than do other public schools. See Constable, Blank, and Caplan, "Rising Rates of Vaccine Exemptions"; Sugerman et al., "Measles Outbreak."
22 Fisher, "Vaccination."
23 Misztal, *Trust in Modern Societies*; Iversen, Napolitano, and Furstenberg, "Middle-Income Families in the Economic Downturn"; Allum et al., "Re-Evaluating the Links."
24 It is worth noting that pediatricians remain important and trusted sources of information about vaccines, and their efforts to partner with families are largely successful. See Freed et al., "Sources and Perceived Credibility'; Kennedy et al., "Confidence about Vaccines"; Gust et al., "Parental Perceptions"; Opel et al., "Architecture of Provider-Parent Vaccine Discussions."
25 See Voices for Vaccines, "From Anti-Vax to Pro-Vax"; Colorado Children's Immunization Coalition, "Parents Talk."
26 C. S. Mott Children's Hospital, "Parents Support Daycare Policies."
27 Kennedy et al., "Confidence about Vaccines."
28 Daley and Glanz, "Straight Talk about Vaccination."

APPENDIX A: METHODS
1 Merck Manuals, "Vegetative State and Minimally Conscious State."
2 Naples, "Towards Comparative Analyses of Women's Political Praxis."
3 Reich, "Old Methods and New Technologies."
4 Reich, *Fixing Families.*
5 Some parents wanted the tetanus vaccine without the pertussis or diphtheria vaccine. They are passionately opposed to vaccination otherwise, and so I treat them the same as having received no vaccines.
6 Smith, Chu, and Barker, "Children Who Have Received No Vaccines."
7 Pneumococcal vaccine was added in 2000. Rotavirus vaccine was introduced in 1996, withdrawn from the market, and relicensed in 2006. Hepatitis A vaccine also became required in 2006.
8 Charmaz, "Qualitative Interviewing," 678.

REFERENCES

"Acid Reflux Meds on Rise in Babies, but Are They Effective?" *Cedar Rapids Gazette*, October 15, 2010.

Albrecht, Paul, Francis A. Ennis, Edward J. Saltzman, and Saul Krugman. "Persistence of Maternal Antibody in Infants beyond 12 Months: Mechanism of Measles Vaccine Failure." *Journal of Pediatrics* 91, no. 5 (1977): 715–18.

Alexander, James P., Kristen Ehresmann, Jane Seward, Gary Wax, Kathleen Harriman, Susan Fuller, Elizabeth A. Cebelinski, Qi Chen, Olen M. Kew, and Mark A. Pallansch. "Transmission of Imported Vaccine-Derived Poliovirus in an Undervaccinated Community in Minnesota." *Journal of Infectious Diseases* 199, no. 3 (2009): 391–97.

Allen, Arthur. "Shingles & Chickenpox: What's the Link?" WebMD, March 15, 2011. http://www.webmd.com/vaccines/features/shingles-chickenpox.

———. *Vaccine: The Controversial Story of Medicine's Greatest Lifesaver*. New York: Norton, 2007.

Allum, Nick, Roger Patulny, Sanna Read, and Patrick Sturgis. "Re-Evaluating the Links between Social Trust, Institutional Trust and Civic Association." In *Spatial and Social Disparities*, edited by John Stillwell et al., 199–215. Dordrecht: Springer Netherlands, 2010.

American Academy of Pediatrics. "Breastfeeding Benefits Your Baby's Immune System." HealthyChildren.org, November 21, 2015. Cited November 24, 2015. http://www.healthychildren.org/English/ages-stages/baby/breastfeeding/pages/Breastfeeding-Benefits-Your-Baby's-Immune-System.aspx.

———. "Chicken Pox Immunity: How Long It Lasts." HealthyChildren.org, August 7, 2013. Cited September 30, 2014. http://www.healthychildren.org/English/safety-prevention/immunizations/Pages/Chicken-Pox-Immunity-How-Long-It-Lasts.aspx.

———. "Documenting Parental Refusal to Have Their Children Vaccinated." Elk Grove Village, IL: American Academy of Pediatrics, 2013.

———. "Immunization Training Guide and Practice Procedure Manual for Pediatricians, Physicians, Nurse Practitioners, Physician Assistants, Nurses, Medical Assistants, and Office Managers." Elk Grove Village, IL: American Academy of Pediatrics, 2012.

———. *Red Book: 2009 Report of the Committee on Infectious Diseases*. 28th ed. Elk Grove Village, IL: American Academy of Pediatrics, 2009.

Amin-Zaki, Laman, Sami Elhassani, Mohamed A. Majeed, Thomas W. Clarkson, Richard A. Doherty, and Michael Greenwood. "Intra-Uterine Methylmercury Poisoning in Iraq." *Pediatrics* 54, no. 5 (1974): 587–95.

Anderson, Benedict. *Imagined Communities: Reflections on the Origin and Spread of Nationalism*. London: Verso, 1991.

Anderson, Joan M. "Empowering Patients: Issues and Strategies." *Social Science & Medicine* 43, no. 5 (1996): 697–705.

Apple, Rima. *Perfect Motherhood: Science and Childrearing in America*. New Brunswick: Rutgers University Press, 2006.

Associated Press. "Measles Outbreak Traced to Disneyland Is Declared Over." April 17, 2015. Cited May 21, 2015. http://www.nbcnews.com/storyline/measles-outbreak/measles-outbreak-traced-disneyland-declared-over-n343686.

Attachment Parenting International. "API's Eight Principles of Parenting." AttachmentParenting.org, 2015. Cited May 31, 2015. http://www.attachmentparenting.org/principles/api.

Autism Speaks. "Jenny McCarthy and Jim Carrey Lead 'Green Our Vaccines' Rally." AutismSpeaks.org, May 11, 2008. http://www.autismspeaks.org/news/news-item/jenny-mccarthy-and-jim-carrey-lead-%E2%80%9Cgreen-our-vaccines-rally%E2%80%9D.

Avishai, Orit. "Managing the Lactating Body: The Breast-Feeding Project and Privileged Motherhood." *Qualitative Sociology* 30 (2007): 135–52.

Baker, Jeffrey P. "Immunization and the American Way: 4 Childhood Vaccines." *American Journal of Public Health* 90, no. 2 (2000): 199–207.

——. "Mercury, Vaccines, and Autism: One Controversy, Three Histories." *American Journal of Public Health* 98, no. 2 (2008): 244–53.

Bakir, F., S. F. Damlugi, L. Amin-Zaki, M. Murtadha, A. Khalidi, N. Y. Al-Rawi, S. Tikriti, H. I. Dhahir, T. W. Clarkson, J. C. Smith, and R. A. Doherty. "Methylmercury Poisoning in Iraq." *Science* 181 (1973): 230–41.

Baldwin, Peter. *Contagion and the State in Europe, 1830–1930*. London: Cambridge University Press, 2005.

Barker, Kristin. "Women Physicians and the Gendered System of Professions: An Analysis of the Sheppard-Towner Act of 1921." *Work and Occupations* 25, no. 2 (1998): 229–55.

Barlow, William E., Robert L. Davis, John W. Glasser, Phillip H. Rhodes, Robert S. Thompson, John P. Mullooly, Steven B. Black, Henry R. Shinefield, Joel I. Ward, and S. Michael Marcy. "The Risk of Seizures after Receipt of Whole-Cell Pertussis or Measles, Mumps, and Rubella Vaccine." *New England Journal of Medicine* 345, no. 9 (2001): 656–61.

Barry, John. *The Great Influenza: The Story of the Deadliest Pandemic in History*. New York: Penguin, 2005.

Becker, Howard S., Blanche Geer, Everett C. Hughes, and Anselm Strauss. *Boys in White: Student Culture in Medical School*. Chicago: University of Chicago Press, 1961.

Benin, Andrea L., Daryl J. Wisler-Scher, Eve Colson, Eugene D. Shapiro, and Eric S. Holmboe. "Qualitative Analysis of Mothers' Decision-Making about Vaccines for Infants: The Importance of Trust." *Pediatrics* 117, no. 5 (2006): 1532–41.

Berlin, Isaiah. *Liberty: Incorporating Four Essays on Liberty.* Edited by Henry Hardy. Oxford: Oxford University Press, 2002.

Blum, Linda. *At the Breast: Ideologies of Breastfeeding and Motherhood in the Contemporary United States.* Boston: Beacon, 1999.

———. "Mother-Blame in the Prozac Nation: Raising Kids with Invisible Disabilities." *Gender & Society* 21, no. 2 (2007): 202–26.

Blume, Stuart S. "Lock In, the State and Vaccine Development: Lessons from the History of the Polio Vaccines." *Research Policy* 34, no. 2 (2005): 159–73.

Bobel, Chris. *The Paradox of Natural Mothering.* Philadelphia: Temple University Press, 2002.

Booth, Michael. "Colorado Parents Rank Second in Nation for Vaccine Refusals." *Denver Post*, November 29, 2011.

Boulis, Ann, Susan Goold, and Peter A. Ubel. "Responding to the Immunoglobulin Shortage: A Case Study." *Journal of Health Politics, Policy and Law* 27, no. 6 (2002): 977–1000.

Bowen, Sarah, Sinikka Elliott, and Joslyn Brenton. "The Joy of Cooking?" *Contexts* 13, no. 3 (2014): 20–25.

Branches, Fernando J .P., Timothy B. Erickson, Steven E. Aks, and Daniel O. Hryhorczuk. "The Price of Gold: Mercury Exposure in the Amazonian Rain Forest." *Clinical Toxicology* 31, no. 2 (1993): 295–306.

Brandt, Alan. *No Magic Bullet: A Social History of Venereal Disease in the United States since 1880.* London: Oxford University Press, 1987.

Brisson, Marc, Nicolas van de Velde, Eduardo L. Franco, Mélanie Drolet, and Marie-Claude Boily. "Incremental Impact of Adding Boys to Current Human Papillomavirus Vaccination Programs: Role of Herd Immunity." *Journal of Infectious Diseases* 204, no. 3 (2011): 372–76. %R 10.1093/infdis/jir285.

Brown, Katrina F., J. Simon Kroll, Michael J. Hudson, Mary Ramsay, John Green, Charles A. Vincent, Graham Fraser, and Nick Sevdalis. "Omission Bias and Vaccine Rejection by Parents of Healthy Children: Implications for the Influenza A/H1N1 Vaccination Programme." *Vaccine* 28, no. 25 (2010): 4181–85.

Brubaker, Sarah Jane, and Heather E. Dillaway. "Medicalization, Natural Childbirth and Birthing Experiences." *Sociology Compass* 3, no. 1 (2009): 31–48.

Bryant, Joanne, Maree Porter, Sally K. Tracy, and Elizabeth A. Sullivan. "Caesarean Birth: Consumption, Safety, Order, and Good Mothering." *Social Science & Medicine* 65, no. 6 (2007): 1192–201.

Buck v. Bell. 274 U.S. 200 (1927).

Business Wire. "National Vaccine Information Center Launches Research Fund to Study Health and Vaccination." 2009.

Buttenheim, Alison M., Karthik Sethuraman, Saad B. Omer, Alexandra L. Hanlon, Michael Z. Levy, and Daniel Salmon. "MMR Vaccination Status of Children

Exempted from School-Entry Immunization Mandates." *Vaccine* 33, no. 46 (2015): 6250–56.

Byington, Carrie L. "Vaccines: Can Transparency Increase Confidence and Reduce Hesitancy?" *Pediatrics* 134, no. 2 (2014): 377–79. %R 10.1542/peds.2014–1494.

Canterbury v. Spence. 464 F.2d 772 (D.C. Cir. 1972).

Carpenter, D. "Can Expedited FDA Drug Approval without Expedited Follow-Up Be Trusted?" *JAMA Internal Medicine* 174, no. 1 (2014): 95–97.

Casiday, Rachel Elizabeth. "Children's Health and the Social Theory of Risk: Insights from the British Measles, Mumps and Rubella (MMR) Controversy." *Social Science & Medicine* 65, no. 5 (2007): 1059–70.

Casper, Monica J., and Laura M. Carpenter. "Sex, Drugs, and Politics: The HPV Vaccine for Cervical Cancer." *Sociology of Health & Illness* 30, no. 6 (2008): 886–99.

Centers for Disease Control and Prevention (CDC). "2015 Measles Cases in the U.S." CDC.gov, 2015. Cited May 21, 2015. http://www.cdc.gov/measles/cases-outbreaks.html.

———. "About Tetanus." CDC.gov, January 9, 2013. Cited September 29, 2014. http://www.cdc.gov/tetanus/about/index.html.

———. "Achievements in Public Health, 1900–1999 Impact of Vaccines Universally Recommended for Children—United States, 1990–1998." *Morbidity and Mortality Weekly Report (MMWR)* 48, no. 12 (1999): 243–48.

———. "Advisory Committee on Immunization Practices (ACIP)." CDC.gov, 2011. Cited May 18, 2011. http://www.cdc.gov/vaccines/acip/index.html.

———. "Autism Spectrum Disorder." CDC.gov, March 24, 2014. Cited June 24, 2014. http://www.cdc.gov/ncbddd/autism/data.html.

———. "Benefits from Immunization during the Vaccines for Children Program Era—United States, 1994–2013." *Morbidity and Mortality Weekly Report (MMWR)* 63, no. 16 (2014): 352–55.

———. "Cases of Ebola Diagnosed in the United States." CDC.gov, December 16, 2014. Cited May 26, 2015. http://www.cdc.gov/vhf/ebola/outbreaks/2014-west-africa/united-states-imported-case.html.

———. "CDC Reports About 90 Percent of Children Who Died from Flu This Season Not Vaccinated." CDC.gov, March 22, 2013. Cited November 23, 2014. http://www.cdc.gov/flu/spotlights/children-flu-deaths.htm.

———. "Chicken Pox (Varicella)." CDC.gov, 2012. http://www.cdc.gov/chickenpox/surveillance.html.

———. "Diphtheria." CDC.gov, 2013. Cited April 14, 2014. http://www.cdc.gov/diphtheria/clinicians.html.

———. "Enterovirus D68 in the United States." CDC.gov, December 4, 2014. Cited December 9, 2014. http://www.cdc.gov/non-polio-enterovirus/outbreaks/EV-D68-outbreaks.html.

———. "Estimates of Deaths Associated with Seasonal Influenza—United States, 1976–2007." *Morbidity and Mortality Weekly Report (MMWR)* 59, no. 33 (2010): 1057–62.

———. "Estimating Seasonal Influenza-Associated Deaths in the United States: CDC Study Confirms Variability of Flu." CDC.gov, 2010. Cited June 6, 2011. http://www.cdc.gov/flu/about/disease/us_flu-related_deaths.htm.

———. "Frequently Asked Questions about Multiple Vaccinations and the Immune System." CDC.gov, December 7, 2012. Cited September 15, 2013. http://www.cdc.gov/vaccinesafety/Vaccines/multiplevaccines.html.

———. "Joint Statement of the American Academy of Pediatrics (AAP) and the United States Public Health Service." Bethesda, MD: Centers for Disease Control and Prevention, 1999.

———. "Measles (Rubeola)." CDC.gov, April 27, 2015. Cited June 5, 2015. http://www.cdc.gov/measles/about/complications.html.

———. "National Infant Immunization Week." CDC.gov, 2011. http://www.cdc.gov/vaccines/events/niiw/index.html.

———. "National, State, and Local Area Vaccination Coverage among Children Aged 19–35 Months—United States, 2011." *Morbidity and Mortality Weekly Report (MMWR)* 61, no. 35 (2013): 689–96. Atlanta, GA

———. "Pertussis Outbreak Trends." CDC.gov, March 11, 2015. Cited May 31, 2015. http://www.cdc.gov/pertussis/outbreaks/trends.html.

———. "Polio Vaccine: What You Need to Know." CDC.gov, January 1, 2000. Cited May 22, 2009. http://www.cdc.gov/vaccines/pubs/VIS/downloads/vis-IPV.pdf.

———. "Possible Side Effects of Vaccines." CDC.gov, February 1, 2014. Cited July 15, 2014. http://www.cdc.gov/vaccines/vac-gen/side-effects.htm.

———. "Rotashield' (Rotavirus) Vaccine and Intussusception." Atlanta: National Center for Infectious Diseases, U.S. Centers for Disease Control and Prevention, 2004.

———. "Rotavirus Vaccine (Rotashield®) and Intussusception: Historical Information as Rotashield® Was Taken Off U.S. Market in 1999." CDC.gov, June 23, 2010. Cited May 23, 2011. http://www.cdc.gov/vaccines/vpd-vac/rotavirus/vac-rotashield-historical.htm.

———. "Rubella: Epidemiology and Prevention of Vaccine-Preventable Diseases." CDC.gov, May 7, 2012. http://www.cdc.gov/vaccines/pubs/pinkbook/rubella.html.

———. "Talking with Parents about Vaccines for Infants: Strategies for Health Care Professionals." CDC.gov, March 2012. Cited June 25, 2014. http://www.cdc.gov/vaccines/hcp/patient-ed/conversations/downloads/talk-infants-bw-office.pdf.

———. "Tetanus: For Clinicians." CDC.gov, January 9, 2013. Cited September 29, 2014. http://www.cdc.gov/tetanus/clinicians.html.

———. "Viral Hepatitis: Statistics and Surveillance." CDC.gov, May 31, 2015. Cited June 4, 2015. http://www.cdc.gov/hepatitis/statistics/.

Charmaz, Kathy. "Qualitative Interviewing and Grounded Theory Analysis." In *Handbook of Interview Research: Context and Method*, edited by J. Gubrium and J. A. Holstein, 675–94. Thousand Oaks, CA: Sage, 2002.

Chaves, Sandra S., Paul Gargiullo, John X. Zhang, Rachel Civen, Dalya Guris, Laurene Mascola, and Jane F. Seward. "Loss of Vaccine-Induced Immunity to Varicella over Time." *New England Journal of Medicine* 356, no. 11 (2007): 1121–29.

Cheal, David. *Family and the State of Theory*. Toronto: University of Toronto Press, 1991.

Cherry, James D. "Historical Review of Pertussis and the Classical Vaccine." *Journal of Infectious Diseases* 174, Supplement 3 (1996): S259–S63.

Cheslack-Postava, Keely, Kayuet Liu, and Peter S. Bearman. "Closely Spaced Pregnancies Are Associated with Increased Odds of Autism in California Sibling Births." *Pediatrics* 127, no. 2 (2011): 246–53.

Children's Hospital of Philadelphia. "General Vaccine Safety Concerns: Is Natural Infection Better Than Immunization?" CHOP.edu, 2013. Cited September 30, 2014. http://www.chop.edu/service/vaccine-education-center/vaccine-safety/general-safety-concerns.html.

———. "History of Vaccine Schedule." CHOP.edu, April 2013. Cited May 22, 2015. http://vec.chop.edu/service/vaccine-education-center/vaccine-schedule/history-of-vaccine-schedule.html.

———. "How Are Vaccines Made?" CHOP.edu, April 2013. Cited January 10, 2014. http://www.chop.edu/service/vaccine-education-center/vaccine-science/how-are-vaccines-made.html.

———. "Too Many Vaccines? What You Should Know." Philadelphia: Vaccine Education Center, Children's Hospital of Philadelphia, 2012.

Clarke, Adele E., Janet K. Shim, Laura Mamo, Jennifer Ruth Fosket, and Jennifer R. Fishman. "Biomedicalization: Technoscientific Transformations of Health, Illness, and U.S. Biomedicine." *American Sociological Review* 68, no. 2 (2003): 161–94.

Cohen, Elizabeth. "Should I Vaccinate My Baby?" *CNN*, June 19, 2008.

Cohen, Elizabeth, and Debra Goldschmidt. "Arizona Measles Exposure Worries Parents of At-Risk Kids." *CNN*, February 2, 2015.

Colgrove, James. "Immunity for the People: The Challenge of Achieving High Vaccine Coverage in American History." *Public Health Reports* 122, no. 2 (2007): 248–57.

———. *State of Immunity: The Politics of Vaccination in Twentieth-Century America.* Berkeley: University of California Press, 2006.

College of Physicians of Philadelphia. "The Development of the Immunization Schedule." HistoryofVaccines.org, 2015. http://www.historyofvaccines.org/content/articles/development-immunization-schedule.

———. "The History of Vaccines Timeline." HistoryofVaccines.org, 2015. Cited May 9, 2015. http://www.historyofvaccines.org/content/timelines/diseases-and-vaccines#EVT_000045.

———. "Top 20 Questions about Vaccination." HistoryofVaccines.org, 2015. http://www.historyofvaccines.org/content/articles/top-20-questions-about-vaccination#2.

Collier, Roger. "No End in Sight for Adult Hepatitis B Vaccine Shortage." *Canadian Medical Association Journal* 182, no. 12 (2010): E580.

Colorado Children's Immunization Coalition. "Parents Talk: Written Testimonials." ImmunizeForGood.com, 2015. http://www.immunizeforgood.com/parents-talk/written-testimonials.

Colorado Department of Public Health and the Environment. "Youngest Children Are at Greatest Risk When Parents Choose Delayed Vaccination Schedules." Edited by Mark Salley. Denver: Colorado Department of Public Health and the Environment Office of Communications, 2012. http://www.prweb.com/releases/2012/4/prweb9441986.htm.

Committee on Community Health Services. "The Pediatrician's Role in Community Pediatrics." Pediatrics 115, no. 4 (2005): 1092–94. %R 10.542/peds.2004–680.

Committee on Hospital Care, and Institute for Patient- and Family-Centered Care. "Patient- and Family-Centered Care and the Pediatrician's Role." Pediatrics 129, no. 2 (2012): 394–404. %R 10.1542/peds.2011–3084.

Conis, Elena. Vaccine Nation: America's Changing Relationship with Immunization. Chicago: University of Chicago Press, 2015.

Conrad, Peter. "The Meaning of Medications: Another Look at Compliance." Social Science in Medicine 20, no. 1 (1985): 29–37.

Constable, Catherine, Nina R. Blank, and Arthur L. Caplan. "Rising Rates of Vaccine Exemptions: Problems with Current Policy and More Promising Remedies." Vaccine 32, no. 16 (2014): 1793–97.

Copelton, Denise A. "'You Are What You Eat': Nutritional Norms, Maternal Deviance, and Neutralization of Women's Prenatal Diets." Deviant Behavior 28, no. 5 (2007): 467–94.

Crawford, Robert. "Healthism and the Medicalization of Everyday Life." International Journal of Health Services 10, no. 3 (1980): 365–88.

C. S. Mott Children's Hospital. "Parents Support Daycare Policies to Get Kids Up-to-Date on Vaccines." National Poll on Children's Health 22, no. 4 (November 17, 2014). http://mottnpch.org/reports-surveys/parents-support-daycare-policies-get-kids-date-vaccines.

Dachel, Anne. "Moms in Charge Presents Dr. Andrew Wakefield on CDC Whistleblower." AgeofAutism.com, May 21, 2015. Cited June 4, 2015. http://www.ageofautism.com/2015/05/moms-in-charge-presents-dr-andrew-wakefield-on-cdc-whistleblower.html.

Daley, Matthew F., and Jason M. Glanz. "Straight Talk about Vaccination." Scientific American 305, no. 3 (2011): 32–34.

Davis, Kathy. The Making of Our Bodies, Ourselves: How Feminism Travels across Borders. Durham: Duke University Press, 2007.

DeHovitz, Ross E. "The 1901 St Louis Incident: The First Modern Medical Disaster." Pediatrics 133, no. 6 (2014): 964–65. %R 10.1542/peds.2013–817.

Demicheli, V., Tom Jefferson, Lubria Al-Ansary, Eliana Ferroni, Alessandro Rivetti, Carlo Di Pietrantonj. "Vaccines for Preventing Influenza in Healthy Adults." Cochrane Database of Systematic Reviews, no. 3 (2014). http://onlinelibrary.wiley.com/doi/10.1002/14651858.CD001269.pub5/epdf/standard

Dempsey, Amanda F., Sarah Schaffer, Dianne Singer, Amy Butchart, Matthew Davis, and Gary L. Freed. "Alternative Vaccination Schedule Preferences among Parents of

Young Children." *Pediatrics* 128, no. 5 (2011): 848–56. http://pediatrics.aappublications.org/content/pediatrics/128/5/848.full.pdf.

Dennehy, Penelope H. "Rotavirus Vaccines: An Overview." *Clinical Microbiology Reviews* 21, no. 1 (2008): 198–208.

Department of Health and Human Services. "Immunization and Infectious Diseases." HealthyPeople.gov, September 6, 2012. Cited December 12, 2012. http://www.healthypeople.gov/2020/topicsobjectives2020/overview.aspx?topicid=23.

DeVault, Marjorie. *Feeding the Family: The Social Organization of Caring as Gendered Work*. Women in Culture and Society Series. Chicago: University of Chicago Press, 1991.

DeWeerdt, Sarah. "Vaccines: An Age-Old Problem." *Nature* 502, no. 7470 (2013): S8–S9.

Diekema, Douglas S., and the Committee on Bioethics. "Responding to Parental Refusals of Immunization of Children." *Pediatrics* 115, no. 5 (2005): 1428–31.

Dinzey-Flores, Zaire Zenit. *Locked In, Locked Out: Gated Communities in a Puerto Rican City*. Philadelphia: University of Pennsylvania Press, 2013.

Elliott, Sinikka. *Not My Kid: What Parents Believe about the Sex Lives of Their Teenagers*. New York: New York University Press, 2012.

Elliott, Sinikka, Rachel Powell, and Joslyn Brenton. "Being a Good Mom: Low-Income, Black Single Mothers Negotiate Intensive Mothering." *Journal of Family Issues* 36, no. 3 (2013): 351–70.

Epstein, Steven. *Impure Science: AIDS, Activism, and the Politics of Knowledge*. Berkeley: University of California Press, 1996.

Fairbrother, Gerry, Amy Cassedy, Ismael R. Ortega-Sanchez, Peter G. Szilagyi, Kathryn M. Edwards, Noelle-Angelique Molinari, Stephanie Donauer, Diana Henderson, Sandra Ambrose, Diane Kent, Katherine Poehling, Geoffrey A. Weinberg, Marie R. Griffin, Caroline B. Hall, Lyn Finelli, Carolyn Bridges, and Mary Allen Staat. "High Costs of Influenza: Direct Medical Costs of Influenza Disease in Young Children." *Vaccine* 28, no. 31 (2010): 4913–19.

Families Fighting Flu. "The Booth Family." FamiliesFightingFlu.org, n.d. Cited May 28, 2015. http://www.familiesfightingflu.org/member-families/the-booth-family/.

Fenton, J. J., A. F. Jerant, K. D. Bertakis, and P. Franks. "The Cost of Satisfaction: A National Study of Patient Satisfaction, Health Care Utilization, Expenditures, and Mortality." *Archives of Internal Medicine* 172, no. 5 (2012): 405–11.

Fisher, Barbara Loe. "Influenza Deaths: The Hype vs. the Evidence." Mercola.com, October 3, 2012. Cited June 25, 2014. http://articles.mercola.com/sites/articles/archive/2012/10/03/hype-vs-evidence-of-influenza-deaths.aspx#_edn32.

———. "Vaccination: Defending Your Right to Know and Freedom to Choose." NVIC.org, November 30, 2014. http://www.nvic.org/nvic-vaccine-news/november-2014/vaccination—defending-your-right-to-know-and-free.aspx.

———. "Vaccines: Doctor Judges & Juries Hanging Their Own." NVIC.org, January 29, 2010. http://www.nvic.org/NVIC-Vaccine-News/January-2010/Vaccines-Doctor-Judges-Juries-Hanging-Their-Own.aspx.

Flavin, Jeanne. *Our Bodies, Our Crimes: The Policing of Women's Reproduction in America.* New York: New York University Press, 2008.

Food and Drug Administration. "Inspections, Compliance, Enforcement, and Criminal Investigations: Sanofi Pasteur Warning Letter." 2012. http://www.fda.gov/ICECI/EnforcementActions/WarningLetters/2012/ucm312929.htm.

———. "Thimerosal in Vaccines." 2010. http://www.fda.gov/BiologicsBloodVaccines/SafetyAvailability/VaccineSafety/UCM096228.

———. "Vaccines, Blood & Biologics." FDA.gov, 2009. Cited August 2, 2014. http://www.fda.gov/biologicsbloodvaccines/developmentapprovalprocess/biologicslicenseapplicationsblaprocess/ucm133096.htm.

Fountain, Christine, Marissa D. King, and Peter S. Bearman. "Age of Diagnosis for Autism: Individual and Community Factors across 10 Birth Cohorts." *Journal of Epidemiology and Community Health* 65, no. 6 (2011): 503–10.

Fox, Maggie. "Teen's Death Shows How Flu Can Kill in a Flash." NBCNews.com, October 18, 2012. http://www.nbcnews.com/id/49465633/ns/health-cold_and_flu/t/teens-death-shows-how-flu-can-kill-flash/.

Freed, Gary L., Sarah J. Clark, Amy T. Butchart, Dianne C. Singer, and Matthew M. Davis. "Parental Vaccine Safety Concerns in 2009." *Pediatrics* 125 (2010): 654–59.

———. "Sources and Perceived Credibility of Vaccine-Safety Information for Parents." *Pediatrics* 127, Supplement 1 (2011): S107-S12. %R 10.1542/peds.2010–1722P.

Freedman, David. "Mailing 'Chickenpox Lollipops' Called Illegal, Risky." CBSNews.com, November 7, 2011. http://www.cbsnews.com/news/mailing-chickenpox-lollipops-called-illegal-risky/.

Freeman, Bradley, and Richard L. Frierson. "Court-Mandated, Long-Acting Antipsychotic Medication as a Condition of Supervised Release." *Journal of the American Academy of Psychiatry and the Law Online* 37, no. 2 (2009): 268–70.

Frizell, Sam. "Tylenol Maker Admits to Selling Liquid Medicine Contaminated with Metal." *Time*, March 11, 2015.

Fulginiti, Vincent A. "A New Pertussis Vaccine: Hope for the Future?" *Journal of Infectious Diseases* 148, no. 1 (1983): 146–47.

Fulton, April. "Bioterrorism Bill Includes Provision Renewing Drug User-Fee Law." *Government Executive*, May 28, 2002.

Gagne, J. J., and N. K. Choudhry. "How Many 'Me-Too' Drugs Is Too Many?" *JAMA* 305, no. 7 (2011): 711–12.

Gellin, Bruce G., and William Schaffner. "The Risk of Vaccination—The Importance of 'Negative' Studies." *New England Journal of Medicine* 344, no. 5 (2001): 372–73.

General Accounting Office. "Report to Congressional Requesters: Welfare Reform: State Sanction Policies and Number of Families Affected." Washington, D.C.: General Accounting Office, 2000.

Gilliom, John. *Overseers of the Poor: Surveillance, Resistance, and the Limits of Privacy.* Chicago: University of Chicago Press, 2001.

Glanz, J. M., S. R. Newcomer, K. J. Narwaney, S. J. Hambidge, M. F. Daley, N. M. Wagner, D. L. McClure, S. Xu, A. Rowhani-Rahbar, G. M. Lee, J. C. Nelson, J. G. Donahue, A. L. Naleway, J. D. Nordin, M. M. Lugg, and E. S. Weintraub. "A Population-Based Cohort Study of Undervaccination in 8 Managed Care Organizations across the United States." *JAMA Pediatrics* 167, no. 2 (2013): 274–81.

Goffman, Erving. *Stigma: Notes on the Management of Spoiled Identity.* New York: Simon and Schuster, 1986.

Gormley, William T., Jr. "A Test of the Revolving Door Hypothesis at the FCC." *American Journal of Political Science* 23, no. 4 (1979): 665–83.

Grandjean, Philippe, Pal Weihe, Roberta F. White, Frodi Debes, Shunichi Araki, Kazuhito Yokoyama, Katsuyuki Murata, Nicolina Sørensen, Rasmus Dahl, and Poul J. Jørgensen. "Cognitive Deficit in 7-Year-Old Children with Prenatal Exposure to Methylmercury." *Neurotoxicology and Teratology* 19, no. 6 (1997): 417–28.

Greenwood, Veronica. "Curing the Common Cold." *Scientific American*, December 27, 2010.

Gust, Deborah A., Natalie Darling, Allison Kennedy, and Ben Schwartz. "Parents with Doubts about Vaccines: Which Vaccines and Reasons Why." *Pediatrics* 122, no. 4 (2008): 718–25. http://pediatrics.aappublications.org/content/122/4/718.

Gust, Deborah A., Tara W. Strine, Emmanuel Maurice, Philip Smith, Hussain Yusuf, Marilyn Wilkinson, Michael Battaglia, Robert Wright, and Benjamin Schwartz. "Underimmunization among Children: Effects of Vaccine Safety Concerns on Immunization Status." *Pediatrics* 114, no. 1 (2004): e16-e22. http://pediatrics.aappublications.org/content/114/1/e16.

Gust, D. A., R. Woodruff, A. Kennedy, C. Brown, K. Sheedy, and B. Hibbs. "Parental Perceptions Surrounding Risks and Benefits of Immunization." *Seminars in Pediatric Infectious Diseases* 14, no. 3 (2003): 207–12.

Haber, G., R. M. Malow, and G. D. Zimet. "The HPV Vaccine Mandate Controversy." *Journal of Pediatric and Adolescent Gynecology* 20, no. 6 (2007): 325–31.

Hales, Craig M., Rafael Harpaz, M. Riduan Joesoef, and Stephanie R. Bialek. "Examination of Links between Herpes Zoster Incidence and Childhood Varicella Vaccination." *Annals of Internal Medicine* 159, no. 11 (2013): 739–45.

Halpern, Sydney Ann. *American Pediatrics: The Social Dynamics of Professionalism, 1880–1980.* Berkeley: University of California Press, 1988.

Hancock, Bronwyn. "Vitamin K: Is This Really Safe or Necessary?" Vaccination Information Service website, October 2003. http://www.vaccination.inoz.com/VitaminK.html.

Harada, M. "Minamata Disease: Methylmercury Poisoning in Japan Caused by Environmental Pollution." *Critical Reviews in Toxicology* 25, no. 1 (1995): 1–24.

Harris, Gardiner, and Duff Wilson. "Glaxo to Pay $750 Million for Sale of Bad Products." *New York Times*, October 26, 2010.

Hays, Sharon. *Cultural Contradictions of Motherhood.* New Haven: Yale University Press, 1996.

Health Resources and Services Administration. "Countermeasures Injury Compensation." HRSA.gov, 2015. http://www.hrsa.gov/cicp/.

Hedgecoe, Adam. *The Politics of Personalised Medicine: Pharmacogenetics in the Clinic.* Cambridge Studies in Society and the Life Sciences. Cambridge, UK: Cambridge University Press, 2004.

Heimer, Megan. "Meet Megan." LivingWhole.org, 2015. http://www.livingwhole.org/about/.

———. "To the Parent of the Immunocompromised Child Who Thinks My Kid Is a Threat." LivingWhole.org, February 9, 2015. http://www.livingwhole.org/to-the-parent-of-an-immunocompromised-child-who-thinks-my-kid-is-a-threat/.

Heininger, Ulrich. "An Internet-Based Survey on Parental Attitudes towards Immunization." *Vaccine* 24, nos. 37–39 (2006): 6351–55.

Heller, Jacob. "The Social Meanings of Vaccines." PhD diss., State University of New York, Stony Brook, 2002.

———. *The Vaccine Narrative.* Nashville: Vanderbilt University Press, 2008.

Hilton, Shona, Mark Petticrew, and Kate Hunt. "'Combined Vaccines Are Like a Sudden Onslaught to the Body's Immune System': Parental Concerns about Vaccine 'Overload' and 'Immune-Vulnerability.'" *Vaccine* 24, no. 20 (2006): 4321–27.

Hinman, Alan R., Jeffrey P. Koplan, Walter A. Orenstein, Edward W. Brink, and Benjamin M. Nkowane. "Live or Inactivated Poliomyelitis Vaccine: An Analysis of Benefits and Risks." *American Journal of Public Health* 78, no. 3 (1988): 291–95.

Hochschild, Arlie Russell. "Emotion Work, Feeling Rules, and Social Structure." *American Journal of Sociology* 85, no. 3 (1979): 551–75.

Hodge, James G. Jr., and Lawrence O. Gostin. "School Vaccination Requirements: Historical, Social, and Legal Perspectives." *Kentucky Law Journal* 90 (2001): 831.

Hunt, Linda M., and Meta J. Kreiner. "Pharmacogenetics in Primary Care: The Promise of Personalized Medicine and the Reality of Racial Profiling." *Culture, Medicine, and Psychiatry* 37, no. 1 (2013): 226–35.

Immunization Action Coalition. "Ask the Experts." *Needling Tips*, July 2009.

———. "Hepatitis B Shots Are Recommended for All New Babies." Saint Paul: Immunization Action Coalition, 2010.

———. "State Information." Immunize.org, February 24, 2015. http://www.immunize.org/laws/.

Immunize Colorado. "Fact or Fiction? Natural Immunity." ImmunizeForGood.com, 2014. http://www.immunizeforgood.com/fact-or-fiction/natural-immunity.

Immunize for Public Health. "Varicella (Chickenpox)." ImmunizationInfo.org, 2014. http://www.immunizationinfo.org/vaccines/varicella-chickenpox.

Informed Parents of Vaccinated Children. Facebook group. 2015. Cited May 21, 2015. https://www.facebook.com/pages/Informed-Parents-of-Vaccinated-Children/236107336440146.

Institute of Medicine. "About the Institute of Medicine." IOM.NationalAcademies.org, 2011. http://iom.nationalacademies.org/About-IOM.aspx.

———. "Member Profiles: Julie Gerberding." IOM.edu, 2014. http://www.iom.edu/Activities/PublicHealth/MedPrep/Member%20Profiles/Julie%20Gerberding.aspx.

Iversen, Roberta Rehner, Laura Napolitano, and Frank F. Furstenberg. "Middle-Income Families in the Economic Downturn: Challenges and Management Strategies over Time." *Longitudinal and Life Course Studies* 2, no. 3 (2011): 15.

Jacks, Tim. "To the Parent of the Unvaccinated Child Who Exposed My Family to Measles." *Mother Jones*, February 2, 2015.

Jacobson v. Massachusetts. 197 U.S. 11 (1905).

Jenner House and Museum. "What Is Small Pox?" JennerMuseum.com, 2015. http://www.jennermuseum.com/vaccination.html.

Johnson, Steven. *The Ghost Map: The Story of London's Most Terrifying Epidemic—and How It Changed Science, Cities, and the Modern World*. New York: Penguin, 2006.

Juffer, Jane. "Dirty Diapers and the New Organic Intellectual." *Cultural Studies* 17, no. 2 (2003): 168–92.

Just the Vax. "Still No Independent Confirmation of Wakefield's Claims." JustTheVax.com, May 8, 2011. http://justthevax.blogspot.com/2011/05/still-no-independent-confirmation-of.html.

Kaddar, Miloud. "Global Vaccine Market Features and Trends." Geneva: World Health Organization, 2013.

Kao, Audiey C., Diane C. Green, Alan M. Zaslavsky, Jeffrey P. Koplan, and Paul D. Cleary. "The Relationship between Method of Physician Payment and Patient Trust." *JAMA* 280, no. 19 (1998): 1708–14.

Kaufman, Sharon R. "Regarding the Rise in Autism: Vaccine Safety Doubt, Conditions of Inquiry, and the Shape of Freedom." *Ethos* 38, no. 1 (2010): 8–32.

Kennedy, Allison, Michelle Basket, and Kristine Sheedy. "Vaccine Attitudes, Concerns, and Information Sources Reported by Parents of Young Children: Results from the 2009 Healthstyles Survey." *Pediatrics* 127, Supplement 1 (2011): S92–S99.

Kennedy, Allison, Katherine LaVail, Glen Nowak, Michelle Basket, and Sarah Landry. "Confidence about Vaccines in the United States: Understanding Parents' Perceptions." *Health Affairs* 30, no. 6 (2011): 1151–59. http://content.healthaffairs.org/content/30/6/1151.full.

Kids Play Safe. Website. 2015. http://kidsplaysafe.net/results.php.

King, Marissa, and Peter Bearman. "Diagnostic Change and the Increased Prevalence of Autism." *International Journal of Epidemiology* 38, no. 5 (2009): 1224–34.

Kirby, David. *Evidence of Harm: Mercury in Vaccines and the Autism Epidemic; A Medical Controversy*. New York: Macmillan, 2007.

Kirkland, Anna. "Credibility Battles in the Autism Litigation." *Social Studies of Science* 42, no. 2 (2012): 237–61.

———. "The Legitimacy of Vaccine Critics: What Is Left after the Autism Hypothesis?" *Journal of Health Politics, Policy and Law* 37, no. 1 (2012): 69–97.

Kivits, Joelle. "Researching the 'Informed Patient.'" *Information, Communication & Society* 7, no. 4 (2004): 510—30.

Kolata, Gina. *Flu: The Story of the Great Influenza Pandemic of 1918 and the Search for the Virus That Caused It.* New York: Touchstone, 2001.

Koprowski, Hilary. "First Decade (1950–1960) of Studies and Trials with the Polio Vaccine." *Biologicals* 34, no. 2 (2006): 81–86.

Lakhani, Sunil. "Early Clinical Pathologists: Edward Jenner (1749–1823)." *Journal of Clinical Pathology* 45, no. 9 (1992): 756.

Lareau, Annette. *Unequal Childhoods: Class, Race, and Family Life.* Berkeley: University of California Press, 2003.

Lareau, Annette, and Vanessa Lopes Muñoz. "'You're Not Going to Call the Shots': Structural Conflicts between the Principal and the PTO at a Suburban Public Elementary School." *Sociology of Education* 85, no. 3 (2012): 201–18.

Largent, Mark. *Vaccine: The Debate in Modern America.* Baltimore: Johns Hopkins University Press, 2012.

Lee, Bruce Y., Shawn T. Brown, Rachel R. Bailey, Richard K. Zimmerman, Margaret A. Potter, Sarah M. McGlone, Philip C. Cooley, John J. Grefenstette, Shanta M. Zimmer, and William D. Wheaton. "The Benefits to All of Ensuring Equal and Timely Access to Influenza Vaccines in Poor Communities." *Health Affairs* 30, no. 6 (2011): 1141–50.

Lee, Ellie, Jan MacVarish, and Jennie Bristow. "Risk, Health and Parenting Culture." *Health, Risk & Society* 12, no. 4 (2010): 293–300.

Lemons, J. Stanley. "The Sheppard-Towner Act: Progressivism in the 1920s." *Journal of American History* 55, no. 4 (1969): 776–86.

Leshem, Eyal, Rebecca E. Moritz, Aaron T. Curns, Fangjun Zhou, Jacqueline E. Tate, Benjamin A. Lopman, and Umesh D. Parashar. "Rotavirus Vaccines and Health Care Utilization for Diarrhea in the United States (2007–2011)." *Pediatrics* 134, no. 1 (2014). http://pediatrics.aappublications.org/content/pediatrics/early/2014/06/03/peds.2013-3849.full.pdf.

Limbach, James. "Merck Recalls Gardasil HPV Vaccine: A Small Number of Vials May Contain Glass Particles." *Consumer Affairs*, December 13, 2013.

Litt, Jacquelyn S. *Medicalized Motherhood: Perspectives from the Lives of African-American and Jewish Women.* New Brunswick: Rutgers University Press, 2000.

Liu, Ka-Yuet, Marissa King, and Peter S. Bearman. "Social Influence and the Autism Epidemic." *American Journal of Sociology* 115, no. 5 (2010): 1387.

Lois, Jennifer. *Home Is Where the School Is: The Logic of Homeschooling and the Emotional Labor of Mothering.* New York: New York University Press, 2012.

Lupton, Deborah. "Risk as Moral Danger: The Social and Political Function of Risk Discourse in Public Health." In *Sociology of Health and Illness*, edited by Peter Conrad, 460–67. New York: Worth, 2009.

Ma, Zhenkun, Christian Lienhardt, Helen McIlleron, Andrew J. Nunn, and Xiexiu Wang. "Global Tuberculosis Drug Development Pipeline: The Need and the Reality." *Lancet* 375, no. 9731 (2010): 2100–2109.

MacKendrick, Norah. "More Work for Mother: Chemical Body Burdens as a Maternal Responsibility." *Gender & Society* 28, no. 5 (2014): 705–28.

Malacrida, Claudia, and Tiffany Boulton. "The Best Laid Plans? Women's Choices, Expectations and Experiences in Childbirth." *Health* 18, no. 1 (2014). %R 10.1177/1363459313476964.

March of Dimes. "A History of the March of Dimes." MarchofDimes.org, August 26, 2010. Cited May 8, 2015. http://www.marchofdimes.org/mission/a-history-of-the-march-of-dimes.aspx.

Mariner, Wendy K. "The National Vaccine Injury Compensation Program." *Health Affairs* 11, no. 1 (1992): 255–65.

Markel, Howard. "April 12, 1955—Tommy Francis and the Salk Vaccine." *New England Journal of Medicine* 352, no. 14 (2005): 1408–10.

Markowitz, Lauri E., Paul Albrecht, Philip Rhodes, Ruth Demonteverde, Emmett Swint, Edmond F. Maes, Clydette Powell, Peter A. Patriarca, and Team Kaiser Permanente Measles Vaccine Trial. "Changing Levels of Measles Antibody Titers in Women and Children in the United States: Impact on Response to Vaccination." *Pediatrics* 97, no. 1 (1996): 53–58.

Mayo Clinic. "Egg Allergy." MayoClinic.org, January 23, 2013. Cited September 29, 2014. http://www.mayoclinic.org/diseases-conditions/egg-allergy/basics/prevention/con-20032721.

McCarthy, Jenny. "Green Our Vaccines Rally." Video. 2008. Lighthouse Studios. Uploaded June 5, 2008. https://www.youtube.com/watch?v=ob1fycxZIwI&noredirect=1.

———. *Mother Warriors.* New York: Plume Penguin, 2008.

McCoy, Terrence. "Amid Measles Outbreak, Anti-Vaccine Doctor Revels in His Notoriety." *Washington Post*, January 30, 2015.

McKinlay, John B., and Sonja M. McKinlay. "The Questionable Contribution of Medical Measures to the Decline of Mortality in the United States in the Twentieth Century." *Milbank Memorial Fund Quarterly: Health and Society* (1977): 405–28.

McQuillan, Julia, Arthur L. Greil, Karina M. Shreffler, and Veronica Tichenor. "The Importance of Motherhood among Women in the Contemporary United States." *Gender & Society* 22, no. 4 (2008): 477–96.

Meckel, Richard A. *Save the Babies: American Public Health Reform and the Prevention of Infant Mortality, 1850–1929.* Ann Arbor: University of Michigan Press, 1990.

Meghani, Zahra, and Jennifer Kuzma. "The 'Revolving Door' between Regulatory Agencies and Industry: A Problem That Requires Reconceptualizing Objectivity." *Journal of Agricultural and Environmental Ethics* 24, no. 6 (2010): 575–99.

Meharry, Pamela M., Eve R. Colson, Alexandra P. Grizas, Robert Stiller, and Marietta Vázquez. "Reasons Why Women Accept or Reject the Trivalent Inactivated Influenza Vaccine (TIV) during Pregnancy." *Maternal and Child Health Journal* 17, no. 1 (2012): 156–64.

Merck Manuals. "Vegetative State and Minimally Conscious State." MerckManuals.com, March 2014. http://www.merckmanuals.com/professional/neurologic_disorders/coma_and_impaired_consciousness/vegetative_state_and_minimally_conscious_state.html.

Mercola, Joseph. "Chickenpox (Varicella) Vaccine: This Is Why a Shingles Epidemic Is Bolting Straight at the U.S." Mercola.com, March 2, 2010. http://articles.mercola.com/sites/articles/archive/2010/11/02/chicken-pox-vaccine-creates-shingles-epidemic.aspx.

———. "Flu Vaccine: The Horrible 'Immune System Mistake' Millions Will Make This Year." Mercola.com, January 3, 2012. http://articles.mercola.com/sites/articles/archive/2012/01/03/flu-shot-increase-flu.aspx.

Michaels, Patrick J. "Vaccination and the Social Contract." Cato Institute, Cato.org, February 4, 2015. Cited May 25, 2015. http://www.cato.org/blog/vaccination-social-contract.

Miller, Gregory E., Sheldon Cohen, Sarah Pressman, Anita Barkin, Bruce S. Rabin, and John J. Treanor. "Psychological Stress and Antibody Response to Influenza Vaccination: When Is the Critical Period for Stress, and How Does It Get inside the Body?" *Psychosomatic Medicine* 66, no. 2 (2004): 215–23.

Mintz, Clifford S., and John Liu. "China's Heparin Revisited: What Went Wrong and Has Anything Changed?" *Journal of Commercial Biotechnology* 19, no. 1 (2013). http://commercialbiotechnology.com/index.php/jcb/article/view/579.

Misztal, Barbara. *Trust in Modern Societies: The Search for the Bases of Social Order.* Malden, MA: John Wiley, 2013.

Molinari, Noelle-Angelique M., Ismael R. Ortega-Sanchez, Mark L. Messonnier, William W. Thompson, Pascale M. Wortley, Eric Weintraub, and Carolyn B. Bridges. "The Annual Impact of Seasonal Influenza in the U.S.: Measuring Disease Burden and Costs." *Vaccine* 25, no. 27 (2007): 5086–96.

Mooney, Chris. "Babies Are Getting Brain Bleeds—Are Vaccine Fears to Blame?" *Mother Jones*, July 28, 2014.

Morgen, Sandra. *Into Our Own Hands: The Women's Health Movement in the United States, 1969–1990.* New Brunswick: Rutgers University Press, 2002.

Mullin, R. H. "Recent Advances in the Control of Diphtheria." *Canadian Medical Association Journal* 14, no. 5 (1924): 398.

Murphy, Elizabeth. "Risk, Responsibility, and Rhetoric in Infant Feeding." *Journal of Contemporary Ethnography* 29, no. 3 (2000): 291–325.

Nadeau, Jessica A., Robert A. Bednarczyk, Munyaradzi R. Masawi, Megan D. Meldrum, Loretta Santilli, Shelley M. Zansky, Debra S. Blog, Guthrie S. Birkhead, and Louise-Anne McNutt. "Vaccinating My Way—Use of Alternative Vaccination Schedules in New York State." *Journal of Pediatrics* 166, no. 1 (2015): 151–56e1.

Naples, Nancy A. "Towards Comparative Analyses of Women's Political Praxis: Explicating Multiple Dimensions of Standpoint Epistemology for Feminist Ethnography." *Women and Politics* 20, no. 1 (Winter 1999): 29–31.

National Academies of Science. *Toxicological Effects of Methylmercury.* Washington, D.C.: National Academies Press, 2000.

National Conference of State Legislatures. "States with Religious and Philosophical Exemptions from School Immunization Requirements." NCSL.org, March 3, 2015. http://www.ncsl.org/research/health/school-immunization-exemption-state-laws.aspx.

National Network for Immunization Information. "Hepatitis B." ImmunizationInfo. org, January 27, 2009. Cited April 25, 2011. http://www.immunizationinfo.org/ vaccines/hepatitis-b.

Nelson, Margaret K. *Parenting Out of Control.* New York: New York University Press, 2010.

Nesi, Tom. *Poison Pills: The Untold Story of the Vioxx Drug Scandal.* New York: Thomas Dunne Books, 2008.

Nichol, Kristin L., Kenneth P. Mallon, and Paul M. Mendelman. "Cost Benefit of Influenza Vaccination in Healthy, Working Adults: An Economic Analysis Based on the Results of a Clinical Trial of Trivalent Live Attenuated Influenza Virus Vaccine." *Vaccine* 21, nos. 17–18 (2003): 2207–17.

Nichol, Kristin L., James D. Nordin, David B. Nelson, John P. Mullooly, and Eelko Hak. "Effectiveness of Influenza Vaccine in the Community-Dwelling Elderly." *New England Journal of Medicine* 357, no. 14 (2007): 1373–81. http://www.nejm.org/doi/ pdf/10.1056/NEJMoa070844.

Nkowane, B. M., S. F. Wassilak, W. A. Orenstein, et al. "Vaccine-Associated Paralytic Poliomyelitis: United States: 1973 through 1984." *JAMA* 257, no. 10 (1987): 1335–40.

Offit, Paul A. "The Cutter Incident, 50 Years Later." *New England Journal of Medicine* 352, no. 14 (2005): 1411–12.

———. *Vaccinated: One Man's Quest to Defeat the World's Deadliest Diseases.* New York: HarperCollins, 2008.

———. "Why Are Pharmaceutical Companies Gradually Abandoning Vaccines?" *Health Affairs* 24, no. 3 (2005): 622–30.

Offit, P. A., J. Quarles, M. A. Gerber, C. J. Hackett, E. K. Marcuse, T. R. Kollman, B. G. Gellin, and S. Landry. "Addressing Parents' Concerns: Do Multiple Vaccines Overwhelm or Weaken the Infant's Immune System?" *Pediatrics* 109, no. 1 (2002): 124–29.

O'Leary, Sean T., Mandy A. Allison, Megan C. Lindley, Lori A. Crane, Laura P. Hurley, Michaela Brtnikova, Brenda L. Beaty, Christine I. Babbel, Andrea Jimenez-Zambrano, Stephen Berman, and Allison Kempe. "Vaccine Financing from the Perspective of Primary Care Physicians." *Pediatrics* 133, no. 3 (2014): 367–74.

Olmsted, Dan. "Weekly Wrap: Another Medical Practice with a Sane Vaccine Schedule—and No Autism." AgeofAutism.com, August 23, 2013. Cited May 28, 2015. http://www.ageofautism.com/2013/08/weekly-wrap-another-medical-practice-with-a-sane-vaccine-schedule-and-no-autism-.html.

Omer, S. B., K. S. Enger, L. H. Moulton, N. A. Halsey, S. Stokley, and D. A. Salmon. "Geographic Clustering of Nonmedical Exemptions to School Immunization Requirements and Associations with Geographic Clustering of Pertussis." *American Journal of Epidemiology* 168, no. 15 (2008): 1389–96.

Omer, Saad B., William K. Y. Pan, Neal A. Halsey, Shannon Stokley, Lawrence H. Moulton, Ann Marie Navar, Mathew Pierce, and Daniel A. Salmon. "Nonmedical Exemptions to School Immunization Requirements: Secular Trends and Association of State Policies with Pertussis Incidence." *JAMA* 296, no. 14 (2006): 1757–63.

Omer, Saad B., Daniel Salmon, Walter A. Orenstein, M. Patricia Dehart, and Neal A. Halsey. "Vaccine Refusal, Mandatory Immunization, and the Risks of Vaccine-Preventable Diseases." *New England Journal of Medicine* 360, no. 19 (2009): 1981–88.

Opel, Douglas J., John Heritage, James A. Taylor, Rita Mangione-Smith, Halle Showalter Salas, Victoria DeVere, Chuan Zhou, and Jeffrey D. Robinson. "The Architecture of Provider-Parent Vaccine Discussions at Health Supervision Visits." *Pediatrics* 132, no. 6 (2013): 1037–46. http://pediatrics.aappublications.org/content/pediatrics/early/2013/10/30/peds.2013-2037.full.pdf.

Orenstein, W. A., and A. R. Hinman. "The Immunization System in the United States—The Role of School Immunization Laws." *Vaccine* 17, Supplement 3 (1999): S19–S24.

Orfield, Gary, and Erica Frankenberg. *Educational Delusions? Why Choice Can Deepen Inequality and How to Make Schools Fair*. Berkeley: University of California Press, 2012.

Oshinsky, David M. *Polio: An American Story*. New York: Oxford University Press, 2005.

Palevsky, Lawrence. "About Dr. Palevsky." DrPalevsky.com, 2015. Cited May 28, 2015. http://www.drpalevsky.com/about.asp.

Pan American Health Organization. "Measles and Rubella: Emergency Plan of Action to Be Implemented to Keep the Americas Free of These Diseases." PAHO.org, November 28, 2012. Cited May 21, 2015. http://www.paho.org/hq./index.php?option=com_content&view=article&id=7611%3Ameasles-and-rubella-emergency-plan-of-action-to-be-implemented-to-keep-the-americas-free-of-these-diseases&catid=740%3Anews-press-releases&Itemid=1926&lang=en.

Parmet, W. E., R. A. Goodman, and A. Farber. "Individual Rights versus the Public's Health—100 Years after *Jacobson v. Massachusetts*." *New England Journal of Medicine* 352, no. 7 (2005): 652.

Pediatrics Digest Summary. "Timely versus Delayed Early Childhood Vaccination and Seizures." *Pediatrics* 133, no. 6 (2014): X14.

Petousis-Harris, Helen, Felicity Goodyear-Smith, Nikki Turner, and Ben Soe. "Family Physician Perspectives on Barriers to Childhood Immunisation." *Vaccine* 22, nos. 17–18 (2004): 2340–44.

Pichichero, Michael E., Angela Gentile, Norberto Giglio, Veronica Umido, Thomas Clarkson, Elsa Cernichiari, Grazyna Zareba, Carlos Gotelli, Mariano Gotelli, Lihan Yan, and John Treanor. "Mercury Levels in Newborns and Infants after Receipt of Thimerosal-Containing Vaccines." *Pediatrics* 121, no. 2 (2008): e208–e214.

Pierce, Jennifer L. *Gender Trials: Emotional Lives in Contemporary Law Firms*. Berkeley: University of California Press, 1995.

Poehling, Katherine A., Kathryn M. Edwards, Geoffrey A. Weinberg, Peter Szilagyi, Mary Allen Staat, Marika K. Iwane, Carolyn B. Bridges, Carlos G. Grijalva, Yuwei Zhu, David I. Bernstein, Guillermo Herrera, Dean Erdman, Caroline B. Hall, Ranee Seither, and Marie R. Griffin. "The Underrecognized Burden of Influenza in Young Children." *New England Journal of Medicine* 355, no. 1 (2006): 31–40.

Pope, Sarah. "Six Reasons to Say No to Vaccination." HealthyHo-
meEconomist.com, 2010. http://www.thehealthyhomeeconomist.com/
six-reasons-to-say-no-to-vaccination/.

Powell, Bill. "Heparin's Deadly Side Effects." *Time*, November 13, 2008.

Prifti, Christine. "The Vaccine Industry—An Overview." VaccineEthics.org, July 2010.
Cited October 8, 2013. http://www.vaccineethics.org/issue_briefs/industry.php.

PubMed Health. "Hepatitis B." National Center for Biotechnology Information, U.S.
National Library of Medicine, NCBI.NLM.NIH.gov, November 23, 2010. Cited
April 25, 2011. http://www.ncbi.nlm.nih.gov/pubmedhealth/PMH0001324/.

Reagan, Leslie. *Dangerous Pregnancies: Mothers, Disabilities, and Abortion in Modern
America*. Berkeley: University of California Press, 2010.

Refutations to Anti-Vaccine Memes. "Vaccine Ingredients: Formaldehyde." RTAVM.
com, February 23, 2013. http://rtavm.blogspot.com/2013/02/vaccine-ingredients-
formaldehyde.html.

Reich, Jennifer A. *Fixing Families: Parents, Power, and the Child Welfare System*. New
York: Routledge, 2005.

———. "Old Methods and New Technologies: Social Media and Shifts in Power in
Qualitative Research." *Ethnography* 16, no. 4 (2015): 394–415.

———. "Public Mothers and Private Practices: Breastfeeding as Transgression." In
Embodied Resistance: Breaking the Rules in Public Spaces, edited by Chris Bobel and
Samantha Kwan, 130–42. Nashville: Vanderbilt University Press, 2011.

Reiss, Dorit Rubinstein. "Thou Shalt Not Take the Name of the Lord Thy God in Vain:
Use and Abuse of Religious Exemptions from School Immunization Requirements."
Hastings Law Journal 65, no. 6 (2014): 1551–1602.

Rennels, Margaret B. "The Rotavirus Vaccine Story: A Clinical Investigator's View."
Pediatrics 106, no. 1 (2000): 123–25.

Reuters. "U.S. Firms to Be Given Special Dispensation in Bid to Boost Search for Ebola
Vaccine." *Guardian* online, December 9, 2014.

Revolving Door Working Group. "A Matter of Trust: How the Revolving Door
Undermines Public Confidence in Government—and What to Do about It."
Revolving Door Working Group, October 2005. http://www.policyarchive.org/
handle/10207/10857.

Reynolds, Meredith A., Sandra S. Chaves, Rafael Harpaz, Adriana S. Lopez, and Jane
F. Seward. "The Impact of the Varicella Vaccination Program on Herpes Zoster
Epidemiology in the United States: A Review." *Journal of Infectious Diseases* 197,
Supplement 2 (2008): S224–S227.

Riedel, Stefan. "Edward Jenner and the History of Smallpox and Vaccination." *Proceed-
ings (Baylor University Medical Center)* 18, no. 1 (2005): 21.

Roan, Shari. "Swine Flu 'Debacle' of 1976 Is Recalled." *Los Angeles Times*, April 27, 2009.

Roberts, Dorothy. *Fatal Invention: How Science, Politics, and Big Business Re-Create
Race in the Twenty-First Century*. New York: New Press, 2012.

———. *Killing the Black Body: Race, Reproduction, and the Meaning of Liberty*. New
York: Vintage, 1997.

Robison, Steve G., Holly Groom, and Collette Young. "Frequency of Alternative Immunization Schedule Use in a Metropolitan Area." *Pediatrics* 130, no. 1 (2012): 32–38.

Rose, Nikolas, and Carlos Novas. "Biological Citizenship." In *Global Assemblages: Technology, Politics, and Ethics as Anthropological Problems*, edited by Aihwa Ong and Stephen J. Collier, 439–63. Malden, MA: Wiley-Blackwell, 2004.

Rosenstock, Irwin M. "Why People Use Health Services." *Milbank Memorial Fund Quarterly* 44, no. 3 (1966): 94–127.

Rustam, H., and T. Hamdi. "Methyl Mercury Poisoning in Iraq: A Neurological Study." *Brain* 97, no. 1 (1974): 499–510.

Salganicoff, Alina, Usha R. Ranji, and Roberta Wyn. "Women and Healthcare: A National Profile." Menlo Park, CA: Kaiser Family Foundation, 2005.

Salmon, D. A., M. Haber, E. J. Gangarosa, L. Phillips, N. J. Smith, and R. T. Chen. "Health Consequences of Religious and Philosophical Exemptions from Immunization Laws: Individual and Societal Risk of Measles." *JAMA* 282, no. 1 (1999): 47–53.

Schulte, Rachael, Lori C. Jordan, Anna Morad, Robert P. Naftel, John C. Wellons III, and Robert Sidonio. "Rise in Late Onset Vitamin K Deficiency Bleeding in Young Infants Because of Omission or Refusal of Prophylaxis at Birth." *Pediatric Neurology* 50, no. 6 (2014): 564–68.

Scott, Elizabeth C. "The National Childhood Injury Act Turns Fifteen." *Food and Drug Law Journal* 56 (2001): 351–83.

Scott, Ellen K. "'I Feel as if I Am the One Who Is Disabled': The Emotional Impact of Changed Employment Trajectories of Mothers Caring for Children with Disabilities." *Gender & Society* 24, no. 5 (2010): 672–96.

Sears, Martha. "Attachment Parenting Babies Are Raised the Way Nature Intended." AskDrSears.com, 2015. Cited May 31, 2015. http://www.askdrsears.com/topics/parenting/attachment-parenting/attachment-parenting-babies.

Sears, Robert. "CNN.com & Dr. Bob: Should I Vaccinate?" AskDrSears.com, 2008. Cited May 28, 2015. http://www.askdrsears.com/topics/health-concerns/vaccines/alternative-vaccine-schedule.

———. "Dr. Bob Sears Offers Advice in March 21st New York Times Health Section on Vaccine Choices Parents Make." AskDrSears.com, 2008. http://www.askdrsears.com/topics/health-concerns/vaccines/dr-bob-sears-offers-advice-march-21st-new-york-times-health-section-vaccine-choices.

———. *The Vaccine Book*. New York: Little, Brown, 2007.

Sencer, David J., and J. Donald Millar. "Reflections on the 1976 Swine Flu Vaccination Program." *Emerging Infectious Diseases* 12, no. 1 (2006): 29.

Sheppard–Towner Maternity and Infancy Act, 1921. Cited April 16, 2014. http://history.house.gov/HistoricalHighlight/Detail/36084.

Silverman, Chloe. *Understanding Autism: Parents, Doctors, and the History of a Disorder*. Princeton: Princeton University Press, 2011.

Singh, Ilina. "Doing Their Jobs: Mothering with Ritalin in a Culture of Mother-Blame." *Social Science & Medicine* 59, no. 6 (2004): 1193–205.

Smith, Michael J., and Charles R. Woods. "On-Time Vaccine Receipt in the First Year Does Not Adversely Affect Neuropsychological Outcomes." *Pediatrics* 125, no. 6 (2010): 1134–41.

Smith, Philip J., Susan Y. Chu, and Lawrence E. Barker. "Children Who Have Received No Vaccines: Who Are They and Where Do They Live?" *Pediatrics* 114, no. 1 (2004): 187–95.

Smith, Philip J., Sharon G. Humiston, Trish Parnell, Kirsten S. Vannice, and Daniel A. Salmon. "The Association between Intentional Delay of Vaccine Administration and Timely Childhood Vaccination Coverage." *Public Health Reports* 125, no. 4 (2010): 534.

Soet, Johanna E., William N. Dudley, and Colleen Dilorio. "The Effects of Ethnicity and Perceived Power on Women's Sexual Behavior." *Psychology of Women Quarterly* 23, no. 4 (1999): 707–24.

Solinger, Rickie. *Beggars and Choosers: How the Politics of Choice Shapes Abortion, Adoption, and Welfare in the United States.* New York: Hill and Wang, 2001.

Starr, Paul. *The Social Transformation of American Medicine.* New York: Basic Books, 1982.

Stehr-Green, Paul, Peet Tull, Michael Stellfeld, Preben-Bo Mortenson, and Diane Simpson. "Autism and Thimerosal-Containing Vaccines: Lack of Consistent Evidence for an Association." *American Journal of Preventive Medicine* 25, no. 2 (2003): 101–6.

Steinhauer, Jennifer. "Public Health Risk Seen as Parents Reject Vaccines." *New York Times*, March 21, 2008.

Stern, Alexandra Minna, and Howard Markel. "The History of Vaccines and Immunization: Familiar Patterns, New Challenges." *Health Affairs* 24, no. 3 (2005): 611–21.

St. Lawrence, Janet S., Daniel E. Montaño, Danuta Kasprzyk, William R. Phillips, Keira Armstrong, and Jami S. Leichliter. "STD Screening, Testing, Case Reporting, and Clinical and Partner Notification Practices: A National Survey of U.S. Physicians." *American Journal of Public Health* 92, no. 11 (2002): 1784–88.

Stratton, Kathleen, Alicia Gable, and Marie C. McCormick, eds. *Immunization Safety Review: Thimerosal-Containing Vaccines and Neurodevelopmental Disorders.* Washington, D.C.: Immunization Safety Review Committee Board on Health Promotion and Disease Prevention, 2001.

Streefland, Pieter, A. M. R. Chowdhury, and Pilar Ramos-Jimenez. "Patterns of Vaccination Acceptance." *Social Science & Medicine* 49, no. 12 (1999): 1705–16.

Stuart, Forrest. "From 'Rabble Management' to 'Recovery Management': Policing Homelessness in Marginal Urban Space." *Urban Studies* 51, no. 9 (2014): 1909–25.

Sugerman, David E., Albert E. Barskey, Maryann G. Delea, Ismael R. Ortega-Sanchez, Daoling Bi, Kimberly J. Ralston, Paul A. Rota, Karen Waters-Montijo, and Charles W. LeBaron. "Measles Outbreak in a Highly Vaccinated Population, San Diego, 2008: Role of the Intentionally Undervaccinated." *Pediatrics* 125, no. 4 (2010): 747–55.

Szabo, Liz. "Unexplained, Polio-Like Illness Has Paralyzed 75 Kids." *USA Today*, November 14, 2014.

Taylor, Verta, and Lisa Leitz. "Emotions and Identity in Self-Help Movements." In *Social Movements and the Transformation of American Health Care*, edited by Jane C.

Banaszak-Holl, Sandra R. Levitsky, and Mayer N. Zald, 266–83. New York: Oxford University Press, 2010.

Tenpenny, Sherri. "Order Vaccine Titer Tests." DrTenpenny.org, n.d. Cited November 24, 2015. http://drtenpenny.com/titer-test-information/titer-tests

Tomljenovic, Lucija, and Christopher A. Shaw. "Too Fast or Not Too Fast: The FDA's Approval of Merck's HPV Vaccine Gardasil." *Journal of Law, Medicine & Ethics* 40, no. 3 (2012): 673–81.

Trattner, Walter. *From Poor Law to Welfare State: A History of Social Welfare in America*. 5th ed. New York: Free Press, 1994.

Trouiller, Patrice, Piero Olliaro, Els Torreele, James Orbinski, Richard Laing, and Nathan Ford. "Drug Development for Neglected Diseases: A Deficient Market and a Public-Health Policy Failure." *Lancet* 359, no. 9324 (2002): 2188–94.

Truong, Van-Anh. "The Pediatric Vaccine Stockpiling Problem." *Vaccine* 30, no. 43 (2012): 6175–79.

Ungar, Michael. "Overprotective Parenting: Helping Parents Provide Children the Right Amount of Risk and Responsibility." *American Journal of Family Therapy* 37, no. 3 (2009): 258–71.

U.S. House of Representatives Committee on Governmental Reform. "Conflicts of Interest in Vaccine Policy Making." 2000.

U.S. Senate Committee on Health, Education, Labor, and Pensions. *Testimony of Dr. Timothy Jacks, DO, the Reemergence of Vaccine-Preventable Diseases: Exploring the Public Health Successes and Challenges*. February 10, 2015.

van der Pol, Rachel J., Marije J. Smits, Michiel P. van Wijk, Taher I. Omari, Merit M. Tabbers, and Marc A. Benninga. "Efficacy of Proton-Pump Inhibitors in Children with Gastroesophageal Reflux Disease: A Systematic Review." *Pediatrics* 127, no. 5 (2011): 925–35.

Vesikari, T. "Rotavirus Vaccines against Diarrhoeal Disease." *Lancet* 350, no. 9090 (1997): 1538–41.

Voices for Vaccines. "From Anti-Vax to Pro-Vax: One Mom's Journey." VoicesforVaccines.org, 2014. http://www.voicesforvaccines.org/from-anti-vax-to-pro-vax/.

Volmink, Jimmy, and Paul Garner. "Directly Observed Therapy for Treating Tuberculosis (Review)." *Cochrane Database of Systematic Reviews* no. 4 (2007). Art. No.: CD003343. DOI: 10.1002/14651858.CD003343.pub3.

Volpe, Joseph J. "Intracranial Hemorrhage in Early Infancy—Renewed Importance of Vitamin K Deficiency." *Pediatric Neurology* 50, no. 6 (2014): 545–46.

Waggoner, Miranda. "Expanding the Reproductive Body: The Emergence of Preconception Care, 1980—2010." PhD diss., Brandeis University, 2011.

Wakefield, Andrew. "Dr. Andrew Wakefield, Health Freedom Rally." Santa Monica, CA. AutismOne Media, 2015. Posted July 6, 2015. https://www.youtube.com/watch?v=cF75NIOQARA.

Wakefield, Andrew J., Simon H. Murch, Andrew Anthony, John Linnell, D. M. Casson, Mohsin Malik, Mark Berelowitz, Amar P. Dhillon, Michael A. Thomson, and Peter Harvey. "Retracted: Ileal-Lymphoid-Nodular Hyperplasia, Non-Specific Colitis, and Pervasive Developmental Disorder in Children." *Lancet* 351, no. 9103 (1998): 637–41.

Watkins, Tom. "Rotarix Rotavirus Vaccine Contaminated, Officials Say." CNN. com, March 22, 2010. Cited November 25, 2015. http://www.cnn.com/2010/ HEALTH/03/22/rotavirus.vaccine.

Wechsler, Jill. "Congress Expands Drug Safety Surveillance as Part of Bioterrorism Bill." *Formulary* 37, no. 7 (2002): 368.

Wei, Feifei, John Mullooly, Mike Goodman, Maribet McCarty, Ann Hanson, Bradley Crane, and James Nordin. "Identification and Characteristics of Vaccine Refusers." *BMC Pediatrics* 9, no. 1 (2009): 18.

Weintraub, Karen. "The Prevalence Puzzle: Autism Counts." *Nature* 479 (2011): 22–24.

Welner, Kevin G. "The Dirty Dozen: How Charter Schools Influence Student Enroll-ment." *Teachers College Record* online, April 2013. ID number 17104. http://www. tcrecord.org.

Wightman, Aaron, Douglas J. Opel, Edgar K. Marcuse, and James A. Taylor. "Wash-ington State Pediatricians' Attitudes toward Alternative Childhood Immunization Schedules." *Pediatrics* 128, no. 6 (2011): 1094–99.

Wilde, James A., Julia A. McMillan, Janet Serwint, Jeanne Butta, Mary Ann O'Riordan, and Mark C. Steinhoff. "Effectiveness of Influenza Vaccine in Health Care Profes-sionals." *JAMA: Journal of the American Medical Association* 281, no. 10 (1999): 908–13.

Wilkins, Andrew. "Affective Practices and Neoliberal Fantasies: Mothers' Encounters with School Choice." In *Mothering in the Age of Neoliberalism*, edited by M. Van-denbeld Giles. Bradford, Ontario: Demeter Press, 2014.

Willrich, Michael. *Pox: An American History*. New York: Penguin, 2011.

Wolf, Joan B. "Is Breast Really Best? Risk and Total Motherhood in the National Breastfeeding Awareness Campaign." *Journal of Health Politics, Policy and Law* 32, no. 4 (2007): 595–636.

World Health Organization. "Global Alert and Response: Hepatitis B." WHO.int, 2015. Cited June 4, 2015. http://www.who.int/csr/disease/hepatitis/whocdscsrlyo20022/ en/index3.html.

———. "Hepatitis B: Fact Sheet N°204." WHO.int, March 2015. Cited June 4, 2015. http://www.who.int/mediacentre/factsheets/fs204/en.

———. "Influenza (Seasonal)." 2014. Cited November 24, 2015. http://www.who.int/ mediacentre/factsheets/fs211/en.

Yale Law Journal. "Police Power of Municipal Authorities." *Yale Law Journal* 18, no. 2 (1908): 128–32.

Yih, W. Katherine, Tracy A. Lieu, Martin Kulldorff, David Martin, Cheryl N. McMahill-Walraven, Richard Platt, Nandini Selvam, Mano Selvan, Grace M. Lee, and Michael Nguyen. "Intussusception Risk after Rotavirus Vaccination in U.S. In-fants." *New England Journal of Medicine* 370, no. 6 (2014): 503–12. http://www.nejm. org/doi/pdf/10.1056/NEJMoa1303164.

INDEX

AAP. *See* American Academy of Pediatrics

Abortion: choice, 17; and MMR, 49–50; spontaneous, 49, 77, 111, 277n14. *See also* Ingredients, vaccine: fetal tissue

ACIP. *See* Advisory Committee on Immunization Practices

ADHD. *See* Attention Deficit/Hyperactivity Disorder

Adolescence, 5, 6, 46, 49, 50, 62, 77, 82, 103, 104, 108, 111, 193, 194–96. *See also* Hepatitis: Hepatitis B; Human Papilloma Virus; Meningococcal disease vaccine

Adverse reaction, 4, 7, 33, 57, 59, 61, 68, 73, 79–85, 87, 92, 105, 114, 127, 131, 135, 137–38, 140–41, 144, 167–68, 171, 175, 177, 182, 226, 236–37, 239, 240–56, 259, 261, 265. *See also* Vaccine Adverse Event Reporting System; Vaccines: complications of

Advisory Committee on Immunization Practices (ACIP), 10, 48, 51, 53–54, 112, 140, 141, 167–69, 171, 174–75, 178, 180–82, 187, 245–46, 253, 262. *See also* Schedule of vaccines

Alternative schedule. *See* Sears, Bob; Slow vax

AMA. *See* American Medical Association

American Academy of Pediatrics (AAP), 10, 39, 40, 48, 49, 58, 59, 64, 130–31, 144, 148, 169, 177, 178, 182, 190, 196, 197, 222–24. *See also* Pediatrics

American Medical Association (AMA), 38, 45, 50, 60

Antibiotics, 39–40, 79, 88, 101, 111, 145, 206, 217

Antigenic drift, 146. *See also* Influenza

Anti-vaccine movements, 28, 31–33, 123, 130, 178

Asthma, 16, 97, 159, 200

Attention-deficit/hyperactivity disorder (ADHD), 84, 97, 131

Autism, 6, 20, 67, 79, 80, 84, 90–94, 97, 119, 123, 128–34, 260–62; Age of Autism website, 133, 167; Generation Rescue, 123; HEAL Foundation, 123; Moms Against Mercury, 123; Talking About Curing Autism (TACA), 123; vaccine link, 62–64, 129–30, 131–34, 136, 167, 201. *See also* Burton, Dan; Leaky gut syndrome; Wakefield, Andrew

Autoimmune disorder, 79–80

Bill and Melinda Gates Foundation, 65

Bioterrorism, 136, 247, 257

Bioterrorism Act of 2002, 135–36. *See also* Influenza: H1N1

Birth, 15–16, 18, 38, 71–72, 97–102, 103, 157, 196, 208, 261; midwives, 14, 38, 102; home birth, 71, 208, 220, 238, 258–59; natural, 15, 97–98, 100–102, 248

Blumberg, Baruch, 103. *See also* Hepatitis: B

Bodies, 106; bodily integrity, 8, 29, 73, 143, 237, 252; as unique 7, 12, 19, 73, 96, 170–74, 177, 187. *See also* Natural

Booth, Austin, 145–6; 158. *See also* Influenza

ABOUT THE AUTHOR

Jennifer A. Reich is Associate Professor of Sociology at the University of Colorado Denver. Her publications include the award-winning book *Fixing Families: Parents, Power, and the Child Welfare System*.